Biochemistry
of Dementia

Biochemistry of Dementia

Based on a
Workshop on Biochemistry of the Dementias,
held at
University of Southampton, March 1979

Edited by
P. J. ROBERTS
*School of Biochemical and Physiological Sciences,
Department of Physiology and Pharmacology,
University of Southampton, U.K.*

A Wiley–Interscience Publication

JOHN WILEY & SONS
Chichester · New York · Brisbane · Toronto

British Library Cataloguing in Publication Data:

Workshop on Biochemistry of the Dementias,
  University of Southampton, 1979
  Biochemistry of dementia.
  1. Dementia—Congresses 2. Mental illness
  —Physiological aspects—Congresses
  I. Title II. Roberts, P J
616.8'9   RC524   79-42895

ISBN 0 471 27698 7

Typeset by The Macmillan Co. of India Ltd., Bangalore
Printed in the United States of America by Vail-Ballou Press, Inc.,
Binghamton, N.Y.

'Last scene of all that ends this strange eventful history is second childishness and mere oblivion . . . .'

William Shakespeare,
As You Like It, Act II, Scene 7

List of Contributors

B. H. ANDERTON *Basic Medical Sciences Group, Chelsea College, University of London, Manresa Road, London, SW3 6LX, U.K.*

R. ARMBRUSTER *Department of Preclinical Research, Sandoz Limited, Basel, Switzerland.*

A. ARREGUI *M.R.C. Neurochemical Pharmacology Unit, Medical School, Hills Road, Cambridge, U.K.*

H. S. BACHELARD *Department of Biochemistry, St Thomas's Hospital Medical School, London, SE1 7EH, U.K.*

I. A. BLACKBURN *M.R.C. Brain Metabolism Unit, Department of Pharmacology, University of Edinburgh, 1 George Square, Edinburgh, EH8 9JZ, U.K.*

J. P. BLASS *The Dementia Research Service, Department of Neurology, Cornell University Medical College, The Burke Rehabilitation Center, 785 Mamaroneck Avenue, White Plains, New York 10605, U.S.A.*

G. BLESSED *St Nicholas Hospital, Gosforth, Newcastle upon Tyne, NE3 3XT, U.K.*

D. M. BOWEN *Institute of Neurology, Queen Square, London, WC1N 2NS, U.K.*

J. E. CHRISTIE *M.R.C. Brain Metabolism Unit, Department of Pharmacology, University of Edinburgh, 1 George Square, Edinburgh, EH8 9JZ, U.K.*

J. COHEN *M.R.C. Neuroimmunology Project, Department of Zoology, University College London, Gower Street, London, WC1E 6BT, U.K.*

D. R. CRAPPER *Departments of Physiology and Medicine, University of Toronto, Toronto, Ontario, M5S 1A8, Canada.*

U. DE BONI *Departments of Physiology and Medicine, University of Toronto, Toronto, Ontario, M5S 1A8, Canada.*

A. ENZ

Department of Preclinical Research, Sandoz Limited, Basel, Switzerland.

G. E. GIBSON

The Dementia Research Service, Department of Neurology, Cornell University Medical College, The Burke Rehabilitation Center, 785 Mamaroneck Avvenue, White Plains, New York 10605, U.S.A.

A. I. M. GLEN

M.R.C. Brain Metabolism Unit, Department of Pharmacology, University of Edinburgh, 1 George Square, Edinburgh, EH8 9JZ, U.K.

C. G. GOTTFRIES

University of Göteborg, Psychiatric Research Centre, St Jörgen's Hospital, Hisings Backa, Sweden.

S. HOYER

Department of Pathochemistry and General Neurochemistry, University of Heidelberg, D-6900 Heidelberg, West Germany.

L. L. IVERSEN

M.R.C. Neurochemical Pharmacology Unit, Medical School, Hills Road, Cambridge, U.K.

P. IWANGOFF

Department of Preclinical Research, Sandoz Limited, Basel, Switzerland.

T. KIHARA

Department of Anatomy, Osaka Medical College, 2–7 Daigakumachi, Takatuski City, Osaka 569, Japan.

K. KURINIOTO

Department of Anatomy, Osaka Medical College, 2–7 Daigakumachi, Takatuski City, Osaka 569, Japan.

G. G. LUNT

Department of Biochemistry, University of Bath, Bath, BA2 7AY, U.K.

A. V. P. MACKAY

M.R.C. Neurochemical Pharmacology Unit, Medical School, Hills Road, Cambridge, U.K.

W. MEIER-RUGE

Department of Preclinical Research, Sandoz Limited, Basel, Switzerland.

M. J. PARRY

Pfizer Central Research, Pfizer Limited, Sandwich, Kent, U.K.

E. K. PERRY

Department of Neuropathology, Newcastle General Hospital, Newcastle upon Tyne, NE4 6BE, U.K.

R. H. PERRY

Department of Neuropathology, Newcastle General Hospital, Newcastle upon Tyne, NE4 6BE, U.K.

S. REHNCRONA

Laboratory of Experimental Brain Research, E-Blocket, University of Lund, Lund, Sweden.

P. J. ROBERTS   *University of Southampton, School of Biochemical and Physiological Sciences, Department of Physiology and Pharmacology, Medical and Biological Sciences Building, Bassett Crescent East, Southampton, SO9 3TU, U.K.*

R. W. R. RUSSELL   *St Thomas' Hospital, London, SE1, and The National Hospital for Nervous Diseases, Queen Square, London WC1, U.K.*

P. SANDOZ   *Department of Preclinical Research, Sandoz Limited, Basel, Switzerland.*

S. SELVENDRAN   *M.R.C. Neuroimmunology Project, Department of Zoology, University College London, Gower Street, London, WC1E 6BT, U.K.*

A. SHERING   *M.R.C. Brain Metabolism Unit, Department of Pharmacology, University of Edinburgh, 1 George Square, Edinburgh, EH8 9JZ, U.K.*

M. SHIMADA   *Department of Anatomy, Osaka Medical College, 2–7 Daigakumachi, Takatuski City, Osaka 569, Japan.*

B. K. SIESJÖ   *Laboratory of Experimental Brain Research, E-Blocket, University of Lund, Lund, Sweden.*

J. SIMPSON   *M.R.C. Brain Metabolism Unit, Department of Pharmacology, University of Edinburgh, 1 George Square, Edinburgh, EH8 9JZ, U.K.*

E. G. SPOKES   *M.R.C. Neurochemical Pharmacology Unit, Medical School, Hills Road, Cambridge, U.K.*

R. THORPE   *Basic Medical Sciences Group, Chelsea College, University of London, Manresa Road, London, SW3 6LX, U.K.*

B. E. TOMLINSON   *Department of Pathology, Newcastle General Hospital, Newcastle upon Tyne, NE4 6BE, U.K.*

M. WATANABE   *Department of Anatomy, Osaka Medical College, 2–7 Daigakumachi, Takatuski City, Osaka 569, Japan.*

L. J. WHALLEY   *M.R.C. Brain Metabolism Unit, Department of Pharmacology, University of Edinburgh, 1 George Square, Edinburgh, EH8 9JZ, U.K.*

H. WISE   *Department of Biochemistry, St Thomas's Hospital Medical School, London, SE1 7EH, U.K.*

P. WOODHAMS   *M.R.C. Development Neurobiology Unit, Institute of Neurology, 33 John's Mews, London, WC1N 2NS, U.K.*

C. M. YATES   *M.R.C. Brain Metabolism Unit, Department of Pharmacology, University of Edinburgh, 1 George Square, Edinburgh, EH8 9JZ, U.K.*

S. ZEISEL   *Massachusetts Institute of Technology, Cambridge, Massachusetts, U.S.A.*

Contents

xi

Contents

Preface

Dementia (Literally, 'from the mind'—madness) is one of the oldest diseases known to man, and it is characterized by progressive degeneration of the whole personality. Even today, little is known of the underlying causes of dementia. The disease is progressive, with an average life expectancy after diagnosis of approximately 7 years.

With increased longevity and a low birth rate, it is now the older section of the population that is increasing most rapidly. It is currently estimated that 1 person in 10 over the age of 65 suffers from senile dementia, and by the age of 80 and above, this rises to the alarming figure of more than 20 %.

Dementia represents a disastrous condition for both patient and family; the cause of the disease is not a dignified descent to the grave but is seen as a steadily worsening global impairment of all the individual's functions, of which he or she is rarely aware.

Unless there is significant progress in the treatment and possible prevention of dementia, the legacy for the twenty-first century is likely to be one of enormous economic cost, pressures on the health and social services and the requirement for a vast increase in the range and scope of institutional care.

Despite the period of time since dementia was first known, until comparatively recently there has been incredible neglect in research on dementia, particularly in respect of the basic neurochemistry and possible pharmacology. This lack of progress can undoubtedly be attributed to a number of factors: (i) the general unfashionability of geriatric medicine and the dearth of neuropathologists; (ii) the lack of awareness and involvement by the basic scientist, and (iii) the failure of the clinicians to solicit this involvement from scientific colleagues.

Notwithstanding these problems, another major obstacle has been the lack of sufficiently refined biochemical techniques to investigate brain, and especially synaptic, function. It is only within the last few years that substances such as the amino acids, dopamine, Substance P and the enkephalins have unequivocally been assigned physiological functions at the synapse, and that powerful techniques such as radio-receptor binding assays have become available.

Thus, the time is ripe for close multi-disciplinary cooperation in research into the dementias, and a report by the Medical Research Council (*Senile and Presenile Dementias*—A report of the M.R.C. sub-committee compiled by W. A. Lishman, 1977) has designated this as a priority area.

In the spring of 1979, the Neurochemical Group of the Biochemical Society held an International Workshop on Biochemistry of the Dementias in the School of Biochemical and Physiological Sciences, University of Southampton, England. As has been the aim of previous workshops organized by the Society, we have brought together basic biochemists, pharmacologists, neuropathologists, neurologists and psychiatrists for the purpose of creating an awareness of the problem of dementia. The chapters contained in this volume are based upon the workshop, and provide comprehensive views and discussion of progress to date, and emphasize the need for much solid fundamental research to be done. Additionally, a number of 'hot topics' are presented as short reports at the end of the book.

All who participated in the workshop will, I am sure, testify to its success in promoting the frank and friendly exchange of new experimental results and ideas, and in several cases, the formation of new research collaborations. The organization of any meeting of this size is fraught with problems to confound its smooth running. I am therefore extremely grateful to the enthusiastic and invaluable assistance from my graduate students, Alan Foster, Gethin Rowlands and Najam Sharif. Thanks are also due to the University for providing a reception for the workshop delegates.

Finally, the workshop would not have been possible without the extremely generous financial support that was accorded the meeting. It is therefore a pleasure to express my gratitude to the following organizations: Sandoz Ltd (Basel, Switzerland); Ciba-Geigy (Macclesfield, U.K.); Merck Institute for Therapeutic Research (West Point, U.S.A.); Duphar Laboratories Ltd (Southampton, U.K.); The Wellcome Trust (London, U.K.); Roche Products Ltd (Welwyn Garden City, U.K.); Janssen Pharmaceutical Ltd (Marlow, U.K.); Merck Sharp & Dohme Ltd (Hoddesdon, U.K.); Beecham Pharmaceuticals (Betchworth, U.K.); The Boots Co Ltd (Nottingham, U.K.); I.C.I. Ltd., Pharmaceuticals Division (Macclesfield, U.K.); Abbott Laboratories Ltd., (Queenborough, U.K.).

PETER J. ROBERTS

Biochemistry of Dementia
Edited by P. J. Roberts
© 1980, John Wiley & Sons Ltd.

Chapter 1

Clinical Aspects of the Senile Dementias

G. BLESSED
St. Nicholas Hospital, Gosforth,
Newcastle upon Tyne, NE3, 3XT, U.K.

I. INTRODUCTION

Dementia has been tidily defined by Marsden (1978) as 'The syndrome of global disturbance of higher mental functions in an alert patient'. It is a syndrome frequently found in old people, and its incidence appears to be higher among the very old than among those who have recently passed their sixty-fifth birthday. Thus, Kay, Beamish, and Roth (1964) and Kay and coworkers (1970) found an incidence of 2.4% among 65–69 year-olds, compared with 22% for those aged 80 and above.

Deteriorating intellectual function is normally associated with declining self-care or daily living skills, and for this reason many people suffering from dementia are admitted to the various forms of institutional care. This tendency has again been demonstrated by Kay and coworkers (1970), who showed that when community-based random samples of elderly people were followed up, those suffering from dementia were more likely to enter a geriatric ward, or a residential home.

The dementia syndrome is also responsible for a high proportion of admissions of elderly people to psychiatric hospitals. Below the age of 50 years, organic brain syndromes (of which dementia forms the largest component) are to be found in less than 10% of total admissions, but after that age the proportion of organic to functional psychosyndromes increases dramatically, as shown in Fig. 1 (Kramer, 1969).

Once admitted, patients with dementia have a poorer prognosis, both for survival and discharge home, than do other mentally-ill people of similar age. This fundamental difference in prognosis, which was used by Roth and Morrissey (1952) as the basis for the definition of discrete psychosyndromes within old-age mental disorder, is supported by contemporary experience in a psychogeriatric admission ward (Table 2).

Biochemistry of Dementia

Table 1. Patterns of outcome for groups of elderly people living at home (Hospital and other Institutional care)

	Normals		Functional		CBS**		Total	
	No.	(%)	No.	(%)	No.	(%)	No.	(%)
Acute	57	(16.6)	15	(18.8)	6	(23.1)	78	(17.4)
Geriatric	10	(2.9)	4	(5.0)	12	(46.2)	26	(5.8)
Mental	3	(0.9)	3	(3.8)	2	(7.7)	8	(1.8)
Local Authority homes	1 }	(1.5)	2 }	(2.5)	3 }	(15.4)	6 }	(2.4)
Private homes	4		0		2		6	
Admitted somewhere	66*	(19.2)	20*	(25.0)	16*	(61.5)	102*	(22.7)
Not admitted	277	(80.8)	60	(75.0)	10	(38.5)	347	(77.3)
Total	343	(100.0)	80	(100.0)	26	(100.0)	449	(100.0)

* Some subjects admitted to more than one type of care.
** Equivalent to dementia in this table.

Table 2. Admissions of elderly patients and outcome of treatment (1972)

Diagnosis	Admissions No.	%	Disposal (% in brackets) 1 year after admission				
			Home	Longstay	Died	Res. Care	Trans. Hospital
Senile dementia	125	33.8	28 (22.4)	30 (24)	49 (39.2)	15 (12)	3 (2.4)
A.S. dementia	21	5.7	7 (33.3)	5 (23.8)	6 (28.6)	3 (14.3)	0 —
Other dementia	21	5.7	9 (42.9)	2 (9.5)	6 (28.6)	3 (14.3)	1 (4.8)
All dementia	167	45.1	44 (26.3)	37 (22.2)	61 (36.5)	21 (12.6)	4 (2.4)
Confusional states	67	18.1	31 (46.3)	5 (7.5)	15 (22.4)	12 (17.9)	4 (6.0)
All 'organics'	234	63.2	75 (32.1)	42 (17.9)	76 (32.5)	33 (14.1)	8 (3.4)
Endo-depression	40	10.8	38 (95)	0 —	1 (2.5)	1 (2.5)	0 —
Reactive depression	21	5.7	20 (95.2)	0 —	0 —	0 —	1 (4.8)
Other depression	16	4.3	14 (87.5)	1 (6.3)	1 (6.3)	0 —	0 —
Mania	10	2.7	8 (80)	0 —	0 —	1 (10)	1 (10)
Paraphrenia	35	9.5	26 (74.3)	0 —	3 (8.6)	3 (8.6)	3 (8.6)
Other neurotic	14	3.8	10 (71.4)	1 (7)	1 (7)	1 (7)	1 (7)
All 'functionals'	136	36.8	116 (85.3)	2 (1.5)	6 (4.4)	6 (4.4)	6 (4.4)
Totals	370	100	193 (52.5)	44 (11.9)	82 (22.2)	39 (10.5)	14 (3.8)

Biochemistry of Dementia

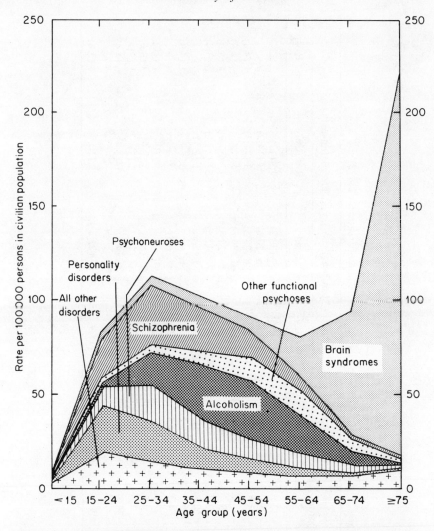

Figure 1. Rates for admission to state and county mental hospitals in the United States in 1965 and specific for age and mental disorder (no previous admission to any in-patient psychiatric facility). From Kramer, 1969. Reproduced by permission of the World Health Organization

II. THE RECOGNITION OF DEMENTIA IN OLD AGE

The dementia syndrome is often concealed, as Williamson and coworkers (1964) discovered. It may be concealed by caring relatives who regard it as an inevitable consequence of ageing, by a frightened patient who fears institutional care, or by the patient whose judgement is impaired and who simply fails to recognize the developing deficits as an illness.

The main patterns of decline are as follows.

A. Slowly Progressive Dementia

The commonest mode of presentation is graphically illustrated in Fig. 2. This pattern of gradual decline with accumulation of handicaps was described by Roth and Morrissey (1952) as being typical of senile psychosis. Typically, such patients are referred for advice some two or three years after the disorder begins, and the syndrome is well established by this time. Patients are vague and forgetful and are seriously disorientated for time, and for less familiar places and persons. Insight is often lacking and seldom complete, so that even when forgetfulness is admitted as a problem, it is usually minimized or simply ascribed to 'old age'. This is the typical presentation of senile dementia but it can be complicated in a number of ways.

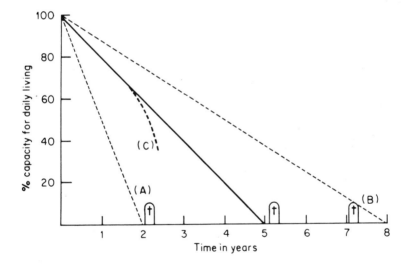

Figure 2. Patterns of psychogeriatric illness—senile dementia. (A)–(B) The speed of decline in function can vary greatly. (C) Associated serious physical disease can accelerate the process of deterioration

1. Depressive Complication

A significant number of demented patients show anxiety and depression, especially in the early stage of the disorder, in what Keet (1978) has described as the first or prodromal stage. The depression is of the reactive type and the patient often shows reduced adaptability to other environmental stresses, and the ability to improve in response to environmental manipulation. Less commonly, more floridly psychotic affective syndromes are seen, but these are clinically incomplete and less sustained than are true late onset affective psychoses. Over a short time-scale, however, the differentiation between severe affective psychosis with 'pseudo-dementia' Kiloh (1961) and dementia with 'pseudo-depression' can prove very difficult.

2. Paranoid Complication

Just as depressive reactions can colour the early stages of dementia, so can paranoid ones. Such reactions can be regarded as neurotic defences which allow the frightened patient to avoid the realization of personal intellectual decline, and to blame their losses upon the ill-will of others—commonly their closest supporters. Such paranoid defences can be very skilfully contrived, so much so that in the absence of a reasonably sensitive test for intellectual decline, these patients can be regarded as suffering from late paraphrenia.

3. The Delirious Complication

Longitudinal observations of patients suffering from senile dementia reveal remarkable variability of course in some 25 % of those with associated physical disease, such as severe chronic bronchitis or cardiac failure syndrome. In other cases the physical disease is less overt, and short-term deterioration in mental functioning, not always associated with clinical clouding of consciousness, may be associated with urinary tract infections, neglected constipation, or intercurrent viral infections. These transient deteriorations may respond quite rapidly to appropriate treatment of the underlying cause, but recovery is incomplete.

4. The 'Alzheimer' Complication

The clinical features of Alzheimer's disease (Alzheimer, 1907) have been reviewed by Sim, Turner, and Smith (1966). Roth and Morrissey (1952) found the focal signs of disturbed parietal and temporal lobe function, so typical of Alzheimer's disease in the presenium, to be rare in patients over 60 years of age, who suffered from progressive dementia; however, in the author's series reported in this paper the incidence is 26.8 %. Patients with aphasia or dyspraxia associated with clear-cut stroke disease are excluded.

Summarizing, elderly patients presenting with slowly progressive dementia may be subclassified as shown in Table 3.

Table 3. Slowly progressive dementia in old age

Condition	No.	Total (%)
Uncomplicated senile dementia	29	40.8
Alzheimer type dementia	19	26.8
S.D. + acute brain syndromes	10	14.1
S.D. + functional brain syndromes	13	18.3
Total	71	100

B. Erratic or Step-like Dementia (Fig. 3)

Roth and Morrissey (1952) regarded dementia of this pattern of development, clearly associated with stroke disease and with signs of focal neurological damage, as being the other major type of dementia found in elderly people. Described as arteriosclerotic or multi-infarct dementia, it occurred in 19 % of the patients in this series.

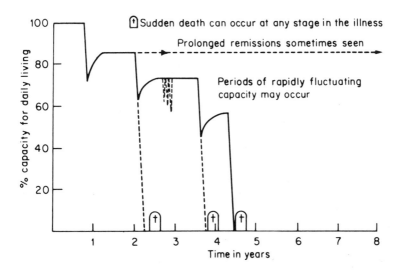

Figure 3. Patterns of psychogeriatric illness—arteriosclerotic dementia

C. Combined Dementia

Neuropathological studies reveal (Tomlinson, Blessed, and Roth, 1970) that vascular lesions and Alzheimer type changes coexist in the brains of some 18 % of demented elderly subjects. Clinically, it is possible to recognize two syndromes which might be expected to result from such a combination. The first is the patient who presents with a major stroke which is not repeated, but who nevertheless suffers from a subsequent progressive intellectual decline. The second pattern, shown in Fig. 4, indicates a clinical combination of erratic steps and steadily progressive deterioration. In the present series, 5 % of demented patients were thought to show this pattern of decline.

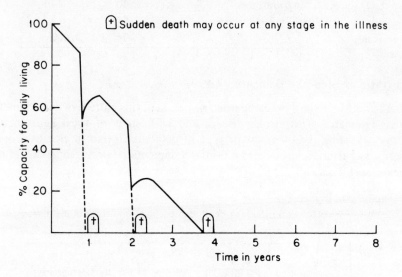

Figure 4. Patterns of psychogeriatric illness—mixed senile and arteriosclerotic dementias

D. Other forms of Dementia

Pick's disease (1892), Jakob–Creutzfeldt disease (Creutzfeldt, 1920; Jakob, 1921) and other forms of dementia are rare in old age, (Roth and Morrissey, 1952). In the present series, five patients were allocated to the following categories:

Secondary dementia, cerebral tumour	1
Korsakow's psychosis	1
Pick's disease	2
Dementia following head injury	1

III. CLINICAL TESTING OF INTELLECTUAL FUNCTION IN THE ELDERLY PATIENT

In 1953, Roth and Hopkins showed that elderly mentally ill people assigned to diagnostic groups, using criteria previously described by Roth and Morrissey

(1952), obtained significantly different scores on a standard test of orientation and information.

Shapiro and coworkers (1956) looked at a number of tests of intellectual performance currently used by both clinical psychiatrists and psychologists, and found that only some were reliable tools for differentiating functionally-ill elderly people from those suffering from organic brain syndrome.

In 1964 (see Blessed, Tomlinson, and Roth, 1968) the author combined four of the tests regarded as reliable by Shapiro and coworkers with items from the Roth–Hopkins tests to produce a mental test battery which was then administered to 244 hospitalized elderly people. The results are shown in Table 4.

Table 4. Mental test score results for groups of hospitalized elderly subjects

Group	*Score	No. of cases	Standard deviations
Medically ill	33.3	46	3.59
Affective disorder	29.7	47	5.63
Paraphrenia	26.6	34	10.71
Acute brain syndrome	20.3	35	7.49
Multi-infarct dementia	13.9	37	7.78
Senile dementia	10.7	45	8.85

* Maximum possible score = 37

Examination of the standard errors of the differences between these mean scores shows that the medically-ill group free from signs of mental confusion or other psychiatric disorder scored significantly better than all other groups ($p < 0.05$ or better).

Patients with functional psychiatric disorder scored better than those with acute or chronic brain syndrome, while the acute brain syndrome cases scored better than those classified as suffering from dementia. Thus, the test not only differentiated between groups of functionally and organically ill elderly people, as did both the Roth–Hopkins and the Shapiro and coworkers' tests, but it was performed significantly better by a control group (not included in the two previous reports) and differentiated an acute brain syndrome group from both the functionally ill and the demented populations tested.

IV. CLINICOPATHOLOGICAL CORRELATIONS OF DEMENTIA

Around the turn of the century, Pick (1892), Alzheimer (1907), and later Simchowicz (1910) found degenerative changes in the brains of demented people. In the 1920s and 1930s, Grunthal (1927) and Gellerstedt (1932) found similar degenerative changes in the brains of elderly people dying in general hospital beds, and threw doubt on the significance of these changes as the principal cause of dementia. In 1942, Rothschild found a poor correlation between the severity of vascular changes in the brain and the presence of, or severity of, dementia and concluded that other factors must be playing an important part in determining whether a person became demented when his brain was damaged by vascular disease. Corsellis (1962) carried out careful semi-quantified studies on the brains of elderly patients dying in mental hospital. He found that moderate or greater degenerative changes occurred in 75 % of patients dying with a diagnosis of dementia, but that changes of comparable severity were to be found in only 25 % of patients who had been allotted the diagnosis of functional psychiatric disorder.

In the late 1960s, a team of research workers (Roth, Tomlinson, and Blessed, 1966; Blessed, Tomlinson, and Roth, 1968; Tomlinson, Blessed, and Roth, 1968, 1970) reported on clinicopathological correlations of dementia and concluded that there was a highly significant relationship between clinical measures of intellectual decline in old people and quantified estimates of the severity of degenerative brain disease found at post-mortem in the same subjects. Finally, Perry and coworkers (1978) have demonstrated a significant relationship between intellectual ability as measured by mental test score, and levels of choline acetyltransferase (CAT) in the post-mortem brain.

Table 5 shows the clinicopathological correlates of 156 elderly people, 100 of whom were clinically demented. The findings can be summarized as follows:

  (i) There is a high level of concordance between a clinical diagnosis of Alzheimer type dementia and Alzheimer pathology.
 (ii) Most cases of senile dementia without typical 'Alzheimer' features nevertheless have Alzheimer pathology, but approximately 10 % have mixed pathology and in a further 10 % no gross pathological lesion is found.
(iii) Only about 50 % of cases regarded as clinical cases of multi-infarct dementia have that pathology alone. A further 20 % have mixed pathology and 10 % have Alzheimer change. 16 % of cases have no more vascular damage to their brains than a control group of subjects.
 (iv) Mixed dementia clinically seems to be dominated by pure Alzheimer pathology, and concordance between clinical diagnosis and morphological classification is poor.
  (v) All cases with both dementia and acute brain syndrome had degenerative brain disease—principally Alzheimer change.
 (vi) Nearly half the cases who showed both functional psychiatric disorder and dementia had morphologically normal brains. The remainder had Alzheimer changes.
(vii) 91 % of 56 people with either pure functional psychiatric disorders, acute brain syndromes without dementia, or physical ill-health without significant psychiatric disorder, had morphologically normal brains, but six patients had morphological changes which were severe in half of these.

Table 5

Pathological Diagnosis

Clinical diagnosis	Alzheimer	Probable Alzheimer	Multi-infarct dementia	Probable mid-dementia	Mixed dementia	Probable mixed dementia	Special lesion	Normal brain	Total clinical cases
Senile dementia	19 (65.5)	4 (13.8)	—	—	—	3 (10.3)	—	3 (10.3)	29
Alzheimer type dementia	18 (94.7)	—	1 (5.3)	—	—	—	—	—	19
Multi-infarct dementia	1 (5.3)	1 (5.3)	8 (42.1)	2 (10.6)	1 (5.3)	3 (15.9)	—	3 (15,9)	19
Mixed dementia	2 (40)	2 (40)	—	—	1 (20)	—	—	—	5
Acute brain syndrome + dementia	2 (20)	4 (40)	1 (10)	1 (10)	2 (20)	—	—	—	10
Functional syndrome + dementia	3 (23.2)	4 (30.5)	—	—	—	—	—	6 (46.2)	13
Special dementia	—	—	—	—	1 (25)	—	4 (75)	—	5
Non-demented	2 (3.4)	2 (3.4)	—	—	—	1 (1.7)	1 (1.7)	50 (91%)	56
Totals	47	17	10	3	5	7	5	62	156

V. DISCUSSION

The hypothesis that dementia in old age is principally due to degenerative brain disease which can be recognized at post-mortem, is supported by the studies reported here. The correlation is not complete, but is sufficiently important to support the need for further careful studies of the brains of patients dying from dementia, and for further exploration of the causes of the 'degenerative' changes found. Where discrepant findings exist these, too, deserve further study. In our material, discrepant cases are comparatively uncommon, but further examination of those with clinical dementia without gross pathological change reveals, firstly, that the severity of the dementia found tends to be less in these cases than in those with typical pathological changes, and secondly, that there is frequently an admixture of functional brain syndrome and dementia clinically. Six patients fell into this last category, and four of these may have been cases of depressive pseudo-dementia (Kiloh, 1961). This finding would seem to call for greater clinical reserve in diagnosing dementia in patients who are also depressed, and a more intensive treatment approach to the depressive component of the apparently combined functional illness dementia.

Looking at the six clinically undemented people who had brain lesions, the pathological changes were of a milder degree of severity in half the cases. Of two patients with typical Alzheimer pathology (one a case of late onset paraphrenic disorder and the other a patient with a recurrent confusional state), it may be significant that neither had neurofibrillary tangles present in the neocortex, although these were extensive in the hippocampal cortex, and both cases showed high plaque counts.

Turning to the question of testing intellectual function in elderly people, it is important that comparatively simple tests of memory, orientation and concentration can both differentiate between diagnostic subgroups of mentally-ill subjects and correlate significantly with measures of brain damage at post-mortem. It is particularly gratifying that they correlate so well with levels of cholinergic neurotransmitter enzymes in the brain, and it may prove to be particularly important that within a diagnostic subgroup of depressed patients, suffering from a condition known to be associated with some reduction in intellectual functioning (Whitehead, 1978), there is a relationship between mental test score and CAT level (Perry and coworkers, 1978).

Nevertheless, performance on these tests is less useful in the individual case than it is in comparing groups of cases because there is a considerable overlap in individual performances between group members. Thus, a demented patient may rarely score 37 (I have seen one such case!), and a depressive may rarely score 10 or less.

Again, although there is a high correlation between test performance and measures of cerebral degeneration when all elderly people are included (normals, functionally ill, delirium cases, and dementia) the level of correlation falls sharply when only dements are considered, and their performance is compared with the severity of degenerative change. Nevertheless, there remains a significant correlation (Blessed, Tomlinson, and Roth, 1968) and in this series patients with full Alzheimer pathology obtained a mean test score of 8.8, while those with probable Alzheimer pathology scored 16.9, i.e. significantly better.

VI. SUMMARY

Dementia is common in old age and frequently leads to institutionalization and early death. Demented elderly people show declining intellectual skills which can be measured using simple tests of orientation and memory, and these tests can be shown to correlate with the severity of the principal types of brain disorder found at post-mortem. Discrepant results do occur but the findings suggest that brain disorder is the most important factor in the development of the senile dementias which may prove to be the major sociomedical problem of the last quarter of this century. Further research into the patterns of brain disorder associated with clinical dementia with the object of more closely defining their causes, and hopefully indicating a method of treatment, is urgently needed.

REFERENCES

Alzheimer, A. (1907). On a peculiar disease of the cerebral cortex. *Allg. Z. Psychiatr*, **64**, 146.
Blessed, G., B. E. Tomlinson, and M. Roth (1968). The association between quantitative measures of dementia and of senile change in the cerebral grey matter of elderly subjects. *Brit. J. Psychiat.* **114**, 797.
Corsellis, J. A. N. (1962). *Mental Illness and the Ageing Brains*. Oxford University Press, London.
Creutzfeldt, H. G. (1920). On a peculiar focal disease of the central nervous system. *Neurol. Psychiat.*, **57**, 1, 462.
Gellerstedt, N. (1932–33). Our knowledge of cerebral changes in normal evolution of old age. *Upsala Lak/Foren Forh.*, **38**, 193.
Grunthal, E. (1927). Clinical and anatomical investigations on senile dementia. *Neurol. Psychiat.*, **111**, 763.
Jakob, A. (1921). On peculiar disease of the central nervous system with pathological findings. *Neurol. Psychiat.*, **163**, 670, 463.
Kay, D. W. K., P. Beamish, and M. Roth (1964). Old age mental disorder in Newcastle upon Tyne 1. A study of prevalence. *Brit. J. Psychiat.*, **110**, 146.
Kay, D. W. K., K. Bergmann, E. M. Foster, A. A. McKechnie, and M. Roth (1970). Mental illness and hospital usage in the elderly: a random sample followed up. *Compr. Psychiat.*, **11**, 26.
Keet, J. P. (1978). The assessment and treatment and mood and affective disturbance in dementia. *Brit. J. Clin. Practice*. A symposium on depression in the elderly, 50–5.
Kiloh, L. G. (1961). Pseudo-dementia, *Acta Psychiat. Scand.*, **37**, 336.
Kramer, M. (1969). Application of mental health statistics. Geneva World Health Organization.

Marsden, C. D. (1978). In Isaacs and F. Post (Eds) *The Diagnosis of Dementia in Studies in Geriatric Psychiatry*, John Wiley & Sons, 99–118.

Perry, E. K., B. E. Tomlinson, G. Blessed, K. Bergmann, P. H. Gibson, and R. H. Perry (1978). Correlation of cholinergic abnormalities in the senile plaques and mental test scores in senile dementia. *Brit. Med. J.*, **2**, 1457.

Pick, A. (1892). On the relation of senile cerebral atrophy and aphasia. *Prag. Med. Wschr.*, **17**, 165, 460.

Roth, M. and B. Hopkins (1953). Psychological test performance in patients over 60. 1. Senile psychosis and the affective disorder of old age. *J. Mental Sci.*, **99**, 439.

Roth, M. and J. D. Morrissey (1952). Problems in the diagnosis and classification of mental disorder in old age. *J. Mental Sci.*, **98**, 66.

Roth, M., B. E. Tomlinson, and G. Blessed (1966). Correlation between scores for dementia and counts of senile plaques in the cerebral grey matter of elderly subjects. *Nature (London)*, **209**, 109.

Rothschild, D. (1942). Neuropathologic changes in arteriosclerotic psychoses and their psychiatric significance. *Arch. Neurol. Psychiat. (Chicago)*, **48**, 417.

Shapiro, M. B., F. Post, B. Lofving, and J. Inglis (1956). Memory function in psychiatric patients over sixty, some methodological and diagnostic implications. *J. of Mental Sci*, **102**, 233.

Sim, M., E. Turner, and W. T. Smith (1966). Cerebral biopsy in the investigation of presenile dementia. 1. Clinical aspects. *Brit. J. Psychiat.*, **112**, 119.

Simchowicz, T. (1910). Histologische Studien über die senile Demenz. *Histopath. Arbeiten*, **4**, 267.

Tomlinson, B. E., G. Blessed, and M. Roth (1968). Observations on the brains of non-demented old people. *J. Neurol. Sci.*, **7**, 331.

Tomlinson, B. E., G. Blessed, and M. Roth (1970). Observations on the brains of demented old people. *J. of Neurol. Sci.*, **11**, 205.

Whitehead, A. (1978). In A. D. Isaacs and F. Post (Eds) *The Clinical Psychologist's Role in Assessment and Management. Studies in Geriatric Psychiatry*, John Wiley & Sons, 153.

Williamson, J., I. H. Stokoe, S. Gray, M. Fisher, A. Smith, A. McGhee, and E. Stephenson (1964). Old people at home—their unreported needs. *Lancet*, **1**, 1117.

Biochemistry of Dementia
Edited by P. J. Roberts
© 1980, John Wiley & Sons Ltd.

Chapter 2

The Structural and Quantitative Aspects of the Dementias

B. E. TOMLINSON

*Department of Pathology, Newcastle General Hospital,
Newcastle upon Tyne, NE46BE, U.K.*

The aim of this chapter is to review briefly the morphological changes which occur in the brains of demented subjects, to indicate some of the numerous gaps in our morphological information about the most common forms of dementia, and to state briefly the evidence which suggests that in the majority of cases in old age quantitative, rather than qualitative, changes in the brain differentiate the demented from the intellectually well-preserved subject. In doing so, most of the pathological causes of dementia will be mentioned, solely to illustrate the many destructive processes which may lead to that clinical state. No attempt will be made to review or even to list all the causes of dementia comprehensively, not only because of space restriction, but because enumeration of all the possible causes lists diseases which will rarely be encountered by a single individual interested in the subject over a lifetime and, also, because such lists usually include disease states which rarely present as dementia. A comprehensive list has been published by Slaby and Wyatt (1974), and Haase (1977) has also discussed numerous causes of dementia.

In any review or, for that matter, in the assessment of any publications which relate to the pathology of dementia, a number of factors should be borne in mind, among which the following are of importance. Firstly, any pathological process which causes sufficient destruction of the cerebral hemispheres will produce dementia; when morphological changes in the brain are severe no doubt usually exists about the relationship between the changes and the clinical picture; this is particularly so in cases of dementia in the pre-senile period when the morphological diagnosis, with thorough examination of the brain, is usually in no doubt. With increasing age, however, the precise morphological diagnosis may be more difficult to reach. Occasional cases present no obvious features beyond a minor or major degree of cerebral atrophy, and some demented subjects in old age only show histological changes of a type and severity which occasionally can be found in subjects who have been proved in life to be intellectually well preserved. Secondly, the great majority of all cases of dementia occur in subjects above the age of 65 years. In surveys of subjects living in the community in different countries, it has been found that more than 5 % of the population show evidence of some degree of dementia over the age of 65 years (Gruenberg, 1961; Nielson, 1962; Kay, Beamish, and Roth, 1964; Bergmann, 1975) and, above the age of 80 years, numbers may reach as high as 20 % (Kay, 1972). There is clearly, therefore, a close relationship between increasing age and the tendency to become demented, and one of the purposes of this chapter will be to examine some of the possible factors which predispose aged individuals to dementia; such factors clearly have major implications for any biochemical studies of demented subjects. Thirdly, it must be remembered that accurate and detailed information about the changes which can occur throughout life in the brains of intellectually well-preserved subjects is incomplete and that, although a great deal is known about the morphological changes in the brains of demented subjects, large gaps exist in our knowledge since, on the whole, attention has usually been paid to the obvious morphological abnormalities. Although the latter is not surprising, we need to know much more about all areas of the brain in dementia, even though on light microscopic grounds they show no apparent significant change. Here it is necessary to emphasize that incomplete or unquantified morphological studies of the brain in demented subjects have and will continue to produce inaccurate diagnoses. Small ischaemic lesions in the brain may produce striking neurological disturbances in life which lead the clinician to attribute an accompanying dementing process to such ischaemic lesions. The finding of small foci of cerebral softening at autopsy may well tempt the pathologist to confirm the diagnosis of arteriosclerotic or multi-infarct dementia, but all such cases need considerable histological study since many intellectually normal old subjects show small areas of cerebral softening, and a considerable number of cases of senile dementia of Alzheimer type (SDAT) suffer some degree of ischaemic cerebral destruction. Even after extensive histological investigation it may be difficult to know whether to classify such cases as SDAT or as mixed senile and arteriosclerotic dementia. As a further example, the most commonly observed coincidentally occurring intracranial neoplasm in old age is the meningioma. Such tumours, sometimes of considerable size, are found in a small proportion of cases of SDAT, and the contribution of the tumour to the symptomatology may be difficult to assess. Diagnostic morphological problems of this kind are much less frequent in the much rarer cases of dementia in middle age. The older the population studied, the more frequent will be the cases in which some doubt exists about their precise morphological diagnosis.

Fourthly, it must also be remembered that old people with confusional states precipitated by relatively minor physical illness, or subjects with severe depression, may still be misdiagnosed as cases of dementia, and any detailed morphological or chemical studies on either supposedly normal or demented subjects are only justified if they are done in collaboration with physicians with major experience and interest in dementia and with the time and facilities to perform psychometric tests. The latter may have to be repeated on a number of occasions during the course of a long dementing illness or in observations of elderly subjects who are initially intellectually well preserved since, quite clearly, the terminal state of such subjects may not be indicated by formal psychometric testing done at a considerable interval prior to death. Also, in almost all the quantitative statements about morphological changes in the brain, whether they be in normal or demented subjects, it must be remembered that terminal illness may produce cerebral changes. Clearly, anoxic or ischaemic lesions are the most frequent complications in the elderly ill subject but we know little about the effects of many terminal illnesses on such important features as brain volume and ventricular size and, perhaps, even on fine neuronal structure. Lastly, there are the effects of post-mortem change: fixation and processing on cerebral tissues can never, in the individual case, be precisely assessed. All that one can do in any investigation of the brains from normal and demented old subjects is to use a well-tried and constant procedure on the assumption, not necessarily justified, that the effects of these factors on the brain will be relatively constant from case to case.

I. DISTRIBUTION AND TYPES OF MORPHOLOGICAL LESIONS ASSOCIATED WITH DEMENTIA

Tables 1 to 5 (at the end of this chapter) list, although not comprehensively, the more important disease processes which are associated with dementia and the distribution of the obvious pathological changes. Some rare disorders are included and it should be noted that a few diseases are mentioned under more than one group. The tables are in no way intended to be interpreted as a pathological classification of dementia, but merely as a reminder of the great variation in distribution of changes which lead to the dementing state. The morphological changes in the majority of the diseases listed will not be detailed in this chapter. Descriptions of many of those conditions mentioned can be found in the accounts of Corsellis (1976a) and Tomlinson (1977).

Table 1 divides the dementing diseases into groups, varying in the site of the predominant pathological change. The fifth category, that of the severe amnestic states is included because of the tendency for subjects with that state to be regarded as demented.

Among those states mentioned in Table 2 as being associated predominantly with diffuse cortical lesions, much the most important numerically is that of Alzheimer's disease occurring in the pre-senile or senile periods. Further details of this condition will be given later in the chapter. All the other processes mentioned there are now uncommon, occur more frequently in the pre-senile than in the senile period and, of course, subacute sclerosing panencephalitis is a disease of children. Pick's disease, although occupying much space in the neuropathological literature, occurs perhaps 50 or 100 times less frequently than Alzheimer's disease. In Pick's disease, cortical neuron loss and severe neuronal abnormality is often widespread in the hemispheres, although it may be much more localized than the changes of Alzheimer's disease and results in severe sclerosis of one or more lobes of the brain. In Alzheimer's disease at any age there is often considerable and sometimes very severe brain atrophy, although absence of this latter phenomenon is not a good or constant guide to the presence of a dementing process in old age. These two disorders are commonly regarded as primary neuronal degenerative conditions and, although they show only inconstant and less severe changes in the white matter and basal ganglia, both conditions are probably associated with major disturbances in the axon or its synaptic terminals either independently or combined with severe abnormalities in the neuron perikaryon. The other five disorders mentioned in this group all show widespread and severe cortical neuron loss and sometimes very severe glial proliferation. Many of the chemical changes in the cortex in such diseases could be predicted in an approximate fashion, and the severe intellectual personality and emotional changes found in these subjects are easy to understand on the basis of the widespread cortical destruction.

Table 3 lists those more common disorders in which the lesions are predominantly within the white matter, often leaving much of the cortex apparently unaffected. As in Table 2, the aetiology of the changes in the conditions listed varies greatly and includes proven infective or suspected infective disorders, lesions which result from ineffective oxygenation of blood supply, mechanical rupture of axons, as well as some conditions of unknown aetiology. The severity of the dementia in this group varies from relatively mild—as in most cases of multiple sclerosis—to profound—as in some instances of post-traumatic and multi-infarct dementia. The predominant factor in the production of the clinical syndrome in these conditions is presumably interference with or destruction of the function of major hemisphere connections and specific white matter tracts, the latter often producing major neurological deficits.

Table 4 lists diseases predominantly associated with subcortical nuclear lesions, although in Huntington's chorea, in which the major pathology is in the caudate head and putamen, there may also be severe cortical involvement. In Wilson's disease, in addition to basal ganglia destruction, considerable white matter degeneration also occurs. In some of the other disorders, however, the observed morphological changes are largely, if not entirely confined to the hypothalamus, thalamus, or brain stem, and lesions in the white matter and cortex may not be demonstrable. In some of these listed disorders, notably progressive supranuclear palsy, many instances of Parkinson's disease and striatonigral degeneration, dementia is relatively mild in character. This may even be so in advanced Huntington's chorea and in this whole group detailed clinicopathological correlation would be of considerable value. It is said, for instance, in Huntington's chorea that some patients exhibit an increasing movement disorder and may die with little evidence of dementia. Others show a progressive dementing process in which abnormal movements may be totally absent and yet others have a progressively severe combination of both these clinical features. I know of no morphological studies which have demonstrated that such variations in the clinical picture are accompanied by major variations in the distribution and severity of the morphological cerebral changes. All cases suffer gross destruction of the caudate nucleus and often its almost total replacement by glial tissue. The state of the cortex or white matter in those cases which dement is surely different from those who terminate with relatively well-preserved intellect. Other diseases in this group would also bear similar detailed clinicopathological investigations. In Parkinson's disease, relatively mild dementia is present in the later stages in most subjects. In most of these, white matter and cortical lesions cannot be demonstrated. Some cases, however, show severe progressive dementia, and a proportion of such cases prove to have the cortical changes of Alzheimer's disease. It is also likely that more cases of corticostriatal nigral degeneration occurs than is suspected in life, and that the clinical syndrome of Parkinsonism in old age is accompanied by very varying histological changes from case to case, with severe destruction of the substantia nigra as the most constant finding. Parkinson's disease, however, and the other conditions in this group demonstrate that we still have much to learn from detailed clinicopathological studies, and illustrate the pitfalls of biochemical studies unaccompanied by extensive morphological investigation.

Table 5 lists a group of disorders in which lesions may be found almost anywhere in the brain. In arteriopathic dementia, dementia following post-subarachnoid haemorrhage, and in post-meningitic dementia a major element is ischaemic cerebral necrosis in varying sites. In post-traumatic dementia a considerable contribution of cerebral destruction may be of similar type, although extensive axonal loss in the hemispheres and elsewhere through tearing of axons at the time of injury and cortical destructive lesions resulting from laceration or contusion may also play a significant role. Inclusion in this group of hydrocephalus is conjectural since no specific morphological features are consistently found in dementing subjects with severe ventricular enlargement although, clearly, the latter may affect particularly cerebral hemisphere white matter, and also basal ganglia, thalamus, and hypothalamus and, to some extent, parts of the cortex by stretching and distortion of tissues. The Parkinsonism dementia complex of Guam and the dementia of boxers are two examples of processes which show extremely severe neurofibrillary degeneration, the former with widespread distribution stretching from the anterior horn cells of the spinal cord through the basal ganglia to the cerebral cortex (Hirano and Kurland, 1961;

Hirano, 1974). In dementia pugilistica, although other lesions are present, neurofibrillary tangles are found in vast numbers in the anteromedial temporal lobes (Corsellis, Bruton, and Freeman-Browne, 1973).

Table 6 lists four situations in which profound memory disturbance may occur as a dominant feature of the illness in the absence of features of a global dementing process. In all of them the predominant morphological changes are in the anterior temporal lobes. The lesions may be present elsewhere in the brain but when the latter are severe, as they may be, for instance, after herpes simplex encephalitis, the clinical picture is likely to involve much more than simply memory disturbance.

Table 7 lists disease states in which neurofibrillary tangle formation is a major morphological feature. Severe neurofibrillary degeneration in the cerebral hemispheres seems always to be accompanied by dementia.

Table 8 has been constructed to illustrate, and by no means completely, the disorders in which cerebral infarction plays a considerable or dominant role.

Finally, and again far from complete, Table 9 lists three disorders for which no firm or consistent morphological changes have been described. Some cases of dementia associated with myxoedema are found at autopsy to have very considerable ischaemic lesions which clearly contribute to the dementing process, and in dialysis dementia aluminium toxicity is likely to be a major factor. In dementia associated with chronic alcoholism, if one eliminates the related disorders, such as the Korsakoff and Marchiafava–Bignami syndromes, no consistent findings have been proved to occur and this, as with the other two conditions listed under this heading, is probably of major significance since in all three conditions considerable and sometimes complete recovery of cerebral function occurs with effective therapy. This group illustrates that dementing processes may, although only in a minority of cases, be unaccompanied by readily recognizable morphological abnormalities.

II. INCIDENCE OF DISEASES PRODUCING DEMENTIA

There are no totally reliable figures which relate to the incidence of dementia produced by different processes previously enumerated. There are several reasons for this. Cases based on clinical diagnosis alone leave an element of doubt about the pathological process involved and even considerable mistakes may occur in the clinical diagnosis of dementia, since depression and confusional states may, in the elderly particularly, without prolonged observation and much experience, be mistaken for dementia. Even when pathological studies are performed, the significance placed on small infarcts or on small numbers of plaques in arriving at a diagnosis, may well be differently interpreted by different observers, with resulting changes in the percentage of cases attributed to arteriosclerotic or Alzheimer type disease. The incidence of dementia reported from neurological clinics is, on the whole, of cases occurring in the pre-senile period, and almost certainly over-represents those diseases presenting with or accompanied by neurological symptomatology; certainly, groups of cases reported from long-term psychiatric institutions would show very considerable differences. The age of the patients being reported on would also make some difference to the percentages of different diseases involved, since before the age of 65 years disorders such as Huntington's chorea and Jakob–Creutzfeldt disease might be found in small, although significant, numbers, whereas over 75 years such diseases are excessively rare and the majority of cases of dementia will be found to be due to senile dementia of Alzheimer type (SDAT), with many of the remainder having either an arteriosclerotic basis or a contribution from multiple infarcts. Also in old age, an increasing number of cases will be found to have no satisfactory morphological explanation for the dementia, although extreme cerebral atrophy might well be present. Two relatively recent studies probably illustrate the position reasonably well. Marsden and Harrison (1972) reported on 106 cases admitted with the diagnosis of pre-senile dementia. The diagnosis of dementia was confirmed in 84 of these (in 7 doubt existed about the diagnosis and 15 proved not to be demented, 8 of these latter being depressed). Of the 84, the final diagnosis was as follows:

Intracranial space occupying masses	8
Arteriosclerotic dementia	8
Dementia in alcoholics	8
Possibly normal pressure communicating hydrocephalus	5
Jakob–Creutzfeldt disease	3
Huntington's chorea	3
Post-traumatic cerebral atrophy	1
Post-subarachnoid haemorrhage	1
Limbic encephalitis	1
Cerebral atrophy of unknown cause	48

The diagnosis in the majority of this group, therefore (those with cerebral atrophy), could only have been made with certainty by biopsy but, as Marsden and Harrison (1972) suggest, the great majority of the latter probably had Alzheimer's disease. This would certainly fit with the findings in series where biopsy has been performed (Sim, Turner, and Smith, 1966; Coblenz and coworkers, 1973).

A consecutive group of 73 cases over the age of 65 years, with a mean age of 77 years, assessed pathologically in our laboratory, produced the following diagnostic groupings:

Senile dementia	33	46%
Probably senile dementia	5	7%
Mixed senile and arteriosclerotic dementia	4	5%
Probably mixed senile and arteriosclerotic dementia	8	11%
Arteriosclerotic dementia	7	10%
Probably arteriosclerotic dementia	5	7%
Other specific disorders	5	– 7%
No histological abnormality	6	– 8%

69% } 33%

Those cases placed in a 'probable' category showed 'senile' changes and/or cerebral softening of a considerable degree, but within the limits of what had been found in the occasional intellectually well-preserved individual. In this group, therefore, senile dementia of Alzheimer type accounted for approximately 50% of the total and contributed to another 20%. Based on the amount of cerebral softening present, multi-infarct dementia probably accounted for approximately 17% but contributed to another group of about the same size so that total multi-infarct and senile dementia of Alzheimer type, alone or together, accounted for between 80 and 85% of all cases. The coexistence of SDAT and significant cerebral softening in a considerable number of elderly subjects is a well-established fact (Corsellis, 1962; Delay and coworkers 1962; Post, 1965; Tomlinson, Blessed, and Roth, 1970). The incidence of SDAT is greater in females than in males and probably accounts for the great majority of cases of dementia in aged females (Tomlinson, Blessed, and Roth, 1970); some authors attribute the great majority of cases of dementia in old age in both sexes to SDAT (Escourolle and Poirier, 1973).

III. PATHOLOGY OF ALZHEIMER'S DISEASE AND SENILE DEMENTIA OF ALZHEIMER TYPE (SDAT)

These two disorders will be discussed together as there is much evidence that they are fundamentally the same disorder differing largely in the age of onset and to some extent in symptomatology, and in the greater severity of the pathological process in the pre-senile group.

1. Macroscopic changes

In Alzheimer's pre-senile dementia the brain at death and probably in the great majority of cases when first referred for clinical opinion, shows considerable or severe atrophy. Fresh brain weight at autopsy is not uncommonly around 1000 g. The most prominent changes are in the cerebral hemispheres where gyral atrophy is usually marked in the frontal and temporal lobes with a considerably lesser degree of involvement of the remainder of the hemispheres. The anterior temporal lobes are usually severely affected, particularly the anterior parts of the middle and superior temporal gyri and the hippocampus and adjacent gyri. Coronal sections show marked broadening of the affected sulci and fissures, and usually moderate or severe dilation of the third and lateral ventricles; white matter appears normal, although it is very much reduced in total volume. A degree of asymmetry in the gyral atrophy is occasionally present, with focal areas of more severe atrophy superimposed on the overall generally shrunken hemispheres. The hind-brain is usually not obviously abnormal.

The above description would fit also for SDAT, although in a considerable number of cases the atrophy is not so severe when compared with normal brains of the same age, since in the latter group a minor degree of generalized atrophy, or a moderate degree of parasagittal gyral atrophy with some ventricular dilatation, is a common occurrence (Tomlinson, Blessed, and Roth, 1968).

2. Microscopic observations

Two features—senile plaque formation and Alzheimer's neurofibrillary change—are to be found throughout the whole of the cerebral cortex in the majority of cases, and in the hippocampus two additional changes—granulovacuolar degeneration and Hirano body formation—are also found in an exceptional degree. In the pre-senile form of the disease, senile plaques and neurofibrillary degeneration, usually occur in great profusion throughout the cerebral cortex, producing a picture which is quite unlike anything ever found in normal subjects of the same age when plaques are either totally absent or few in number and tangles cannot usually be found at all. Plaques, in silver-impregnated preparations, are found by light microscopy to consist of irregular masses 15–200 μm across, of threads and granules, often, and particularly in the larger plaques, with a more uniform densely staining centre (Fig. 1). In some instances they appear to occupy almost 50 % of the cerebral cortex and the intervening tissue is often also abnormal in that twirls and wisps of fibrillary material of varying thickness are commonly seen. Considerable variations are found in the numbers of plaques present in various lobes of the brain and even from gyrus to gyrus in the same area, but no part of the neocortex will be found free of the structures and usually all areas are heavily involved. The hippocampus, the amygdaloid, and the hippocampal gyrus are also usually heavily affected. At an ultrastructural level, plaques (Fig. 2) consist of numerous greatly swollen nerve terminals, the majority axonal in origin, and filled with numerous laminated or dense, round or oval bodies sometimes containing abnormal fibrillary material (Kidd, 1964; Terry, Gonatas, and Weiss, 1964; Wisniewski and Terry, 1976). Between these often densely packed abnormal neurites are occasional normal cell processes, microglia, and astrocytes, but in the large plaques the other prominent feature is a central mass of amyloid fibrils (Fig. 3)

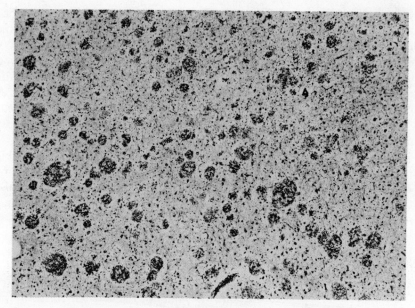

Figure 1. Senile plaques in the neocortex from a case of SDAT. Von Braunmühl (× 70)

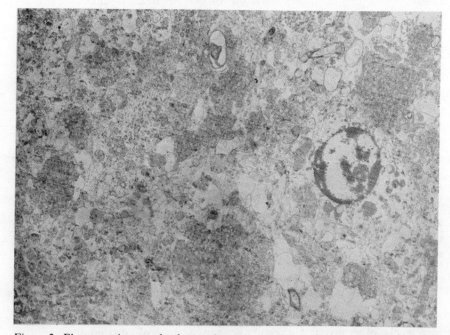

Figure 2. Electron micrograph of part of a senile plaque showing numerous distended neurites filled with round and oval dense bodies (× 4620)

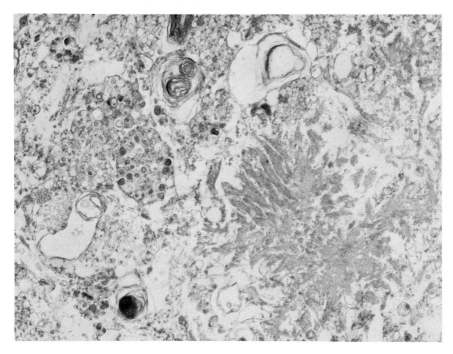

Figure 3. Senile plaque with a central core of amyloid and more peripherally situated distended neurites (× 7960)

with extensions towards the periphery among neurite processes. Although not commonly seen in standard preparations, synapses of normal appearance are said to be present between the abnormal axonal terminals and normal-looking post-synaptic terminals (Wisniewski and Terry, 1976). Of some importance from an aetiological point of view is the statement that when plaques are small, consisting of a cluster of only four or five distended neurites, amyloid fibrils cannot be found among them but, when large, amyloid is a constant element of the plaques (Terry and Wisniewski, 1970). Outside the neocortex and the heavily involved structures of the anteromedial temporal lobes, plaques are found irregularly and in much smaller numbers, particularly in the periventricular tissues of the third ventricle, the mamillary bodies, and the upper stem, but their numbers rarely reach a concentration which would suggest that they are significant in terms of functional disturbance in these latter sites.

The other striking finding is the presence of neurofibrillary tangles, (Fig. 4), again throughout all areas of the cerebral cortex, and particularly numerous in the anteromedial temporal lobes. At light microscopic level, silver impregnation demonstrates these as abnormally thick intracytoplasmic fibrils, which can be seen curving around the nucleus towards the basal dendrite in the larger pyramidal cells or intertwined and twisted in the neuron perikaryon. Electron

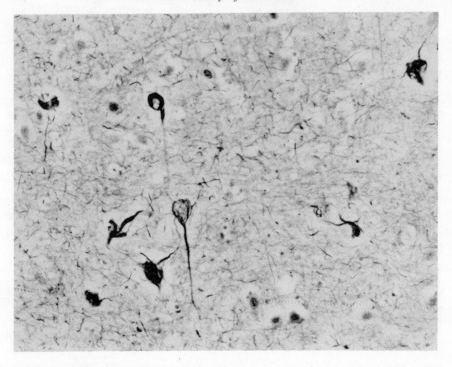

Figure 4. Neurofibrillary tangles in the neocortex from a case of SDAT Glees, Eriksons, and Marsland (× 320)

microscopically (Figs 5 and 6) they consist of a proliferation of abnormal intracellular fibrillary material, for a number of years described as twisted tubules in much of the literature but now regarded as formed from pairs of helically twisted fibrils (Kidd, 1963; Terry, 1963; Wisniewski, Narang, and Terry, 1976). The spiralled fibrils show a maximum diameter between the twists of around 22 nm, with the twists occurring at fairly regular intervals of 65–80 nm, where the diameter diminishes to 10 nm. Within the neuron they appear to displace other cytoplasmic elements, which are normal in appearance and are occasionally found in among the clusters of abnormal fibrils. The fibrils extend into the axon and can be seen in some instances, although in much smaller numbers, in the distended neurites of the plaques. Vast numbers of cells involved by tangle formation can be found in the anterior temporal lobes, particularly in the amygdaloid and Sommer's sector of the hippocampal pyramidal cells, in the adjacent subiculum, and in the hippocampal gyrus, but again, although concentrations may vary from case to case in different areas of the brain, scarcely any gyrus will be found to have escaped totally, and in many instances literally millions of neurons are involved. Again, in the deeper structures of the brain

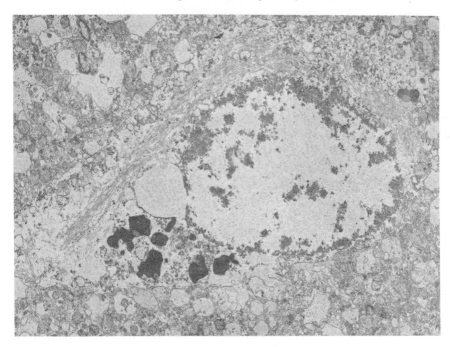

Figure 5. Electron micrograph of a neurofibrillary tangle showing the paired helically wound filaments coursing around the periphery of the nucleus (× 5775)

tangles occur relatively rarely but may be found on careful searching in the same areas in which plaques are present, and in the upper stem may affect occasional pigmented cells in the substantia nigra.

Two other lesions are almost constantly present, these being granulovacuolar degeneration of hippocampal pyramidal cells, and the presence in the same area, of Hirano bodies. Granulovacuolar degeneration consists (Fig. 7), as the name suggests, of the presence of vacuoles (approximately 5 μm in diameter) containing a central haematoxyphylic and argyrophilic granule, in the cytoplasm of the affected cells. The granule is usually around 1 μm across. The process is almost entirely limited to the pyramidal cells of the hippocampus and the adjacent presubiculum and subiculum. In the hippocampus it particularly affects the cells in segments h_1 and h_2 although it may extend into the end-plate. Involved cells may be ballooned by numerous vacuoles: in 6-μm thick sections, up to 15 can be seen in a single cell. Ultrastructurally the lesions consist of roughly spherical translucent areas within the cytoplasm, containing a central, granular electron-dense particle (Hirano and coworkers, 1968). Scattered among, and often apparently within, the perikaryon of the pyramidal cells of the hippocampus, again particularly in sectors h_1 and h_2 and in the stratum lacunosum, here less

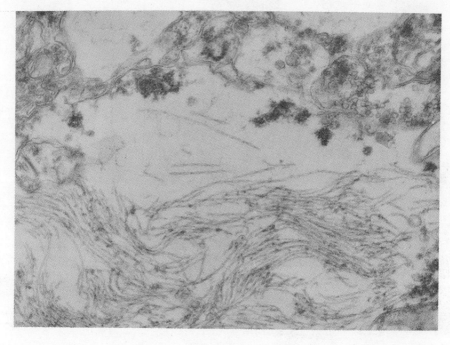

Figure 6. Detail of the fibrillary elements of a tangle showing the regular constriction
along the length of the paired filaments (× 99680)

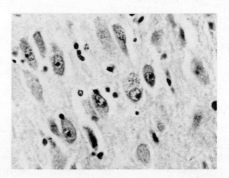

Figure 7. Hippocampal pyramidal cells
with a centrally placed neuron distended by
granulovacuolar degeneration. Haematoxylin and eosin (× 260)

regularly, may be found numerous round, oval or rod-like eosinophilic bodies
varying from 8 to 15 μm across and up to about 30 μm long (Fig. 8). In the larger,
elongated forms, faint longitudinal striations may be visible. These are the so-

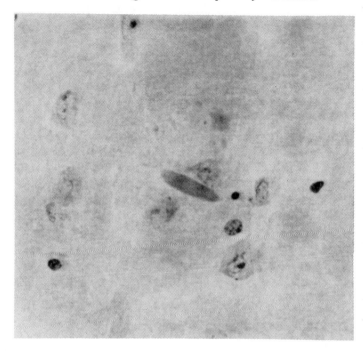

Figure 8. Large elongated Hirano body lying between two pyramidal
neurons in the hippocampus. Haematoxylin and eosin (× 560)

called 'Hirano bodies' (Hirano, 1965) which have usually been interpreted as
being intraneuronal although they certainly can occur in other central nervous
elements (Cavanagh, Blakemore, and Kyu, 1971; Field and Narang, 1972;
Spencer and Thomas, 1974; Gessaga and Anzil, 1975), and even in the
hippocampus their intracytoplasmic neuronal situation has been challenged
(Gibson, 1978). At ultrastructural level they consist of flat plates, 100–150 μm
thick, and parallel rod-like structures, 60–100 nm thick, alternately layered
(Hirano and coworkers, 1968; Schochet and McCormick, 1972). Again, they can
be found in other areas of the cortex but are never a prominent feature outside the
hippocampus.

It has been repeatedly stated in the neuropathological literature that in
Alzheimer's disease there is a major loss of nerve cells throughout the neocortex.
Nerve cell loss in severely affected cases is certainly strikingly visible in the
shrunken hippocampus and other structures of the anterior temporal lobes, but
little objective evidence exists that there is a significant fall in packing density of
the nerve cells throughout the neocortex in this condition by comparison with
age-matched controls, although the reports on small numbers of cases have
suggested that nerve cell loss of significant proportions may be found (Colon,

1973; Shefer, 1973). Some recent studies have, however, failed to identify significant diminution in nerve cell packing density outside the anterior temporal lobes (Tomlinson and Henderson, 1976; Terry and coworkers, 1977). Nerve cell counts, of course, neglect the question of total volume of cerebral cortex in Alzheimer's disease and, again, limited studies suggest that this is significant and considerable in many instances (Corsellis, 1976a) so that, if packing density of neurons remains roughly the same as in normal elderly subjects, total neuron counts could still be substantially reduced.

Greater abnormalities in the dendritic system have also been described in Golgi preparations of the cortex in Alzheimer's disease and SDAT (Mehraein, Yamada, and Tarnowska-Dzidusko, 1975), by comparison with the striking changes which occur in normal old subjects (Scheibel and coworkers, 1975; Scheibel and Scheibel, 1976). Surprisingly in Alzheimer's disease and SDAT, nerve cells in areas of the brain which do not show any characteristic lesions by standard light microscopy may be severely affected with, for instance, greater loss of many of the normally multi-branching dendrites in the Purkinje cells of the cerebellum (Mehraein, Yamada, and Tarnowska-Dzidusko, 1975). Along with this has come the statement that nucleolar volume and RNA production in a number of areas of the brain, some of which are not affected by the characteristic pathological changes of Alzheimer's disease, are significantly reduced in the latter and SDAT (Mann, Yates, and Barton, 1977a; Mann and Sinclair, 1978) (although this has been denied in the recent publication of Vemura and Hartman (1978)). The possibility clearly exists, therefore, that many parts of the central nervous system are affected which do not show the morphological changes that are considered to be characteristic of the disorder, and this needs much further study. Clearly, numerous brain areas might be affected as a result of the cortical changes, but perhaps a more general abnormality, which particularly affects protein synthesis within nerve cells and dendritic arborization, exists.

The very dramatic changes seen in silver-impregnation preparations within neurons and their axonal terminals, produces strangely little glial response. Astrocytic and microglial proliferation around or within plaques is detectable but is not a striking feature and certainly does not suggest any major response or primary involvement of glia in the disease. Occasionally, in severely affected areas, particularly in the outer cortex, there is some degree of vacuolation of the neuropil which is not apparently artefactual, and which presumably reflects distended or vacuolated astrocytic or axonal processes. Histological changes, other than tangle and plaque formation, are so limited that only much experience of the disorder enables one to suspect it in standard cytological stains. The blood vessels in the majority of cases show no unusual features and indeed, in many instances, the cardiovascular system, the major vessels at the base of the brain, and the pial arteries are strikingly normal for elderly subjects, and the intracerebral arterioles only show minor degrees of hyalinization such as is found in many people of similar age groups. In some instances, pial arteries and arterioles and occasional venules show considerable infiltration of walls with amyloid, a condition which has been termed 'congophilic angiopathy', but this condition is usually only present in a small proportion of cases and it occurs in some elderly subjects in the absence of plaque formation.

Everything described above can be found in the brain in SDAT but, on the whole, in subjects dying above the age of 70 years, changes are not so severe and are considerably more varied. Plaque formation may not be so consistent or dense in all areas of cortex and neurofibrillary tangle formation not so severe, although both are usually plentiful. General brain atrophy and ventricular dilatation is usually of considerable and often major degree. Naturally, when plaque and tangle formation in the neocortex are severe, the histological appearance is very similar or identical to that of the pre-senile disorder. When plaque formation is more limited, when it affects, as it does in some instances, predominantly the outer layers of the cortex and the depths of sulci leaving other cortical layers largely uninvolved, or when plaque formation is much less defined, producing in silver impregnations only an irregular fibrillary abnormality with few focal densely staining plaques, the appearances are considerably different from what is commonly found in the pre-senile group, although only in degree. In such cases, however, neurofibrillary tangles are usually present in considerable or great numbers throughout the neocortex, and no doubt about the diagnosis should exist since the latter condition is one which is rarely, if ever, found in intellectually well-preserved subjects. In some demented old subjects, however, the problem in diagnosis, and indeed in the theoretical explanation of the dementia on morphological grounds, arises from the observation that the brain changes may be similar, both qualitatively and quantitatively, to the changes which can be found in the occasional intellectually well-preserved subject. Such cases are not numerous but the situation requires some comment which is best based on a short statement about the findings in the brains of intellectually well-preserved old people.

IV. 'SENILE CHANGE' IN INTELLECTUALLY NORMAL OLD SUBJECTS

It has been established for many years that senile plaques and neurofibrillary tangles occur in the brains of many apparently normal old people. Only in recent years, however, have studies been performed on the brains of subjects who were established by formal examination and testing to be intellectually well-preserved shortly before death. Unquestionably, in many of the earlier studies assumptions on the normality of the subjects were made on the basis of past history and such unsatisfactory criteria as the absence of any known psychological disorder, or death having occurred in a general medical ward, and subjects studied under these circumstances would almost certainly include some cases of early dementia. Up to the age of 60 years it would seem reasonable to accept for studies of normal brains, material coming from patients dying suddenly from ischaemic heart disease, from road accidents, or from rapidly fatal illnesses, without specific intellectual testing, provided they had been in normal health and occupation shortly before death. Above that age, however, and particularly above the age of 70, there is an increasing likelihood that the series will be distorted by cases of early dementia unless specific psychiatric and psychometric investigations have taken place.

Detailed studies of a small group of such tested individuals were made by Tomlinson, Blessed and Roth (1968) and the findings of a much larger group of subjects dying suddenly or rapidly from acute illnesses but without specific testing were also reported (Tomlinson, 1972). The findings in these two groups were not greatly different, except that the latter larger group contained a number of cases in which neurofibrillary tangle formation in the neocortex suggested the subjects concerned were demented. In the larger study, small numbers of plaques were found in the neocortex in about 15 % of subjects in the fourth decade, in 50 % by the seventh decade, and in almost 80 % by the tenth decade. Under the age of 60 years, plaques were almost invariably few in number and widely scattered but, above that age, there was a steady rise in the mean numbers of plaques per field, although even in the highest age group they failed to reach the numbers which can be found in Alzheimer's disease of the pre-senile or senile period. In the intellectually normal old subjects reported in the earlier study, plaques were found in about 65 % above the age of 65 years but never in large numbers. In continuing studies of proven intellectually well-preserved old people two cases have occurred, however, in which plaque formation has been heavy throughout all areas of the cerebral cortex, in a concentration similar to that which occurs in SDAT. Despite the rarity of such cases, no doubt now exists about their occurrence. However, in the great majority of normal or apparently normal old subjects, in which the total numbers of plaques are small, greater concentrations may be found in the outer cortical layers, in the depths of sulci and in the structures of the anterior temporal lobes, particularly the amygdaloid nucleus and overlying cortex and in the hippocampus, and hippocampal gyrus. As in Alzheimer's disease, however, there is an unquestionable tendency for all the so-called senile changes to be concentrated more severely in the anterior temporal lobes than in any other part of the brain. Nevertheless, the plaques in normal subjects are identical at both light and electron microscopic level with the plaques of Alzheimer's disease, the difference between normal and Alzheimer-diseased subjects of the pre-senile or senile period being largely quantitative; Roth, Tomlinson, and Blessed (1966), Blessed, Tomlinson, and Roth (1968), and Tomlinson, Blessed, and Roth (1970) produced evidence that a statistically significant correlation exists between the mean numbers of plaques in the cerebral cortex and tests of cerebral function which relate to the severity of the dementing process, although the correlation ceases to exist when dementia becomes severe.

Cells affected by Alzheimer's neurofibrillary degeneration can also be found in the majority of normal elderly subjects in the structures of the anterior temporal lobes, particularly in the amygdaloid nucleus and the hippocampus, and in the glomerular formation of the hippocampal gyrus. In normal old age, however, tangles are either absent or present in small numbers only in the neocortex. In Tomlinson's study (1972) few normal subjects under the age of 50 years were found to show tangle formation in the hippocampus. The numbers reached 60 % by the sixties and 100 % by the eighties. Tomlinson, Blessed, and Roth (1970) reported that tangle formation was usually much heavier in the hippocampus in Alzheimer's disease, and Ball (1976) showed in very detailed quantitative studies that the number of tangles in the hippocampus was significantly greater in Alzheimer's disease and SDAT than in intellectually well-preserved old subjects. Undoubtedly, in intellectually normal old subjects sparse neurofibrillary tangle formation may be found in some areas of the neocortex, but the author has never seen a proven non-demented case in which neurofibrillary tangle formation was heavy throughout the neocortex. Again on all morphological criteria, the tangles in normal old age and in Alzheimer's disease appear to be identical. The difference is quantitative, once more, but the most important distinction is that numerous neurofibrillary tangles are never found throughout the neocortex in normal old age and their presence in large numbers is confined to the demented population. The chemistry of the neurofibrillary protein, including that of the twisted fibrils of Alzheimer's disease, has recently been reviewed by Iqbal and coworkers (1978).

Granulovacuolar degeneration in hippocampal pyramidal cells was regarded as occurring largely in Alzheimer's disease until Woodard (1962, 1966) showed that here, again, the difference is largely quantitative. He demonstrated that neurons of the inferolateral quadrant of the hippocampus, (approximately Sommer's sector) were more affected in Alzheimer's disease and SDAT than in subjects with non-dementing psychiatric disorders or those dying from non-neurological diseases. Woodard (1962, 1966) found an absolute difference in that no non-demented subject had more than 9 % of cells affected in that quadrant, whereas in Alzheimer's disease more than that number of cells were invariably affected. Woodard's (1962, 1966) findings were largely confirmed by Tomlinson, Blessed, and Roth (1970) and by Tomlinson and Kitchener (1972), although they found that the distinction was not absolute if one examined only a single section from one hippocampus or from both sides. Ball and Lo (1977), however, in a very detailed study, showed a much more severe involvement in a small group of senile dements, compared with controls. Granulovacuolar degeneration was found to occur (Tomlinson, 1972) in a very small number of subjects below the age of 60 years and with increasing numbers from then on, so that by the age of 90 years some 80 % of subjects showed this change. The detailed studies of Ball and Lo (1977), on serial sections of the hippocampus, demonstrated that some cells were affected in all subjects above the age of 49 years, and that there was a slight tendency for the number of cells to increase steadily from that time on in normal subjects. Here again, therefore, the differences appear to be quantitative. Even in the most severely affected cases (Tomlinson, Blessed, and Roth, 1970) it is rare in Alzheimer's disease to find cells outside the hippocampus and the adjacent subiculum affected by granulovacuolar degeneration, and it is clear that changes limited to such a small area of the brain cannot be responsible for any form of global dementia or probably even contribute significantly to it. However, heavy granulovacuolar degeneration in the hippocampus and subiculum appears to be a useful marker for Alzheimer's disease and is further evidence of the tendency for the anterior temporal lobes to be especially, and possibly selectively, involved by senile change in normal old age and particularly heavily affected in this type of dementing process.

Hirano bodies have not been quantitatively studied until very recent years. Gibson and Tomlinson (1977), in a semi-quantitative analysis, showed that again there is a statistical difference in the numbers of bodies to be found among the hippocampal pyramidal cells and in the stratum lacunosum in intellectually well-preserved and demented old subjects, the latter having greater numbers although with a considerable overlap in individual cases. Hirano bodies, however, are certainly present in some subjects in this site from early adult life (Gibson and Tomlinson, 1977) and probably gradually increase in number until the age of 60 years, when they begin to appear in considerable numbers in a few intellectually normal subjects and almost invariably occur in large numbers in subjects with Alzheimer's disease.

There is, therefore, good evidence that at a histological level the differences between Alzheimer's disease and intellectually normal old subjects is quantitative and not qualitative. No structural change is absolutely peculiar to Alzheimer's disease or present in that disorder which cannot be found in intellectually normal old subjects to some degree. This, of course, is very far from saying that the senile changes which are to be found in normal old age are the result of a simple ageing process and that Alzheimer's disease is merely an exaggeration of normal ageing; all that can be said is that the so-called senile changes which in intellectually normal subjects are clearly age-related, occur with much greater severity in Alzheimer's disease and SDAT.

Clearly senile plaques, which consist of grossly abnormal nerve cell processes, and neurofibrillary tangles which result from a massive proliferation of intracytoplasmic fibrillary structures, may interfere with normal synaptic and neuronal function. In the normal elderly subject in which plaque formation is slight or moderate although often widely distributed, and in which neurofibrillary tangle formation is largely limited to the anterior temporal lobes, cerebral function is not affected to a degree which produces an abnormal clinical state, although it clearly seems possible that these changes may contribute to the relatively minor memory, intellectual, and personality changes which are common in normal subjects from middle age onwards. Evidence exists that aluminium-induced neurofibrillary degeneration in animals is associated with abnormal electrophysiological responses (Crapper, 1973; Crapper and Dalton, 1973; Crapper, 1976), and that the tangles in.humans are abnormal fibrillary proteins has been established (Iqbal and coworkers, 1978). Nevertheless, it is clear that in old age a good many other morphological factors may contribute to the development of dementia as well as the specific histological changes which characterize Alzheimer's disease, and some of these known changes will now briefly be stated, for it is possible that variations in factors other than senile plaque and tangle formation are of major significance in determining whether, with varying degrees of the latter abnormalities, any individual subject becomes demented or remains apparently within the non-demented group. It is, of course, entirely possible that both plaque and tangle formation in Alzheimer's disease and SDAT are merely markers of some much more fundamental process which has not yet been defined. Some of the other possible variables which may be factors in the development of dementia will now be briefly described.

A. Changes of Cerebral Volume with Age

It has long been established that the weight and volume of the brain diminishes considerably in old age, with much of the published data suggesting that mean loss of brain weight from youth to extreme old age is between 100 and 150 g from a starting point of around 1380 g in males and 1240 g in females (Korenschevsky, 1961; Blinkov and Glezer, 1968). Decrease in volume is visible at autopsy in many old patients since the cerebral hemispheres commonly lie several milli-metres beneath the inner skull table, whereas in youth there is virtually no defin-able space between the dura and the brain. Individual variation, however, is great, and the brain in some old subjects without any terminal neurological disorder may fill the cranial cavity almost to the same extent as in youth. Further evidence of diminution in cerebral size is visible in narrowed gyri, widened sulci, and fissures, even in intellectually well-preserved subjects. Figures produced from surveys of brain weight have usually contained two main sources of error, although almost all have stressed the wide range of normal values. Firstly, the subjects being investigated have not had any specific examination in life to determine that they were intellectually normal, and many series in the past must have included cases of dementia in the older age groups. Secondly, although this diminution in brain weight has reflected what is clearly an undeniable trend, in the individual case it has been quite impossible to know the original brain weight. A recent publication (Davis and Wright, 1977) has dealt with both these difficulties, and produced figures for loss in brain weight and volume throughout life in normal subjects. The brains examined came from subjects without evidence of dementia or neurological disorder, and the capacity of the cranial cavity as well as the brain volume were accurately obtained. This investigation established that considerable variation does exist in loss of volume and brain weight throughout life but that, as a mean, there is little reduction in the brain volume/cranial cavity volume ratio (BV/CCV), from youth to 50 years. Expressed as a percentage, the BV/CCV has a mean of around 93 % in youth and 92 % in the fifties, but after the age of 65 years it falls off considerably, and in the ninth and tenth decades is around 82 %. Even in extreme old age, however, the BV/CCV percentage may still be in the upper eighties. This investigation took no account of ventricular volume but, again, subjective observation would suggest that ventricular volume in old age is often considerably greater than in youth. Precise estimations of ventricular volume have been few, in the most detailed of which (Last and Tompsett, 1953) casts were produced of the ventricular system. This failed to show any evidence, in a small series, of increasing ventricular size in a group of subjects above the age of 45 years, although a very considerable variation in size was demonstrated. In a less accurate assessment of ventricular size, Tomlinson, Blessed, and Roth (1968) failed to produce evidence of increasing ventricular size in a small group of intellectually normal subjects above the age of 65 years, but again showed that considerable variation existed, and they judged 70 % of the ventricles to be enlarged to a slight or moderate degree. Ventricular volumes in the intellectually normal old subjects averaged only about half that of a demented group, the majority of whom were suffering from SDAT (Tomlinson, Blessed, and Roth, 1970). Messert, Wannamaker, and Dudley (1972) found that over 70 % of the normal old brains in their series possessed small ventricles, although above the age of 60 years a number of 'normal' brains with large ventricles were seen. The problems of estimating ventricular volume in autopsy material and knowing how it relates to what was present in life are very considerable, since terminal illness can almost certainly produce considerable changes in short periods of time and the loss of CSF during removal of the brain and changes in ventricular volume during fixation are largely uncontrollable. The development of computerized transaxial tomography (CTT) shows promise, however, of overcoming all these problems since intellectually normal subjects, of any age, while in totally good health, can be examined without invasive procedures.

Huckman, Fox and Topel (1975), using CTT, found that 50 % of their normal group had small ventricles, but that they were slightly enlarged in 40 %, and moderate or severely enlarged in 10 % of cases. Barron, Jacobs, and Kinkel (1976) and Jacobs and coworkers (1978) have reported on planimetric and computer-produced data from CTT, the latter in a total of 281 normal subjects. Both reports showed only a gradual mean increase in ventricular size from the second to the seventh decades, but a rapid increase from then on. Individual data are unfortunately not given in these papers, but the range of ventricular size was stated to be more narrow in the first six decades and larger in the eighth and ninth decades. Naturally, these studies do not yield absolute values of ventricular volume, but hopefully further development of techniques may enable this to be done. Here then, among the normals, is another variable which, to some extent, reflects loss of cerebral tissue as does the variable of total brain weight and volume. What we still do not know is how much of this volume and weight loss is due to cortical or white matter loss. Again, the impression in the examination of multiple coronal sections is that there is very considerable diminution in cortical volume and probably in white matter in normal old age, but precise figures have yet to be produced. Corsellis (1976b) stated that there is a mean cortical volume loss of some 18 % in the brains of females suffering from SDAT compared with normal females matched for age, but absolute figures for total cerebral volume, both in normal old age and demented subjects, have never been published to my knowledge. An investigation is currently being carried out in the author's laboratories in an attempt to establish absolute values for cortical and white matter volume in brains fixed and examined by a standardized procedure.

B. Neuron Loss in Old Age

Until a few years ago, there was much dispute about the presence or absence of nerve cell loss in the central nervous system in normal people throughout life (Hanley, 1974). The situation has largely been resolved, in my view, in the past 20 years and can briefly be stated as follows. Certain groups of nerve cells, particularly in the brain stem, have stable numbers of neurons throughout life. Those nuclei in which no nerve cell loss has been demonstrated are the facial nerve nucleus (Van Buskirk, 1945), the trochlear nuclei (Vijayashankar and Brody, 1971), the ventral cochlear nucleus (Konigsmark and Murphy, 1972), the abducens nuclei (Vijayashankar and Brody, 1973), and the inferior olive (Monagle and Brody, 1974). There is now, however, good evidence that in many parts of the cerebral cortex (Brody, 1955; Colon, 1972; Shefer, 1973; Tomlinson and Henderson, 1976), in the locus coeruleus (Vijayashankar and Brody, 1973), in the Purkinje cells of the cerebellum (Hall, Miller, and Corsellis, 1975), and in the spinal cord motor neurons (Tomlinson and Irving, 1977), nerve cells are lost in very considerable numbers in many individuals, particularly above the age of 60 years. Again, there is much individual variation from case to case as there seems to be in many of the described changes in normal old age. Of particular relevance to dementia is neuron loss in the cerebral cortex. Brody (1955, 1970), in a detailed study, produced evidence that in the pre-central, superior temporal and superior frontal gyrus, and in the visual cortex there was a mean loss of neurons of around 40 % between youth and old age, although significant cell loss did not occur in the post-central and inferior temporal gyrus. Figures not dissimilar to this have been produced by a number of different authors with much evidence that the variations are considerable in different parts of the brain (Colon, 1972; Shefer, 1973; Tomlinson and Henderson, 1976). Using an automatic particle counting apparatus (the Quantimet 720 Image Analysing Computer), Tomlinson and Henderson (1976) showed that there was a very considerable loss in particles of a size that could only be neurons in a number of different cortical gyri with a mean loss in packing density of these particles of between 40 and 50 % in several areas of the cortex. Extension of these studies, which will be published in detail, has confirmed the preliminary findings and, as with most other parameters, striking variations exist in individual subjects even in extreme old age (Fig. 9). Their studies, as with the majority of others, relate only to the packing density of nerve cells in the cortex and take no account of total cortical volume. Unless cortical volume increases in old age, a proposition which would appear to be absurd, the figures of neuron loss expressed in terms of packing cell density/unit area or volume actually underestimate the number of nerve cells that are lost in the cerebral cortex when cortical volume is taken into account.

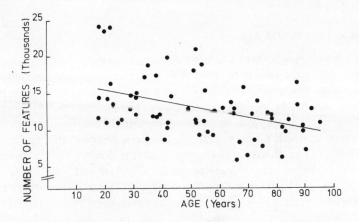

Figure 9. Neuron counts (features lying between 12 and 19 μ per 100 mm^2 in longest cord) in the cerebral cortex at different ages; pooled from 11 selected sites ($r = -0.444$; $p < 0.001$)

C. Changes in Dendritic Arborization

By the use of the Golgi–Cox procedure, which presents considerable technical and interpretational problems in autopsy material, evidence is accumulating, although not yet sufficiently quantified, that the pyramidal neurons of the third layer of the pre-frontal and superior temporal human cortex suffer considerable changes in their dendritic systems in old age. Scheibel and coworkers (1975) and Scheibel and Scheibel (1976) have described globular swelling of the cell body, the appearance of nodules on dendrites, and loss of basilar dendrites and branches. The most severely affected cells eventually possess a deformed cell body with a thickened nodular apical dendrite and a few thick, stunted, or even no basal dendrites. Presumably this process leads eventually to cell death. In further studies, Scheibel (1978), extending observations to the superior and middle frontal gyri, superior and middle temporal gyri, the motor oortex, hippocampus, and subiculum, has concluded that a similar sequence of changes may affect any pyramidal cell, although differences in severity and detail are present in different areas. Horizontal dendritic branches are probably first affected by varicosities occurring at branches and at the junction of the apical shaft and cell body. With progression of the process, the cell body swells and the basilar dendrites, oblique branches of the apical shaft, and terminal arches become distorted and actually lost. Betz cells are particularly severely affected, and by the ninth decade up to 80 % of them have significant dendritic pathology. The above descriptions have been purely qualitative, but Mehraein, Yamada, and Tarnowska-Dzidusko (1975) reported on a quantitative study of the apical dendritic system in the third and fifth pyramidal neurons of the cingulate gyrus. They showed a diminution in spinal density with increasing distances from the cell body, spine loss being greatest in pre-senile Alzheimer's disease, although also significantly more severe in SDAT by comparison with more normal controls. Similar, more severe changes, also occurred in the dendritic systems of cerebellar Purkinje cells in Alzheimer's disease (pre-senile and senile) by comparison with controls. It is clear from the recent investigation of Williams, Ferrante, and Caviness Jr (1978), that all observations using the Golgi method on human material require meticulous care and control, since they demonstrated closely similar changes to those seen in old age by Scheibel and Scheibel (1976) in material from young subjects in which delayed fixation was apparently responsible.

Supporting the reality of the dendritic changes in old age humans however, are observations on ageing animals in which artefact produced by delayed, incomplete, or varying fixation is excluded. Feldman and Dowd (1974) and Feldman (1976) showed a 24 % loss of dendritic spines from the apical tuft, and a 40 % loss from oblique branch dendrites in old compared with young rats. Variations were marked from animal to animal and all the old rats showed numerous normal nerve cells. As in the human observations (Scheibel, 1978; Scheibel and Scheibel, 1976), severely affected cells were limited to old animals and not seen in the young.

Although confirmation and more detailed observations on the human cerebral cortex in both normal old age and in various forms of dementia is needed, the evidence so far strongly suggests that variable dendritic abnormalities and loss of synapses is a feature of the normal human cerebral cortex, and it is probably more severe in Alzheimer's disease and SDAT than in normal old age.

D. Lipofuscin, RNA Production, and Nucleolar Volume

That lipofuscin increases in many cells throughout the body in old age is well known. Indeed, the constancy of this phenomenon in many tissues, including the central nervous system, is such that it might well be regarded as a true phenomenon of ageing, unlike all the other features in the ageing brain so far described which are much more properly regarded as age-related disorders of unknown aetiology. Within the central nervous system, although lipofuscin does occur in small amounts in astrocytes, neurons are particularly affected although different groups to very different degrees. Cells of the brain stem are most severely involved, particularly those of the inferior olive where, from middle life onwards, much of the cytoplasm of the cell appears to be occupied by lipofuscin and in old age the cells are commonly rounded and the cytoplasm apparently completely filled. In some other sites, such as the anterior horn cells of the spinal cord, lipofuscin accumulation in old age results in marked localized bulging of a cell. Mann and Yates (1974), using a quantitative procedure, have demonstrated an almost linear increase in lipofuscin from childhood to old age in the cells of the inferior olive, this increase being accompanied by a progressive decrease in cytoplasmic RNA. These authors put forward the proposition that RNA reduction accompanying lipofuscin accumulation could reach such a degree that essential protein manufacture, with which RNA is concerned, might be so interfered with as to render the cell non-viable. However, evidence that this change produces death in cells in the inferior olive is not forthcoming since this is one of the sites where cell counting has established that neuron numbers are stable into extreme old age (Monagle and Brody, 1974). The possibility, nevertheless, clearly exists that severe reduction in RNA content within any cell may have a significant effect on protein production and hence the flow of axonal material to terminals, and might well, therefore, be deleterious to its physiological activity. Mann, Yates, and Barton (1977b) demonstrated a somewhat similar situation in the pigmented cells of the substantia nigra showing here that cell RNA diminishes as melanin increases throughout life. When pigmentation is at its maximum in the seventh decade, there is some evidence of cell death among the pigmented cells and, again, their proposition was that beyond a particular limit of melanin accumulation, RNA production is so interfered with as to render the cell non-viable.

Pursuing nucleolar volume and RNA measurements further, Mann, Yates, and Barton (1977a) and Mann and Sinclair (1978) have demonstrated that in a number of different sites, some totally unexpected, such as the cells of the inferior olive, thalamus, dentate nucleus, and the cerebellar Purkinje cells, nucleolar volume and RNA content, and hence probably protein metabolism, are diminished in senile dementia by comparison with normal, age-matched controls. That nucleolar volume of cells in the hippocampus containing neurofibrillary tangles was diminished by comparison with normal cells has been established by Dayan and Ball (1973), but the finding of nucleolar volume decrease in cells in sites of the central nervous system other than those affected by the characteristic morphological changes of senile dementia of Alzheimer type does suggest the important possibility that parts of the central nervous system not exhibiting any obvious morphological changes in Alzheimer's disease or SDAT are, nevertheless, affected in a fundamental way which may have considerable significance both for functional performance elsewhere in the CNS in those diseases, and for aetiological considerations. The diminution in nucleolar size at most of these sites is only in the order of 20 % but it nevertheless directs our attention to the function of other parts of the brain in this disease and mirrors to some extent the finding of reduced dendritic arborization in, for instance, the Purkinje cells which Mehraein, Yamada, and Tarnowska-Dzidusko (1975) demonstrated as being quantitatively somewhat reduced in Alzheimer's disease. Indeed, it is not impossible that the two findings could be connected and that cells with diminished nucleolar size and diminished RNA production may well result in a reduction in dendritic arborization, since essential axonal and dendritic metabolism is dependent upon synthesis occurring within the cell perikaryon. Perhaps the most important feature of these observations is that it directs our attention to parts of the brain other than the cerebral cortex on which most observations have been made in relation to Alzheimer's disease and SDAT. It is clear that the severity of change in the cerebral cortex in these diseases must be reflected by changes in function in the numerous subcortical nuclei with which the cortex is directly connected, but that primary changes are possibly occurring in other sites of the brain which are not related to the cortical abnormalities has not previously been emphasized. The reduction in nucleolar volume and cytoplasmic RNA in neurons in SDAT is not due to increased cytoplasmic lipofuscin since the latter is not increased in that disease by comparison with controls (Mann and Sinclair, 1978). Clearly, these possibly important observations require confirmation, particularly since Uemura and Hartman (1978) were unable to identify any significant loss of RNA in cortical cells of the superior frontal gyrus in three cases of dementia (with numerous senile plaques) by comparison with 15 controls, although confirming a considerable diminution in RNA content in extreme old age by comparison with youth and middle age.

E. Cerebral Softening in Old Age and Arteriosclerotic Dementia

On clinical grounds, until the last two decades, dementia in old age has perhaps most frequently been ascribed by physicians, neurologists and psychiatrists to arteriosclerotic disease. The more careful clinical requirements for diagnosing this disorder and detailed morphological studies have shown that the incidence of arteriosclerotic dementia is very considerably less than that of SDAT and, indeed, some authors regard the latter as accounting for 80–90 % of all cases of dementia in old age.

That multiple small or large infarcts, or occasionally single massive infarcts in the cerebral hemispheres may lead to dementia, is an undisputed fact since many carefully detailed and assessed cases of dementia occur in which the only pathological changes within the brain that can be demonstrated are those of cerebral softening and ischaemic scarring. The assessment of the role of cerebral softening in the production of dementia in individual subjects in old age is not, however, infrequently difficult, for the same reason that difficulties arise over the interpretation of plaque formation in many subjects in old age; that is that cerebral softening is not infrequently present in subjects in whom no evidence of clinical dementia has been found and, indeed, the frequency of strokes without dementia is sufficient testimony to that fact. Our knowledge of the incidence of ischaemic lesions and their distribution in the brains of non-demented elderly subjects is by no means as well established as are the changes of so-called senile type. In a detailed study of a small number of proven intellectually normal old subjects Tomlinson, Blessed, and Roth (1968) showed that 65 % had some degree of cerebral softening, varying quantitatively from occasional microscopic lesions to, in the most severely affected case, some 90 ml of destroyed tissue. In that series there were a number of instances of quite widely scattered small infarcts which had produced severe neurological disturbance in which no evidence of dementia was present on detailed examination shortly before death. Clearly, therefore, a considerable number of elderly subjects do have multiple small ischaemic lesions in, for instance, the basal ganglia and brain stem, and occasional lesions in the white matter or cerebral cortex, and yet remain intellectually well preserved. The figure of 65 % of people showing some degree of softening probably overstates the incidence of ischaemic disease in subjects in the community since all the patients examined in that series (Tomlinson, Blessed, and Roth, 1968) had been hospitalized, and some patients with strokes had been included deliberately. In a similar study of demented subjects (Tomlinson, Blessed, and Roth, 1970) it became clear that a similar situation existed quantitatively to that which had been found in relation to the senile changes: that is, ischaemic destruction of cerebral tissue above a particular quantity is usually accompanied by evidence of dementia. To some extent, when large quantities of the brain are destroyed, the actual site of the ischaemic tissue appears to be less important than the quantity of gross destruction. In their series, Tomlinson, Blessed, and Roth (1970) found that no subject with more than 100 ml of destroyed brain tissue (using a uniform if somewhat arbitrary and approximate method of estimating the quantity of destroyed tissue) was non-demented. The conclusion to be reached, therefore, was that, as with the changes of plaque and tangle formation, the relationship of cerebral infarction to the development of dementia is partly and perhaps largely quantitative. Some evidence exists that the severity of the dementia in such cases is significantly correlated with the total quality of brain destroyed by infarction (Blessed, Tomlinson, and Roth, 1968). Much more detailed investigation of a series of cases of dementia attributable to infarction requires to be undertaken, as it would appear that the location of ischaemic softening must be of major significance in producing dementia in those cases in which the amount of infarction is limited. Certainly, bilateral anterior temporal lobe destruction, which quantitatively may not be great, could be confidently anticipated to produce a major amnestic syndrome and unsuspected infero-occipital temporal lobe infarction is the predominant lesion in some instances of dementia, which on clinical grounds have been of unknown aetiology. Also, in the cases described in 1970 (Tomlinson, Blessed, and Roth) considerable destruction of the corpus callosum, which in itself was not volumetrically great, was possibly associated with a higher incidence of dementia than similarly sized lesions in other sites. From a practical point of view, perhaps the most important lesson on pathological grounds is that small ischaemic lesions within the brain must not be regarded at autopsy as explaining the presence of a dementing process without detailed histological examination and, indeed, since infarcts in the brain occur in subjects with all the pathological and often the clinical evidences of SDAT, no case of dementia whatever the gross changes to be found should be attributed to infarction in the absence of thorough histological examination. The most difficult present problem is how much significance to attribute to multiple small or a single large infarct in the brain in a demented subject who also has considerable numbers of senile plaques throughout the cortex, accompanied or unaccompanied by neurofibrillary tangle formation. If the latter is severe, there are good grounds for saying that dementia would have been present even without additional ischaemic lesions; but it seems reasonable to argue that any additional cerebral destruction superimposed on widespread plaque and tangle formation must add to the severity of the dementing process. Detailed analysis of more cases carefully assessed clinically might lead to further elucidation of the role of these quite different components of cerebral morphological change which are not uncommonly present together (between 15 and 20 % of subjects who are demented).

F. Amyloid Deposition in the Ageing Central Nervous System

Detailed observations producing figures for the frequency and severity of amyloid in the human brain are not available. A description of the various sites in which it may occur is given by Lampert (1968). Subpial arteries and intracerebral arterioles and capillaries may be affected, as may the vessels of the choroid plexus and infundibulum, and microscopic nodular deposits may be found in the subpial tissues of the cerebral cortex with small linear extensions into the molecular layer; the subpial layers of the brain stem and spinal cord may be affected, and minute deposits may occur in the septum pellucidum and between ependymal cells. Within arteries and arterioles, both media and adventitia may be involved and in some instances fingers of amyloid appear to extend into adjacent cortical tissue where it may apparently merge with the amyloid of a plaque. The finding of amyloid in plaques and adjacent blood vessels led Schwartz (1970) to propose that plaques formed following the seepage of amyloid from blood vessels into the cortical tissues. Quantitatively, in the majority of aged humans, the greatest amount will be found associated with senile plaques, since all those which are visible on light microscopy will be associated with amyloid (Terry and Wisniewski, 1970). Since plaques occur in more than 60 % of the population above the age of 70 years (Tomlinson, 1972), it follows that at least 60 % of subjects above that age have some cerebral amyloid. Wright and coworkers (1969) demonstrated amyloid in small cerebral blood vessels or plaques or both in 63 % of patients above the age of 70 years, with amyloid in plaques accounting for the largest number. Two patients over the age of 80 years without plaques, however, showed amyloid within blood vessels. Morimatsu and coworkers (1975) found vascular involvement by amyloid to be much less frequent than amyloid-containing plaques, only 24 % of patients over 70 years showing amyloid in vessels; their tables suggest that demented subjects probably had a higher incidence of vascular amyloid than non-demented cases. Amyloid in plaques therefore appears to occur with much greater frequency than amyloid in vessels; and amyloid within vessels may occur without plaque formation. The presence of amyloid in blood vessels in Alzheimer's disease was studied by Mandybur (1975); again, although both sites were commonly involved, the severity of the vascular deposition varied greatly; it was not detected within vessels in 13 % of cases and was extremely severe in others. The presence of severe amyloid deposition within blood vessels, termed 'congophilic angiopathy' by Pantelakis (1954) may also be unassociated or associated with plaque formation of any severity, so that, overall there is little to support the proposition that they are of identical origin in these two principal sites. Indeed, Glenner (1978) suggests, on the basis of localization, that the amyloid within plaques probably results from proteolysis of locally secreted protein, whereas that within blood vessel walls is more likely derived from circulating serum proteins. Ishii and Haga (1976) have, by immunohistochemical procedures, demonstrated immunoglobulins within the amyloid of plaques; the possibility exists that the microglia associated with plaques are responsible for proteolytic degradation of immunoglobins to amyloid fibrils (Glenner and coworkers, 1971, 1976).

Whatever the origins of amyloid within vessels and plaques—and, clearly, clarification of the possibilities could have major implications for the aetiology of plaque formation—it is difficult to conceive that its presence within blood vessel walls and within the extracellular cortical tissues can have anything but a deleterious effect on the function of the affected tissues. In small quantity the effects appear to be unimportant in relation to cerebral function; but in large amounts it seems likely that the amyloid itself can only be an additional added interference with a number of different aspects of cerebral function.

V. EVIDENCE FOR A MULTI-FACTORIAL ORIGIN OF DEMENTIA IN OLD AGE

The preceding statements have been intended to indicate that in the great majority of demented subjects in old age, numerous morphological changes may well be involved in contributing to the intellectual and personality changes which are present. In extremes of morphological change, where plaque formation is severe and neurofibrillary tangles are present throughout the neocortex in considerable numbers, or when multiple infarcts have destroyed large quantities of cerebral tissue (in excess of 100 ml), dementia appears to be inevitable, but with lesser degrees of change, the results are much more variable. Cases undoubtedly exist of proven demented old subjects in whom, on morphological grounds, no satisfactory explanation for dementia exists using conventional neuropathological techniques. Perhaps extensive studies, including cortical volume and neuron counting, electron microscopy, quantitative Golgi, and RNA studies, would reduce the numbers in that category. Occasionally the reverse is true, and cases with, for instance, heavy plaque formation occur in subjects in whom intellectual performance has been adequate shortly before death. In this relatively small group, in which clinical and pathological observations are discrepant, it appears very likely that other factors, some of which have been described, which have not been assessed in those instances, may well be the deciding morphological contribution. Thus, in a brain in which much cortical neuron loss has occurred in old age and which later develops considerable numbers of plaques (abnormalities of axon terminals), the numbers of the latter may need to be considerably less for the production of dementia than in a brain in which nerve cell loss has been minimal. Similarly, a subject in whom dendritic abnormality, as demonstrated by Golgi preparations, has been very considerable, or in whom multiple small silent ischaemic infarctions have occurred, will probably be more susceptible to the development of dementia with relatively minor or moderate plaque and tangle formation. An individual in whom considerable plaques have occurred throughout the neocortex may again be much more susceptible to the onset of dementia after a single or several small ischaemic incidents than a subject whose brain has remained free of plaque formation. Clearly, what has been described is probably only part of a much more complicated situation. Thus, we do not know what is happening to the numbers and efficiency of synapses in the brain with increasing age, although loss of dendritic spines clearly indicates loss of synapses. With increasing axonal and dendritic abnormalities occurring in many subjects, it would appear very unlikely that the numbers of functioning synapses would not significantly decrease in later years, and one would expect that they are fewer in subjects with Alzheimer's disease and SDAT than in age-matched controls. Perhaps most importantly we do not know that enzymic abnormalities and other biochemical disturbances are not present in demented old subjects which are not reflected by the major morphological changes that are present in Alzheimer's disease and SDAT. In relation to arteriosclerotic or multi-infarct dementia we do not even have quantitative information about the numbers of neurons present in the cortex in areas not obviously affected by ischaemic change. There have been many proponents of the view that loss of total nerve cell numbers in the cortex is of fundamental importance in the production of dementia in old age, and it is possible that in arteriosclerotic dementia, in addition to the gross or microscopic ischaemic lesions which are obvious, there could be a significant overall loss of neurons between the obviously damaged tissue. On subjective grounds this appears unlikely, but quantitative studies are needed to establish the facts. The present intensive investigations into neurotransmitter abnormalities in the central nervous system in normal and demented old subjects may yet reveal that in Alzheimer's disease and SDAT, abnormalities in specific systems, but particularly in the cholinergic system, are more evident at the onset of dementia than the morphological abnormalities. Already, in a small group of cases, some evidence exists that plaque formation correlates statistically with loss of choline acetyltransferase (Perry and coworkers, 1978). Whatever is established about the chemical status of the brain in demented old subjects will not eliminate the probability that in many circumstances in old age some of the multiple changes which we now know to occur in many intellectually normal old subjects have contributed in an additive way to the final demented state.

Table 1. Pathological processes producing dementia

1. Predominantly cortical and diffuse
2. Predominantly white matter
3. Mainly subcortical nuclear masses
4. Generalized or widespread lesions
5. Profound memory disturbances—
   Bilateral hippocampal destruction

Table 2. Dementia associated with predominantly diffuse cortical lesions

1. Alzheimer's disease—pre-senile or senile
2. Pick's disease
3. Jakob–Creutzfeldt disease
4. Subacute sclerosing panencephalitis
5. GPI
6. Post-anoxic cerebral destruction
7. Hypertensive (small vessel) ischaemic disease

Table 3. Dementia associated with predominantly white matter lesions

1. Multiple white matter infarcts
2. Multiple sclerosis
3. Leucodystrophies
4. Progressive multi-focal leucoencephalopathy
5. Post-traumatic (some cases)
6. Subcortical gliosis of Neumann

Table 4. Dementia associated with lesions of subcortical nuclear masses

1. Huntington's chorea (? with cortical involvement)
2. Wilson's disease (? with white matter destruction)
3. Wernicke's encephalopathy
4. Progressive supranuclear palsy
5. Parkinson's disease
6. Bilateral thalamic degeneration
7. Bilateral thalamic ischaemia
8. (Cortico) striatonigral degeneration

Table 5. Dementia associated with widespread lesions

1. Arteriopathic
2. Post-traumatic
3. Post-subarachnoid haemorrhage
4. Parkinsonism dementia complex of Guam
5. Post-meningitis
6. Hydrocephalus
7. Diffuse tumours
8. Dementia of boxers

Table 6. Profound memory disturbances

1. Bilateral temporal lobectomy
2. Bilateral hippocampal infarction
3. Herpes simplex encephalitis
4. Limbic encephalitis

Table 7. Dementia associated with neurofibrillary tangles

1. Alzheimer's disease —pre-senile or senile
                        + senile plaques
2. Parkinsonism dementia complex of Guam
3. Progressive supranuclear palsy
4. Dementia in boxers
5. Dementia in mongols

Table 8. Dementias associated with cerebral
information

1. Arteriosclerotic or multi-infarct
2. Post-anoxic
3. Post-brain injury
4. Post-subarachnoid haemorrhage
5. Post-meningitis and encephalitis
6. Some cases of 'myxoedematous dementia'
7. Congophilic angiopathy

Table 9. Dementia associated with no or
ill-defined morphological changes

1. Myxoedema
2. Chronic alcoholism (excluding specific
related disorders such as Wernicke's
encephalopathy)
3. Dialysis

REFERENCES

Ball, M. J. (1976). Neurofibrillary tangles and the pathogenesis of dementia: a quantitative study. *Neuropath. Appl. Neurobiol.*, **2**, 395–410.

Ball, M. J. and P. Lo (1977). Granulovacuolar degeneration in the aging brain and in dementia. *J. Neuropath. Exp. Neurol.*, **36**, 474–87.

Barron, S. A., L. Jacobs, and W. R. Kinkel (1976). Changes in size of normal lateral ventricles during aging determined by computerized tomography. *Neurology (Minneap.)*, **26**, 1011–3.

Bergmann, K. (1975). The epidemiology of senile dementia. *Brit. J. Psychiat.* (Spec. Publ.), **9**, 100.

Blessed, G., B. E. Tomlinson, and M. Roth (1968). The association between quantitative measures of dementia and senile changes in the cerebral grey matter of elderly subjects. *Brit. J. Psychiat.*, **114**, 797–811.

Blinkov, S. M. and I. I. Glezer (1968). *The Human Brain in Figures and Tables*, Basic Books, Plenum Press, New York.

Brody, H. (1955). Organisation of the cerebral cortex. 3. A study of aging in the human cerebral cortex. *J. Comp. Neurol.*, **102**, 511–56.

Brody, H. (1970). Structural changes in the aging nervous system. In H. T. Blumenthal (Ed.) *Interdisciplinary Topics in Gerontology*, Vol. 7, Karger, New York. pp. 7–21.

Cavanagh, J. B., W. F. Blakemore, and M. H. Kyu (1971). Fibrillary accumulation in oligodendroglia processes of rats subjected to portocaval anastomosis. *J. Neurol. Sci.*, **14**, 143–52.

Coblenz, J. M., S. Mattis, L. H. Zingesser, S. S. Kasoff, H. M. Wisniewski, and R. Katzman (1973). Presenile Dementia. *Arch. Neurol.*, **29**, 299.

Colon, E. J. (1972). The elderly brain: a quantitative analysis of cerebral cortex in two cases. *Psychiat. Neurol. Neurochir.*, **75**, 261–70.

Colon, E. J. (1973). The cerebral cortex in presenile dementia. A quantitative analysis. *Acta neuropath. (Berl).*, **28**, 281–90.

Corsellis, J. A. N. (1962). *Mental Illness and the Ageing Brain.* Oxford University Press, Oxford.

Corsellis, J. A. N. (1976a). Ageing and the Dementias. In W. Blackwood and J. A. N. Corsellis (Eds) *Greenfield's Neuropathology*, 3rd edn, Edward Arnold, London. pp. 796–848.

Corsellis, J. A. N. (1976b). Some observations on the Purkinje cell population and on brain volume in human aging. In R. D. Terry and S. Gershon (Eds) *Neurobiology of Aging*, Vol. 3, Raven Press, New York. p. 205.

Corsellis, J. A. N., C. J. Bruton, and D. Freeman-Browne (1973). The aftermath of boxing. *Psychol. Med.*, **3**, 270.

Crapper, D. R. (1973). Experimental neurofibrillary degeneration and altered electrical activity. *Electroencephalogr. Clin. Neurophysiol.*, **35**, 575.

Crapper, D. R. (1976). Functional consequences of neurofibrillary degeneration. In R. D. Terry and S. Gershon (Eds) *Neurobiology of Aging*, Vol. 3, Raven Press, New York. pp. 405–32.

Crapper, D. R. and A. J. Dalton (1973). Aluminium-induced neurofibrillary degeneration, brain electrical activity and alterations in acquisition and retention. *Physiol. Behav.*, **10**, 935–45.

Davis, P. M. J. and E. A. Wright (1977). A new method for measuring cranial cavity volume and its application to the assessment of cerebral atrophy at autopsy. *Neuropath. Appl. Neurobiol.*, **3**, 341–58.

Dayan, A. D. and M. J. Ball (1973). Histometric observations on the metabolism of tangle-bearing neurones. *J. Neurol. Sci.*, **19**, 433–6.

Delay, J., S. Brion, R. Escourolle and L. Dujarier (1962). Étude anatomique des artères carotides et vertébrales en cours des démences séniles. *Rev. Neurol. (Paris)*, **106**, 772.

Escourolle, R. and J. Poirier (1973). *Manual of Basic Neuropathology*, W. B. Saunders, Philadelphia.

Feldman, M. L. (1976). Aging changes in the morphology of cortical dendrites. In R. D. Terry and S. Gershon (Eds) *Neurobiology of Aging*, Vol. 3, Raven Press, New York. pp. 211–27.

Feldman, M. L. and C. Dowd (1974). Aging in rat visual cortex: light microscopic observations on layer V pyramidal apical dendrites. *Anat. Rec.*, **178**, 355.

Field, E. J. and H. K. Narang (1972). An electronmicroscopic study in the rat. Further observations on 'Inclusion bodies' and virus-like particles. *J. Neurol. Sci.*, **17**, 347–64.

Gessaga, E. C. and A. P. Anzil (1975). Rod-shaped filamentous inclusions and other ultrastructural features in a cerebellar astrocytoma. *Acta. Neuropath. (Berl.)*, **33**, 119–27.

Gibson, P. (1978). Light and electronmicroscopic observations on the relationship between Hirano bodies, neuron and glial perikarya in the human hippocampus. *Acta. Neuropath. (Berl.)*, **42**, 165–71.

Gibson, P. and B. E. Tomlinson (1977). The numbers of Hirano bodies in the hippocampus of normal and demented subjects with Alzheimer's disease. *J. Neurol. Sci.*, **33**, 199–206.

Glenner, G. G. (1978). Current knowledge of amyloid deposits as applied to senile plaques and congophilic angiopathy. In R. Katzman, R. D. Terry, and K. L. Bick (Eds) *Alzheimer's Senile Dementia and Related Disorders* (Aging Vol. 7), Raven Press, New York. pp. 493–501.

Glenner, G. G., D. Ein, E. D. Eames, H. A. Bladen, W. Terry, and D. Page (1971). The creation of amyloid fibrils from Bence–Jones proteins *in vitro*. *Science*, **174**, 712–4.

Glenner, G. G., W. Terry, M. Harada, C. Isersky and D. Page (1976). Amyloidosis and amyloidogenesis. In G. W. Richter and M. A. Epstein (Eds) *International Review of*

Experimental Pathology, Vol. 15, Academic Press, New York. pp. 1–92.

Gruenberg, E. M. (1961). *A Mental Health Survey of Older People*, Utica, New York.

Haase, G. R. (1977). Diseases presenting as dementia. In C. E. Wells (Ed.) *Dementia*, 2nd edn, F. A. Davis Co., Philadelphia. pp. 27–68.

Hall, T. C., A. K. H. Miller, and J. A. N. Corsellis (1975). Variations in the human Purkinje cell population according to age and sex. *Neuropath. Appl. Neurobiol.*, **1**, 267–92.

Hanley, T. (1974). Neuronal fall-out in the aging brain: a critical review of the quantitative data. *Age and Aging*, **3**, 133–51.

Hirano, A. (1965). Slow, latent and temporate virus infections. In D. C. Gajdusek and C. J. Gibbs (Eds) *Monograph*, No. 2, National Institute of Health. pp. 23–7.

Hirano, A. (1974). Parkinsonism-dementia complex on Guam: current states of the problem. In A. Subirana and J. M. Espadaler (Eds) *Proceedings of the 10th International Congress of Neurology, Barcelona, 1973*, Excerpta Medica, Amsterdam. p. 348.

Hirano, A., H. M. Dembitzer, L. T. Kurland and H. M. Zimmerman (1968). The fine structure of some intraganglionic alterations. *J. Neuropath. Ex. Neurol.*, **26**, 167–82.

Hirano, A. and L. T. Kurland (1961). Parkinsonism-dementia complex, an endemic disease on the island of Guam. 2. Pathological features. *Brain*, **84**, 662.

Huckman, M. S., J. Fox, and J. Topel (1975). The validity of criteria for the evaluation of cerebral atrophy by computerised tomography. *Radiology*, **116**, 85–92.

Iqbal, K., I. Grundke-Iqbal, H. M. Wisniewski, and R. D. Terry (1978). Neurofibres in Alzheimer's disease and other conditions. In R. Katzman, R. D. Terry, and K. L. Bick (Eds) *Alzheimer's Disease: Senile Dementia and Related Disorders*, Raven Press, New York. pp. 409–20.

Ishii, T. and S. Haga (1976). Immuno-electron microscopic localization of immunoglobulin in amyloid fibrils of senile plaques. *Acta Neuropath. (Berl.)*, **36**, 243–9.

Jacobs, L., W. R. Kinkel, F. Painter, J. Murawski, and R. R. Heffner (1978). Computerised tomography in dementia with special reference to changes in size of normal ventricles during aging and normal pressure hydrocephalus. In R. Katzman, R. D. Terry, and K. L. Bick (Eds) *Alzheimer's Disease: Senile Dementia and Related Disorders (Aging*, Vol. 7), Raven Press, New York. pp. 241–60.

Kay, D. W. K. (1972). Epidemiological aspects of organic brain disease in the elderly. In G. M. Gaitz (Ed.) *Aging and the Brain*, Plenum, New York. pp. 15–27.

Kay, D. W. K., P. Beamish, and M. Roth (1964). Old age mental disorders in Newcastle upon Tyne. Part 1: A study of prevalence. *Brit. J. Psychiat.*, **110**, 146.

Kidd, M. (1963). Paired helical filaments in electronmicroscopy in Alzheimer's disease. *Nature (London)*, **197**, 192.

Kidd, M. (1964). Alzheimer's disease—an electron microscopic study. *Brain*, **87**, 307–21.

Konigsmark, B. W. and E. A. Murphy (1972). Volume of ventral cochlear nucleus in man: its relationship to neuronal population and age. *J. Neuropath. Exp. Neurol.*, **31**, 304–16.

Korenschevsky, V. (1961). In G. H. Bourne (Ed.) *Physiological and Pathological Aging*, Karger, Basel and New York.

Lampert, P. (1968). Amyloid and amyloid-like deposits. In J. Minckler (Ed.) *Pathology of the Nervous System*, Vol. 1, McGraw-Hill, New York. pp. 1113–21.

Last, R. J. and D. H. Tompsett (1953). Casts of the cerebral ventricles. *Brit. J. Surg.*, **40**, 525–43.

Mandybar, T. I. (1975). The incidence of cerebral amyloid angiopathy in Alzheimer's disease. *Neurology* (Minneap.), **25**, 120–6.

Mann, D. M. A. and P. O. Yates (1974). Lipoprotein pigments—their relationship to aging in the human nervous system. I. The lipofuscin content of nerve cells. *Brain*, **97**, 481–8.

Mann, D. M. A., P. O. Yates, and C. M. Barton (1977a). Cytophotometric mapping of neuronal changes in senile dementia. *J. Neurol., Neurosurg. Psychiat.*, **40**, 299–302.

Mann, D. M. A., P. O. Yates, and C. M. Barton (1977b). Neuromelanin and RNA in cells of the substantia nigra. *J. Neuropath. Exp. Neurol.*, **36**, 379–83.

Mann, D. M. A. and K. G. A. Sinclair (1978). The quantitative assessment of lipofuscin pigment, cytoplasmic RNA, and nucleolar volume in senile dementia. *Neuropath. Appl. Neurobiol.*, **4**, 129–35.

Marsden, C. G. and M. J. G. Harrison (1972). Outcome of investigation of patients with presenile dementia. *Brit. Med. J.*, **2**, 249.

Mehraein, P., M. Yamada, and E. Tarnowska-Dzidusko (1975). Quantitative studies on dendrites in Alzheimer's disease and senile dementia. In G. W. Kreutzberg (Ed.) *Physiology and Pathology of Dendrites*, Raven Press, New York. pp. 453–8.

Messert, B., B. B. Wannamaker, and A. W. Dudley (1972). Revaluation of the size of the lateral ventricle of the brain. *Neurology (Minneap.)*, **22**, 941–51.

Monagle, R. D. and H. Brody (1974). The effects of age upon the main nucleus of the inferior olive in the human. *J. Comp. Neurol.*, **155**, 61–6.

Morimatsu, M., S. Hirai, A. Muramatsu, and M. Yoshikawa (1975). Senile degenerative brain lesions and dementia. *J. Amer. Geriat. Soc.*, **23**, 390–406.

Nielson, J. (1962). Geronto-psychiatric period-prevalence investigation in a geographically delimited population. *Acta Psychiat. Scand.*, **38**, 307.

Pantelakis, S. (1954). Un type particulier d'angiopathie sénile du système nerveux central: l'angiopathie congophile. Topographie et frequence. *Monatsschr. Psychiatr. Neurol.*, **128**, 219.

Perry, E. K., B. E. Tomlinson, G. Blessed, K. Bergmann, P. H. Gibson and R. H. Perry (1978). Correlation of cholinergic abnormalities with senile plaques and mental test scores in senile dementia. *Brit. Med. J.*, **2**, 1457–9.

Post, F. (1965). *The Clinical Psychiatry of Late Life*. Pergamon Press, Oxford.

Roth, M., B. E. Tomlinson, and G. Blessed (1966). Correlation between scores for dementia and counts of 'senile plaques' in cerebral grey matter of elderly subjects. *Nature (London)*, **209**, 109.

Scheibel, A. B. (1978). Structural aspects of the aging brain: spine systems and the dendritic arbor. In R. Katzman, R. D. Terry, and K. L. Bick (Eds) *Alzheimer's Disease: Senile Dementia and Related Disorders (Aging, Vol. 7)*, Raven Press, New York. pp. 353–73.

Scheibel, M. E., R. D. Lindsay, U. Tomiyasu, and A. B. Scheibel (1975). Progressive dendritic changes in aging human cortex. *Exp. Neurol.*, **47**, 392–403.

Scheibel, M. E. and A. B. Scheibel (1976). Structural changes in the aging brain. In H. Brody, D. Harmon, and J. M. Ordy (Eds) *Aging, Clinical, Morphological and Neurochemical Aspects of the Aging Central Nervous System*, Vol. 1, Raven Press, New York. pp. 11–37.

Schochet, S. S. Jr. and W. F. McCormick (1972). Ultrastructure of Hirano bodies. *Acta Neuropath. (Berl.)*, **21**, 50–60.

Schwartz, P. (1970). *Amyloidosis: Cause and Manifestations of Senile Deterioration*, C. C. Thomas, Springfield, Illinois.

Shefer, V. F. (1973). Absolute numbers of neurons and thickness of cerebral cortex during aging, senile and vascular dementia and Pick's and Alzheimer's disease. *Neurosci. Behav. Physiol.*, **6**, 319–24.

Sim, M., E. Turner, and W. T. Smith (1966). Cerebral biopsy in the investigation of presenile dementia. 2. Pathological aspects. *Brit. J. Psychiat.*, **112**, 127.

Slaby, A. E. and R. J. Wyatt (1974). *Dementia in the Presenium*. C. C. Thomas, Springfield, Illinois.

Spencer, P. S. and P. K. Thomas (1974). Ultrastructural studies of the dying-back process. II. The sequestration and removal by Schwann cells, and oligodendrocytes of organelles from normal and diseased axons. *J. Neurocyt.*, **3**, 763–83.

Terry, R. D. (1963). The fine structure of neurofibrillary tangles in Alzheimer's disease. *J. Neuropath. Exp. Neurol.*, **22**, 629–42.

Terry, R. D., C. Fitzgerald, A. Pack, J. Millner, and P. Farmer (1977). Cortical cell counts in senile dementia. (abstr.). *J. Neuropath. Exp. Neurol.*, **36**, 633.

Terry, R. D.,N. K. Gonatas, and M. Weiss (1964). Ultrastructural studies in Alzheimer's presenile dementia. *Amer. J. Path.*, **44**, 269–97.

Terry, R. D. and H. M. Wisniewski (1970). The ultrastructure of the neurofibrillary tangle and the senile plaque. In G. E. M. Wolstenholme and M. A. O'Connor (Eds) *Alzheimer's Disease and Related Conditions*, Ciba Foundation Symposium. pp. 145–68.

Tomlinson, B. E. (1972). Morphological brain changes in non-demented old people. In H. M. von Praag and A. F. Kalverboer (Eds) *Aging of the Central Nervous System*, De Ervon F. Bohn, New York. pp. 38–57.

Tomlinson, B. E. (1977). Pathology of dementia. In C. E. Wells (Ed.) *Dementia*, 2nd edn, F. A. Davis, Philadelphia, pp. 113–54.

Tomlinson, B. E., G. Blessed, and M. Roth (1968). Observations on the brains of non-demented old people. *J. Neurol. Sci.*, **7**, 331–56.

Tomlinson, B. E., G. Blessed, and M. Roth (1970). Observations on the brains of demented old people. *J. Neurol. Sci.*, **11**, 205.

Tomlinson, B. E. and G. Henderson (1976). Some quantitative cerebral findings in normal and demented old people. In R. D. Terry and S. Gershon (Eds) *Neurobiology of Aging*, Raven Press, New York.

Tomlinson, B. E. and D. Irving (1977). The numbers of limb motor neurons in the human lumbosacral cord throughout life. *J. Neurol. Sci.*, **34**, 213–9.

Tomlinson, B. E. and D. Kitchener (1972). Granulovacuolar degeneration in hippocampal pyramidal cells. *J. Path.*, **106**, 165–85.

Uemura, E. and H. A. Hartman (1978). RNA content and volume of nerve cell bodies in human brains. 1. Prefrontal cortex in aging and demented subjects. *J. Neuropath. Exp. Neurol.*, **37**, 487–97.

Van Buskirk, C. (1945). The seventh nerve complex. *J. Comp. Neurol.*, **82**, 303–33.

Vijayashankar, N. and H. Brody (1971). Neuronal population of the human abducens nucleus. *Anat. Rec.*, **169**, 447.

Vijayashankar, N. and H. Brody (1973). The neuronal population of the nuclei of the trochlear nerve and the locus coeruleus in the human. *Anat. Rec.*, **172**, 421–2.

Williams, R. S., R. J. Ferrante, and V. S. Caviness Jr (1978). The Golgi rapid method in clinical neuropathology. The morphologic consequences of suboptimal fixation. *J. Neuropath. Exp. Neurol.*, **37**, 13–33.

Wisniewski, H. M., H. K. Narang, and R. D. Terry (1976). Neurofibrillary tangles of paired helical filaments. *J. Neurol. Sci.*, **27**, 173–81.

Wisniewski, H. M. and R. D. Terry (1976). Neuropathology of the aging brain. In R. D. Terry and S. Gershon (Eds) Neurobiology of Aging, Vol. 3, Raven Press, New York. pp. 265–80.

Woodard, J. S. (1962). Clinico-pathological significance of granulovacuolar degeneration in Alzheimer's disease. *J. Neuropath. Exp. Neurol.*, **21**, 85–91.

Woodard, J. S. (1966). Alzheimer's disease in late adult life. *Amer. J. Path.*, **49**, 1157–69.

Wright, J. R., E. Calkins, W. T. Breen, G. Stolte, and R. T. Schultz (1969). Relationship of amyloid to aging. Review of the literature and a systematic study of 83 patients derived from a general hospital population. *Medicine*, **48**, 39–60.

Chapter 3

Models for the Biochemical Study of Dementia

D. R. CRAPPER and U. DE BONI

*Departments of Physiology and Medicine,
University of Toronto, Toronto, Ontario, M5S 1A8, Canada*

I. DEMENTIA

Dementia is an altered state of brain function characterized by acquired deficits in higher intellectual activity, with preservation of feeling and movement. Acquisition and retrieval of auditory, visual, and spatial events is altered together with judgment, insight, impulse control, calculation, and the organization of complex motor acts. The major pathophysiological insults are upon the more recently evolved neocortical association or polysensory regions of the frontal, parietal, temporal, and occipital lobes. A dementia process results in a global disconnection of neocortical regions and their brain stem projections. Virtually any brain insult may result in dementia. Such diverse conditions as head injury, stroke, multiple sclerosis, endocrine dysfunction, brain infections, and vitamin deficiencies may be associated with dementia. It is therefore mandatory that biochemical studies of the dementias be accompanied by detailed clinical and exhaustive neuropathological examination. Since the functional state of dementia is a continuum from mild to profound, and since brains exhibit pathologically a wide range of changes, studies employing data acquired by chemical techniques must involve appropriate methods for correlation with the ante-mortem functional state and pathological changes in the brains from which the data was obtained. Many laboratories bisect brains in the sagittal plane, reserving one half for detailed pathological study and the other half, after gross inspection by a pathologist, for chemical analysis.

II. SELECTION OF 'CONTROLS'

Chemical studies on the senile dementias are particularly difficult because

53

interpretable data require consideration of several factors which may influence the results. Experimental data should be matched to at least the following categories:

(i) Age-matched to brains of patients who were intellectually intact.
(ii) Age-matched to dementias of a type other than that under study to exclude a relation to altered neuronal discharge patterns unique to the dementia under investigation.
(iii) Matched in the events which resulted in death of the donor. Prolonged hypoxia, hypotension, sepsis, or seizures are important variables which alter the metabolic state of the brain.
(iv) Matched in the manner in which the donor was processed after death including refrigeration, transport, time to autopsy, and length of storage of brain.
(v) Data compared to brains of younger individuals who died acutely from extraneuronal causes.

III. MODELS OF DEMENTIA

As outlined elsewhere in this book, Alzheimer's disease is the most common cause of senile dementia. Suitable laboratory models for the study of other common causes of senile dementia including multi-infarct dementia, hypertensive encephalopathy, and alcohol-related dementias are also available. Animal models for Jakob–Creutzfeldt disease and kuru are now well established (Gajdusek, 1977). However, laboratory models for certain other conditions which may be associated with dementia, such as Parkinson's disease with Lewy bodies, Pick's disease with Pick bodies, low-pressure hydrocephalus, or Huntington's chorea are not yet available.

IV. ALZHEIMER'S DISEASE

Alzheimer's disease is well suited to intensive laboratory investigation at this time because some of the major histological manifestations of the disease may be reproduced in the laboratory. Alzheimer's disease is a slowly progressive, fatal global encephalopathy that cannot be diagnosed with certainty in the living subject without tissue examination following a brain biopsy. The disease usually begins with learning-memory deficits and slowly progresses to involve all aspects of intellectual activity including judgement, calculation, and language. With progression, difficulties in recognition of common sensory stimuli, together with difficulty in organization of complex motor acts, become apparent. There are changes in muscle tone, the appearance of abnormal reflexes, myoclonic jerks, and sometimes general seizures. As the terminal stages approach, urinary incontinence and loss of all useful motor control necessitates total nursing care and predisposes to the usual terminal events: cachexia and bronchopneumonia.

The disease may have a course as short as 18 months or as long as 19 years, with an average duration of illness of about 8 years. The condition is untreatable and the factors responsible for the condition are unknown. Tissues outside the central nervous system do not seem to be directly involved by the degenerative process which affects the brain.

The brain pathology of Alzheimer's disease is outlined in Table 1. There are a remarkably large number of changes in this condition. It would seem most productive to select laboratory models which investigate some component of either the dementia or the several histopathological manifestations of this disease. No known agent is capable of reproducing in the laboratory all the tissue changes characteristic of Alzheimer's disease. A list of agents and animal models which may be useful for this purpose are given in Table 2. Some of the more promising areas for research into this common disease include the following.

Table 1. Neuropathological changes
associated with Alzheimer's disease

1. Cerebral atrophy
2. Neuron loss
3. Altered dendritic configuration
4. Hippocampal granulovacuolar degeneration
5. Neuritic (senile) plaques
6. Neurofibrillary degeneration
7. Perivascular amyloid deposits
8. Hirano bodies
9. Spongioform change

Table 2. Models for the study of Alzheimer's disease and related conditions

Histopathological change		Agent	Animal
Neuritic (senile) plaques	Amyloid cores	Scrapie	Mouse
	'Early' plaques	Aluminium and trauma	Rabbit, cat
Neurofibrillary degeneration	Paired helical 10-nm filaments	Alzheimer brain extract	Human neuron explant
	10-nm Single filaments	Colchicine	Most species
		Aluminium	Cat, rabbit
	15-nm Single filaments (supranuclear palsy)	Elevated Mg^{2+}	Catfish photoreceptor
		Dengue virus	Mouse brain
Spongioform change		Scrapie	Several species
		Kuru–Jakob–Creutzfeldt extract	Several species

A. Neuritic (senile) Plaques

Perhaps the most useful laboratory model of human senile plaques results from the intracranial injection of certain strains of scrapie agent into certain strains of mice (Bruce and Fraser, 1975; Wisniewski, Bruce, and Fraser, 1975). These plaques contain amyloid cores, a change which has not been observed in neuritic plaques induced by aluminium. As in Alzheimer's disease, perivascular amyloid deposits were also observed in the scrapie-affected mouse brain. The scrapie-mouse model is the only laboratory preparation in which amyloid is known to occur in the brain. There are several reasons why the scrapie model may be useful in the study of Alzheimer's disease. Scrapie is caused by a replicating agent considered to be a member of a group of unconventional viruses (Gajdusek, 1977). These agents differ in several ways from conventional viruses: they do not induce viral-associated inflammatory responses in the brain, nor do they alter cerebrospinal fluid cell counts and protein concentration. Furthermore, these agents are not associated with viral particles nor do they induce a systemic immune response. The aetiological factor in Alzheimer's disease also appears to have these characteristics. In addition, the histopathology of scrapie involves vacuolar degeneration that may attain severe spongy change. Ultrastructural changes are characterized by membrane whirls. Recently, two independent workers have reported electron microscopic evidence of spongioform change in brain biopsy material from Alzheimer's disease. Flament-Durand (1978) reported the changes in three of six brain biopsies with a clinical history and pathological change compatible with the diagnosis of Alzheimer's disease. Rewcastle, Gibbs, and Gajdusek (1978) also reported that in biopsy material from a case considered to be familial Alzheimer's disease, spongioform changes identical to those seen in Jakob–Creutzfeldt disease, a condition closely related to the sheep and goat disease of scrapie, were encountered. Importantly, brain material from the case reported by Rewcastle injected into primates by the N.I.H. group resulted in a progressive spongioform encephalopathy. While the interpretation of these findings is currently a matter for speculation, the possibility remains that a component of the Alzheimer aetiological factor has cytotoxic manifestations similar to those of the scrapie agent.

Characterization of the scrapie agent is in the initial stages. Prusiner and coworkers (1978a, 1978b) have reported that the scrapie particles may be as small as 40 S ($S_{20,w}$). These workers have also suggested the agent may have a surface coat with hydrophobic regions, which could explain some of the unusual properties of the agent. The stability of the agent to heating is consistent with such a view since hydrophobic interactions are stabilized at high temperatures. The apparent association of the scrapie agent with membrane fractions would also be expected since hydrophobic proteins could insert themselves into membranes. The scrapie agents are poor antigenic agents and resemble many lipoproteins in this regard. Finally, Prusiner argues that the apparent discrepancy in the size of the agent (2×10^5 daltons) as determined by ultrafiltration and by ionizing radiation, might be due to the ability of the agent to undergo aggregation and dissociation as a consequence of the hydrophobic surface.

The infective component of the scrapie agent appears to be sensitive to enzymes which destroy DNA. Marsh and coworkers (1978), employing a high-speed supernatant free of membranes, reported that infectivity of the agent was markedly reduced by treatment with DNase I but resistant to RNase. Pre-treatment with proteinase K led to a tenfold increase in the amount of infective agent bound to a hydroxyapatite column and a greater inactivation by DNase. These workers argue that the scrapie agent may contain low-molecular weight DNA of about 2000 nucleotides. The heat resistance of the scrapie agent also suggests the possibility that the genetic information may exist as a single strand of DNA. This would be in keeping with other heat-resistant small single-stranded DNA viruses, such as the parvoviruses (Prusiner and coworkers, 1978a, 1978b). While there is no direct evidence that a transmissible agent capable of neuritic plaque formation exists in Alzheimer-affected brain, all of the above circumstantial evidence should stimulate an intensive search for such an agent.

B. Neurofibrillary Degeneration

The electron microscope reveals the accumulation of arrays of pairs of 10 nm diameter solid filaments which form a helical structure termed the 'paired helical filament' (PHFs), (Kidd, ·1964; Wisniewski, Narang, and Terry, 1976). Neurofibrillary degeneration of the Alzheimer type occurs in a variety of diseases with apparently different aetiological factors. Repeated head trauma resulting in dementia pugilistica, liposomal disorders with lipid storage such as Kufs' disease and Neiman Pick's disease, may exhibit neurons with neurofibrillary degeneration (Horoupian and Yang, 1978). In addition, one of the events responsible for neurofibrillary degeneration may be the delayed expression of a conventional viral infection. Neurofibrillary degeneration occurred in brain stem nuclei, particularly in the substantia nigra, many years after epidemic encephalitis lethargica (Hallervorden, 1933). While a pathogenic agent in this condition has not been identified, the neuropathology of acute cases was typical of a viral encephalitis. Two other types of viral infections may also be accompanied by neurofibrillary degeneration in brains of young patients: progressive multi-focal leukoencephalopathy (Hadfield, Martinez, and Gilmartin, 1974) and subacute sclerosing panencephalitis (Mandybur and coworkers, 1977). In the former condition, alterations in the immune system of the host appear to permit the proliferation of an otherwise benign virus. In subacute sclerosing panencephalitis there is an apparently incomplete suppression of a measles-like paramyxovirus which permits slow replication of the agent. Some of these conditions may be adaptable to laboratory models for further study. In addition, PHF formation may occur in spinal cord in Guam amyotrophic lateral sclerosis cases (Hirano and Zimmerman, 1962) and in a similar condition found in certain prefectures in the Kii peninsula of Japan (Yoshimasu and coworkers, 1976; Yase, 1977). Whether these various conditions permit the expression of a class of closely related agents to form paired helical filaments, or whether PHFs are a non-specific morphological response to a diverse group of agents, cannot be answered at present. Paired helical filaments are not known to occur in animal brain diseases.

The only laboratory model of PHFs so far reported resulted from the addition of extracts from Alzheimer-affected brain to human fetal cerebral neurons in tissue culture (De Boni and Crapper, 1978).

Explanted fragments ($0.5 mm^3$) of cerebral cortex derived from human fetuses of approximately 12–14 weeks' gestation were employed. Explant cultures were maintained on collagen-coated coverslips in a medium composed of 35 % Simm's balanced salt solution, 40 % heat-inactivated human cord· serum, and 25 % medium 199 (Gibco), with 600 mg % glucose (final concentration). The coverslips with cultures were placed in plastic Petri dishes and incubated at 36 °C in a water-saturated atmosphere of 95 % air and 5 % CO_2. The culture medium was changed twice weekly.

Material from four patients' brains has been employed. Each patient had· a well-documented history of slowly progressive intellectual decline ending in profound dementia. None of the patients had a family history of Alzheimer's disease. At necropsy, each brain contained large numbers of neuritic plaques and neurons with neurofibrillary degeneration in the hippocampus, neocortex, and brain stem. Case 1 was a carpenter with the onset of the disease at age 56 and death at age 63 years. Case 2 was a veteran and business man who first sought medical advice for memory loss at age 59 and who died with profound dementia at age 78 years. Cases 3 and 4 were housewives, one of whom developed symptoms at age 51 and died at age 60 years, and the other had an onset at about age 58 and died at age 65 years. As yet, no brain with Alzheimer's disease has failed to induce PHF in explanted neurons.

Several types of extract have been prepared from these brains. A crude saline extract was prepared from a homogenate of $2 cm^3$ of the tip of the temporal lobe. The homogenate was first spun at 1500 r.p.m. on a bench-top centrifuge and the cell-free supernatant passed through a Millipore filter of 250-nm pore size. Ultrastructural examination of this extract did not reveal fragments of paired helical filaments. An extract from Alzheimer-affected brain was also prepared from a neuron-enriched fraction collected on discontinuous sucrose gradients (Crapper, Quittkat, and De Boni, 1979). This fraction contained 10–12 % neurons with neurofibrillary degeneration when stained with congo red and viewed under polarized light in the light microscope. The neurons were then broken by osmotic shock and the nuclei and mitochondria were spun into ·a pellet. Aliquots of the supernatant were spun at 55 000 r.p.m. for various lengths of time in an IEC SB-405 rotor and were considered cleared of particles corresponding to 10 S, 20 S, 40 S, 80 S, 150 S, and 200 S ($S_{20,w}$). The supernatants were added to the explanted neurons for the first six days in culture.

Detailed ulstrastructural examination of cultures exposed to the crude saline extract and fixed at 4, 8, and 11 days of incubation revealed no paired helical filaments, and the morphological characteristics of the cells were identical to control cultures. However, after 14 days' incubation, occasional paired helical filaments were observed, and after 21–35 days of incubation paired helical filaments were found in many cell processes. Approximately 3 % of all cell processes at 35 days' incubation contained one or more paired helical filaments. Synaptic contacts established that the paired helical filaments occurred in neurons. Generally, the PHFs were found in distended processes in which the density of organelles was reduced and microtubules fragmented. Many of the PHFs appear to be assembled from separate, morphologically normal-appearing individual filaments of about 10 nm in diameter (Fig. 1). The major difference in ultrastructural configuration between the induced PHFs and the naturally occurring PHFs is that the induced PHFs are more open and wider in transverse diameter. In addition, processes with large parallel arrays of PHFs, such as those found in Alzheimer's disease, were not encountered in the *in vitro* model.

Supernatant preparations from Alzheimer-affected neurons cleared of $S_{20,w}$ 10 S, 20 S, and 40 S particles failed to reveal PHFs after exhaustive electron microscopic examination. Cultures exposed to solutions cleared of 80 S particles required extensive searching but PHFs were encountered (Table 3). Supernatants cleared of particles ranging to 200 S or larger, invariably resulted in numerous PHFs in cultured neurons (Table 4). Thus, the Alzheimer PHF-inducing factor resembles the particle size distribution of the scrapie agent as reported by Prusiner and coworkers (1978a, 1978b).

The PHF-inducing agent also appears to have a sensitivity to ultraviolet light, similar to that reported for the scrapie agent (Table 5). A 1-mm thick solution of high-speed supernatant, demonstrated to induce PHFs, was irradiated at 254 nm on a shaker platform. PHF formation was completely blocked at irradiation levels of 2×10^5, 5.0×10^5, and 11.5×10^5 ergs mm^{-2}. Paired helical filaments were present in the cultured cells following the addition of supernatant which received 1×10^5 ergs mm^{-2} irradiation. The inactivation dose at 254 nm for scrapie is reported to be 2.4×10^5 ergs mm^{-2} (Haig and coworkers, 1969). Experiments to determine whether the PHF assembly agent contains genetic information employing DNase, RNase, and proteinases are in progress in our laboratory.

Before instituting rigorous biohazard control in our laboratory, an occasional control culture exhibited PHFs. However, in the past ten months, meticulous attention to the prevention of cross-contamination and the use of sodium hypochlorite and prolonged high-temperature sterilization, HEPA filters, and revised pipetting techniques, have resulted in no examples of control cultures exhibiting PHFs. Furthermore, a wide range of challenges has been delivered to

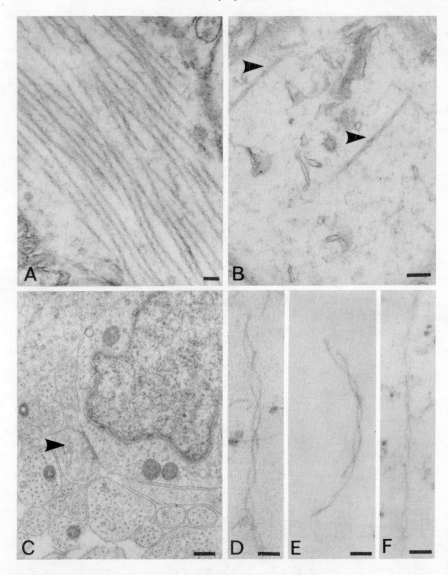

Figure 1. Paired helical filaments (PHFs) in Alzheimer's disease and induced in cultured, human neurons. A, B: Brain biopsy of patient with Alzheimer's disease, showing aggregate (A) and single (B, arrowheads) PHFs. C: Normal, human cerebral cortical neuron, representative of cells in culture, 32 days *in vitro*. Synaptic contact (arrowhead) identifies cell as neuron. D, E, F: Representative PHFs induced in cultured human neurons, 35 days following inoculation with extract from Alzheimer-affected brain. Magnification: A, B, D, E, bar = 0.1 μm; C, bar = 0.25 μm; F, bar = 0.2 μm

Table 3. Properties of PHF-inducing agent

Particle size cleared (S_{20}, w)	$\log_{10} w^2 t$ IEC B60 (SB 405)	Paired helical filaments
10 S	11.7	Absent
20 S	11.4	Absent
40 S	11.1	Absent
80 S	10.8	Rare
150 S	10.5	Rare
200 S	10.2	Present
200 S		Abundant

Table 4. Patient material employed in PHF induction

Patient	Sex	Age of onset (years)	Age of death (years)	Occupation	Familial history	Preparations
162	Male	56	63	Carpenter	Nil	Crude extract
203	Female	?58	65	Housewife	Nil	Crude extract
250	Male	59	78	Veteran; business man	Nil	Crude extract 200 S Supernatant 200 S Pellet
263	Female	51	60	Housewife	Nil	High-speed supernatants

Table 5. PHF induction—sensitivity to ultraviolet irradiation

ergs mm^{-2} $\times 10^5$ (254 nm)	PHFs
1.0	Present
2.1	Absent
5.0	Absent
11.5	Absent

control cultures to stimulate filament formation, including aluminium and hormone treatment; no PHF formation has been observed in the absence of Alzheimer extract. Finally, all the Alzheimer-affected brains from which extracts were prepared induced PHF formation in cultured brain cells.

The induction of paired helical filaments in cultured neurons suggest several possibilities. Firstly, fragments or subunits of PHFs from the Alzheimer donor brain may have been ingested from the extracts and assembled into PHFs after

3–4 weeks *in vitro*. The delay in appearance may be related to altered metabolic states as the survival limits of neurons in explant are approached. Since PHF fragments were not observed in the extract and many of the PHFs appear to be assembled from long segments of normal-appearing neurofilaments, this possibility seems unlikely. Secondly, the Alzheimer donor extract may contain metabolic products which are capable of assembling neurofilaments into paired helical filaments, resulting in cross-bonding and twisting of the naturally occurring filaments. Thirdly, the assembly of PHFs may result from a small fragment of genetic information contained in a particle size less than 80 S and resistant to 10^5 ergs mm^{-2} at 254 nm, which is transcribed and translated within 15 days in the brain explant system. Fourthly, the widespread prevalence of PHFs in all ageing human brains leads to the speculation that a factor extracted from Alzheimer-affected brain is capable of releasing, in the cultured cells, genetic information which is normally suppressed.

As yet, there is no evidence upon which to judge whether the postulated agent extracted from Alzheimer brains has replicated within the survival time of neurons in explant.

Although the induction of PHFs *in vitro* offers many avenues for future research, methods are not yet available which would permit the *in vitro* model to replicate exactly the high density of PHFs seen in the naturally occurring disease.

C. Aluminium: A model of a dementia process with neurofibrillary degeneration

The progressive encephalopathy following intracranial injection of trace amounts of a soluble salt of aluminium offers a suitable model for the study of both a dementia process and the biochemistry of intermediate neurofilaments (Klatzo, Wisniewski, and Streicher, 1965; Terry and Peña, 1965). The aluminium model is of particular interest since elevated aluminium concentrations occur in: human brain with Alzheimer's disease (Crapper and coworkers, 1973, 1976; Trapp and coworkers, 1978), in aged brains (McDermott and coworkers, 1977), in association with neurons with neurofibrillary degeneration (Liss, Ebner, and Couri, 1979), and in the brains and spinal cords of Guam and Kii peninsula amyotrophic lateral sclerosis, and Parkinson-dementia complex with Alzheimer type neurofibrillary degeneration (Yoshimasu and coworkers, 1976; Yase, 1977, 1978).

Intracranial injection in cats or rabbits, of a carefully selected amount of aluminium as the chloride or lactate salt, is followed by an asymptomatic period of about 8–10 days. Signs of a progressive encephalopathy begin with changes in learning-memory performance, followed by impairment in the organization of complex motor acts (motor dyspraxia), the appearance of apathy, changes in motor tone, myoclonic jerks, and general convulsions (Crapper and Dalton, 1973). The entire course of the encephalopathy is about four weeks and the brains contain numerous neurons with 10-nm diameter neurofibrillary degeneration but never PHFs. This model is well suited to the study of behavioural and learning-memory changes resembling those found in a human dementia process. Furthermore, the model offers a unique opportunity to examine changes in neuronal spike and slow wave activity as the dementia evolves (Crapper and Tomko, 1975). Unfortunately, neither monkeys nor rats develop an encephalopathy which resembles that seen in the cat aluminium model (King, De Boni, and Crapper, 1975; Crapper, Quittkat, and De Boni, 1979).

Perhaps one of the most important applications of the aluminium model is to test the hypothesis that this trace element may contribute to processes associated with the filamentous component of the paired helical filaments of the Alzheimer type of neurofibrillary degeneration. Since serum levels of aluminium are not elevated in Alzheimer's disease, this hypothesis requires the operation of an antecedent pathogenic process which alters brain aluminium metabolism such that this neurotoxic metal gains access to brain tissue compartments from which it is normally excluded. This would suggest that aluminium would act as a compounding factor in the pathogenesis of the disease. The issue is of some practical importance, since chelation of the metal might alter the course of the disease.

Aluminium content of brain increases with age. The human fetal and infant brain contains about 0.7 μg Al per g dry weight. In the age range, 50–65 years, several laboratories have reported aluminium contents of between 1.5 and 2.2 μg per g dry weight. In Alzheimer's disease and in several human diseases associated with neurofibrillary degeneration, several groups have reported increased aluminium content. Using a small sample size of 10–15 mg, material assayed in our laboratory indicates that about 30 % of neocortical regions from brains of patients with a clinical history of dementia and widespread neocortical neurofibrillary degeneration had aluminium concentrations greater than 4 μg per g dry weight. Control brains from patients between 50 and 65 years of age, had an average value of 1.9 $\pm$ 0.7 μg per g dry weight (Crapper, Krishnan, and Quittkat, 1976). Several animal studies suggest that the toxic concentration lies between 4 and 8 μg per g dry weight (Crapper and Tomko, 1975; Crapper, 1976; De Boni and coworkers, 1976). Furthermore, human fetal cerebral neurons in culture develop neurofibrillary degeneration of the single 10-nm filament type and die at concentrations of aluminium in the growth medium which are also lethal, *in vivo*, to cats and rabbits (6 μg ml$^-$, Crapper, Karlik, and De Boni, 1978). In both Alzheimer's disease and the experimental encephalopathy in cats, aluminium accumulated on intranuclear structures (De Boni and coworkers, 1974, 1976). Several studies suggest that protein synthesis is altered in Alzheimer's disease. Suzuki, Katzman, and Korey (1965) reported a selective decrease in the ratio of proteins to lipids. Nucleolar size, a useful index of protein synthesis, is decreased in Alzheimer's disease (Dayan and Ball, 1973; Mann and Sinclair, 1978) and is also reduced in brain cell cultures exposed to aluminium (Crapper and De Boni, 1977). A decrease in RNA to DNA ratio was observed by Bowen and coworkers

(1977a, 1977b) in cerebral cortex of brains of patients with senile dementia, and these workers reported a decrease in the percentage of total protein accounted for by microsomal proteins. Decreased RNA content has also been observed by histological techniques in senile dementia (Mann and Sinclair, 1978). Aluminium has been observed to reduce RNA in neuroblastoma cells in tissue culture (Miller and Levine, 1974).

Chromatin, separated by sonication from isolated nuclei from Alzheimer-affected brains, exhibits a statistically significant increase in aluminium content on the heterochromatin compared to age-matched controls (Crapper and De Boni, 1977). While the functional significance of these observations cannot be assessed at present, aluminium has been shown to block steroid (ecdysterone)-induced conformational changes in the polytene chromosomes of the salivary gland cells of *Simulium vittatum*, a black fly (Sanderson, Crapper and De Boni, 1979). Furthermore, aluminium, even at low concentrations, alters sister-chromatid exchange in human cells in culture (De Boni, Seger and Crapper, 1980).

Recent work in our laboratory indicates that aluminium interacts with DNA in a complex manner dependent upon the interaction with hydrating water molecule (Crapper, Karlik, and De Boni, 1978). The multiple equilibria which are generated between aluminium, DNA, water, and available ligands, may be shifted by changes in concentration and pH. These equilibria involve the binding of free and ligand-bound aluminium to DNA and the interconnection between molecular forms. Lowering pH produces 'free' aluminium species in solution. However, the addition of ligand with a high affinity for aluminium favours the formation of 'bound' species for the metal. Under intracellular conditions, many ligands may be present which could bind this element. Aluminium interactions with DNA have been examined by thermal denaturation, circular dichroism, and fluorescent dye binding. These studies indicate that a variety of ionic species is produced when aluminium is dissolved in water, including free cation $Al(H_2O)_6^{3+}$, called complex A, and the monohydroxylated $Al(H_2O)_5 OH^{2+}$, complex B. Below pH 6 and between Al:DNA phosphate mole ratios of 0.3 and 0.7, two distinguishable DNA–Al complexes are produced. Complex I increases the DNA melting temperature. Complex II reduces the DNA T_m while producing interstrand cross-links. These are reversible in the presence of salt or EDTA and permit DNA renaturation. The data are consistent with the existence of two forms of aluminium: (A) and (B), producing complexes II and I, respectively. The concentrations of aluminium employed in these *in vitro* experiments approach those found in association with DNA extracted from some brains from Alzheimer-affected patients. Overall, the available evidence supports the possibility that a major action of aluminium is upon the genetic apparatus.

Nevertheless, before aluminium is assigned a role in Alzheimer's disease, several investigations must be undertaken including: (a) the chemical identification of both the aluminium-induced filaments and the PHFs of Alzheimer's disease, and (b) the characterization of changes in protein synthesis in both the aluminium encephalopathy and in Alzheimer's disease. It is anticipated that the various hydrated states of aluminium will affect many steps in protein synthesis in model systems, and it will be necessary to establish which are likely to be important in Alzheimer's disease. The issue is of some importance because if aluminium is shown to be of cytotoxic significance in Alzheimer's disease, aluminium chelation therapy may be useful in the management of this otherwise untreatable condition.

V. PROGRESSIVE SUPRANUCLEAR PALSY

Progressive supranuclear palsy, first described by Steele, Richardson, and Olszewski (1964), may be associated with dementia. The histopathology of this condition indicates the presence of brain stem neurons with neurofibrillary degeneration. The electron microscope reveals the neurofibrillary material to be composed of 15-nm diameter straight filaments distinctly different from other forms of neurofibrillary degeneration (Tellez-Nagel and Wisniewski, 1973). Similar appearing filaments have been reported to occur reversibly in catfish photoreceptors exposed to 25 mmol Mg^{2+} in the bathing medium (Ryan and Potter, 1978). This suggests that under conditions of altered ionic environment, certain naturally occurring proteins are capable of assembly into structures resembling those found in progressive supranuclear palsy, perhaps offering a useful model for the further investigation of this disease. Alternatively, the proteins of the 15-nm filaments may be induced by an agent important in the pathogenesis of the disease and foreign to human neurons. Structures of 15–20 nm in diameter, and bearing some resemblance to the filaments of human supranuclear palsy, have been reported to occur in mouse neurons infected with the arbor virus Dengue, type 3 (Spiurairatna, Bhamaropravati, and Onishi, 1974).

VI. CONCLUSION

Despite the human tragedy associated with the dementias, these degenerative brain conditions have remained refractory to treatment. In the past 20 years, a critical step has been achieved: these diseases have been brought from the clinic to the laboray bench through the development of several useful models. As the powerful tools of basic science begin to investigate these mind-destroying conditions, the biology of dementia will become one of the most rewarding endeavours of modern medicine.

ACKNOWLEDGEMENTS

This work was supported by the Ontario Mental Health Foundation and the Medical Research Council of Canada. Special thanks are extended to S. Karlik, A. Rodriguez, O. Augustinas, and C. Karlik.

REFERENCES

Bowen, D. M., C. B. Smith, P. White, M. J. Goodhardt, J. A. Spellane, R. H. A. Flack, and A. N. Davison (1977a). Chemical pathology of the organic dementias. I. Validity of biochemical measurements on human post-mortem brain specimens. *Brain*, **100**, 397–426.

Bowen, D. M., C. B. Smith, P. White, R. H. A. Flack, L. H. Carrasco, J. L. Gedye, and A. N. Davison (1977b). Chemical pathology of the organic dementias. II. Quantitative estimation of cellular changes in post-mortem brains. *Brain*, **100**, 427–53.

Bruce, M. A. and H. Fraser, (1975). Amyloid plaques in the brains of mice injected with scrapie: Morphological variation and staining properties. *Neuropath. Appl. Neurobiol.*, **1**, 189.

Crapper, D. R. (1973). Experimental neurofibrillary degeneration and altered electrical activity. *Electroencephl. Clin. Neurophysiol.*, **35**, 575–88.

Crapper, D. R. (1976). Functional consequences of neurofibrillary degeneration. In R. D. Terry and S. Gershon (Eds) *Neurobiology of Aging*, Raven Press, New York, pp. 405–32.

Crapper, D. R. and A. J. Dalton (1973). Alterations in short-term retention, conditioned avoidance response acquisition and motivation following aluminium-induced neurofibrillary degeneration. *Physiol. Behav.*, **10**, 925–33.

Crapper, D. R. and U. De Boni (1977). Aluminium and the genetic apparatus in Alzheimer disease. In K. Nanely (Ed.) *Symposium on The Ageing Brain and Senile Dementia*, Plenum Press, New York, pp. 229–46.

Crapper, D. R., S. S. Krishnan, and A. J. Dalton (1973). Brain aluminum distribution in Alzheimer's disease and experimental neurofibrillary degeneration. *Science (Washington)*, **180**, 511.

Crapper, D. R., S. Karlik, and U. De Boni (1978). Aluminum and other metals in senile (Alzheimer) dementia. In R. Katzman, R. D. Terry, and K. L. Bick (Eds) *Alzheimer's Disease: Senile Dementia and Related Disorders (Aging*, Vol. 7), Raven Press, New York. p. 471.

Crapper, D. R., S. S. Krishnan and S. Quittkat (1976). Aluminum, neurofibrillary degeneration and Alzheimer's disease. *Brain*, **99**, 67–80.

Crapper, D. R., S. Quittkat, and U. De Boni (1979). Altered chromatin conformation in Alzheimer's disease. *Brain.* **102**, 483–495.

Crapper, D. R. and G. J. Tomko (1975). Neuronal correlates of an encephalopathy induced by aluminum neurofibrillary degeneration. *Brain Res.*, **971**, 253–64.

Dayan, A. D. and M. J. Ball (1973). Histometric observations on the metabolism of tangle-bearing neurons. *J. Neurol. Sci.*, **19**, 422–6.

De Boni, U. and D. R. Crapper (1978). Paired helical filaments of the Alzheimer type in cultured neurones. *Nature (London)*, **271**, 566–8.

De Boni, U., Seger, M. and D. R. Crapper (1980). Functional consequences of chromatin bound aluminium in cultured human cells. *Neurotoxicology*, In press.

De Boni, U., A. Otvos, J. W. Scott, and D. R. Crapper (1976). Neurofibrillary degeneration induced by systemic aluminum. *Acta Neuropath. (Berl.)*, **35**, 285–94.

De Boni, U., J. W. Scott, and D. R. Crapper (1974). Intracellular aluminum binding; a histochemical study. *Histochemie*, **40**, 31–7.

Flament-Durand, J. (1978). Ultrastructural observations in brain biopsies of Alzheimer's dementia. VIII. *International Congress of Neuropathology*. Abst. No. 99.

Gajdusek, D. C. (1977). Unconventional viruses and the origin and disappearance of Kuru. *Science*, **197**, 943–60.

Hadfield, M. G., A. H. Martinez, and R. C. Gilmartin (1974). Progressive multifocal leukoencephalopathy with paramyro-virus-like structures. Hirano bodies and neurofibrillary tangles. *Acta Neuropathol. (Bul.)*, **27**, 277–88.

Haig, D. A., M. C. Clarke, E. Blum, and T. Alper (1969). Further studies on the inactivation of the scrapie agent by ultraviolet light. *J. Gen. Virol.*, **5**, 455–7.

Hallervorden, J. (1933). Zur pathogenese des post-encephalitischen Parkinsonismus. *Klin. Wochenschr.*, **12**, 692–5.

Hirano, A. and H. Zimmerman (1962). Alzheimer neurofibrillary changes. *Arch. Neurol.*, **7**, 227–42.

Horoupian, D. S. and S. S. Yang (1978). Paired helical filaments in neurovisceral lipidosis (juvenile dystonic lipidosis). *Ann. Neurol.*, **4**, 404–11.

Kidd, M. (1964). Alzheimer's disease, an electron microscopical study. *Brain*, **87**, 307–19.

King, G. A., U. De Boni, and D. R. Crapper (1975). Effect of aluminum upon conditioned avoidance response acquisition in the absence of neurofibrillary degeneration. *Pharmacol. Biochem. Behav.*, **3**, 1003–9.

Klatzo, I., H. Wisniewski, and E. Streicher (1965). Experimental mental production of neurofibrillary degeneration. I. Light microscopic observations. *Neuropath. Exp. Neurol.*, **24**, 187.

Liss, L., K. Ebner, and D. Couri (1979). Neurofibrillary tangles induced by a sclerosing angioma. *Human Path.*, **10**, 104–8.

Mandybur, T. I., A. S. Nagpaul, Z. Pappos, and W. J. Niklowitz (1977). Alzheimer neurofibrillary changes in subacute sclerosing panencephalitis. *Ann. Neurol.*, **1**, 103–7.

Mann, D. M. A. and K. G. A. Sinclair (1978). The quantitative assessment of lipofuscin pigment, cytoplasmic RNA and nucleolar volume in senile dementia. *Neuropath. Appl. Neurobiol.*, **4**, 129–35.

Marsh, R. F., T. Malone, J. Semaneik, W. D. Lancaster, and R. P. Hanson (1978). Evidence for an essential DNA component in the scrapie agent. *Nature (London)*, **275**, 146–7.

McDermott, J. R., A. I. Smith, K. Igbal, and H. M. Wisniewski (1977). Aluminium and Alzheimer's disease. *Lancet*, **11**, 710.

Miller, C. A., and E. M. Levine (1974). Effect of aluminum gels on cultured neuroblastoma cells. *J. Neurochem.*, **22**, 751–8.

Prusiner, S. B., W. J. Hadlow, C. M. Eklund, R. E. Race, and S. P. Cochran (1978a). Sedimentation characteristics of the scrapie agent from spleen and brain. *Biochemistry*, **17**, 4987–92.

Prusiner, S. B., W. J. Hadlow, D. E. Garfin, P. Cochran, J. R. Baringer, R. E. Race, and C. M. Eklund (1978b). Partial purification and evidence for multiple molecular forms of the scrapie agent. *Biochemistry*, **17**, 4993–9.

Rewcastle, N. B., C. A. Gibbs, and C. D. Gajdusek (1978). Transmission of familial Alzheimer's disease to primates. VIII. *International Congress of Neuropathology*, Abst. No. 295.

Ryan, T. and H. D. Potter (1978). A Mg^{2+}-dependent class of thick filaments and correlated nuclear chromatin in catfish photoreceptors. *J. Neurocytol.*, **7**, 313–21.

Sanderson, C. I., Crapper, D. R., and U. De Boni (1979). Altered response to ecdysterone by chromatin bound aluminium in a polytene chromosome of Simulium Vittatum. *J. Cell Biol.*, **83**, 1529.

Spiurairatna, S., N. Bhamaropravati, and S. Onishi (1974). Filamentous structures in Dengue type 3 virus-infected mouse neurons. *Bikem. J.*, **17**, 183–91.

Steele, J. C., J. C. Richardson, and J. Olszewski (1964). Progressive supranuclear palsy: A heterogeneous degeneration involving the brain stem, basal ganglia and cerebellum with vertical gaze and pseudobulbar palsy, nuchal dystonia and dementia. *Arch. Neurol.*, **10**, 333–59.

Susuki, K., R. Katzman, and S. R. Korey (1965). Chemical studies on Alzheimer's Disease. *J. Neuropath. Exp. Neurol.*, **24**, 211–24.

Tellez-Nagel, I. and H. M. Wisniewski (1973). Ultrastructure of neurofibrillary tangles in Steele–Richardson–Olszewski syndrome. *Arch. Neurol.*, **29**, 324–7.

Terry, R. D. and C. Peña (1965). Experimental production of neurofibrillary degeneration. II. Electron microscopy, phosphatase histochemistry and electron probe analysis. *J. Neuropath. Exp. Neurol.*, **24**, 200.

Trapp, G. A., G. D. Miner, R. L. Zimmerman, A. R. Mastri, and L. L. Heston (1978). Aluminium levels in brain in Alzheimer's disease. *Biol. Psych.*, **13**, 709–18.

Wisniewski, H. M., M. E. Bruce, and H. Fraser (1975). Infectious etiology of neuritic (senile) plaques in mice. *Science*, **190**, 1108–10.

Wisniewski, H., H. Narang, and R. D. Terry (1976). Neurofibrillary tangles of paired helical filaments. *J. Neurol. Sci.*, **27**, 173–81.

Yase, Y. (1977). The basic process of amyotrophic lateral sclerosis as reflected in Kii peninsula and Guam. Excerpta. Med. Int. Congr. Series, No. 434. *Neurology*, 413.

Yase, Y. (1978). *Kii Peninsula Amyotrophic Lateral Sclerosis*. USPHS, NIW CDS, NIH Guam Alz/PD Workshop.

Yoshimasu, F., Y. Uebayashi, Y. Yase, S. Iwata, and K. Sasajima (1976). Studies on amyotrophic lateral sclerosis by neutron activation analysis. *Folia Psych. Neurol. Jap.*, **30**, 49.

Biochemistry of Dementia
Edited by P. J. Roberts
© 1980, John Wiley & Sons Ltd.

Chapter 4

Cerebral Blood Flow in Dementia

R. W. Ross Russell

*St Thomas' Hospital, London, SE1, and The National Hospital
for Nervous Diseases, Queen Square, London, WC1, U.K.*

To the neurologist a patient with dementia presents a number of problems in diagnosis as well as in treatment. Where in the central nervous system is the lesion responsible for his altered mental state? What type of pathological process is present? Is it structural or functional? Can it be reversed? These questions are made more difficult by the variety of causes of organic dementia which include the effects of trauma, chronic infection, alcoholism and vascular disease, as well as of primary degeneration or ageing of neurones. In this review I shall restrict attention to two questions: firstly, how often and by what means does degenerative arterial disease cause senile or pre-senile dementia; secondly, can anything be done to prevent or reverse the vascular lesion?

I. DEMENTIA CAUSED BY VASCULAR DISEASE

On the first point there is ample clinical evidence that successive strokes may result in mental as well as physical incapacity. Only the most massive strokes are fatal but a series of minor non-fatal ischaemic lesions may affect different parts of the brain producing aphasia, visuospatial disturbances, amnesia, or emotional change. This cumulative deficit may appear to be a global dementia although it is, in fact, a succession of small focal lesions. It should be noted, in passing, that in some patients a localized defect, such as dysphasia or amnesia, or a physical impairment, such as pseudobulbar palsy or Parkinsonism, may be wrongly diagnosed as a degenerative dementia.

The underlying pathological mechanism in patients with multiple infarcts is usually one of a series of acute vascular occlusions affecting the small or large intracranial arteries. Occlusion may result from local arterial disease or from embolism. Small-vessel disease is characterized by focal regions of lipohyaline change, microaneurysm formation, segmental disorganization, vascular thrombosis, and finally by lacunar infarction (Fisher, 1969). Such patients nearly always suffer from hypertension or diabetes, but similar changes may also sometimes be found in elderly subjects (Cole and Yates, 1967). The other important cause of multiple infarction is embolism, the emboli originating either in the heart or on the surface of large arteries, and consisting either of fragments of thrombus or of atheromatous debris containing cholesterol (Jorgensen and Torvig, 1966). In only a few patients with multiple infarction is the vascular lesion truly atherosclerotic due to atheroma of the major vessels, such as the middle cerebral artery.

A. Not all Dementias are due to Vascular Disease

Thus, vascular occlusion is capable of producing a type of dementia; is it possible that many other forms of pre-senile and senile dementia might have a vascular cause due not to discrete infarcts but to an overall restriction of blood to the brain from generalized atherosclerosis? The evidence is not in favour of this. Pathological studies show no more vascular change in patients with Alzheimer's disease than in normal subjects dying at the same age (Corsellis and Evans, 1965). The characteristic pathology of Alzheimer's disease is not found in relation to ischaemic lesions (Fisher, 1968) and has not been produced experimentally by ischaemia. Clinical evidence of arterial disease, such as myocardial infarction, angina, hypertension, or intermittent claudication, are not found in greater prevalence in Alzheimer's disease. The diagnosis of arteriopathic dementia should, therefore, be restricted to those patients having clinical features of multiple small infarcts. These are a history of sudden irregular transient cerebral events with a step-wise cumulative deficit, both physical and mental, the frequent presence of abnormal physical signs such as hemiparesis, sensory loss, visual field defect, vertigo, ataxia, or disordered ocular movement. Dysphasia, apraxia, extrapyramidal rigidity, and emotional lability of pseudobulbar type are also frequently found. The purely mental symptoms are less useful in diagnosis; amnesia, paranoid ideas, confusion, deteriorated habits, restlessness, and hallucinations are found in both types of organic dementia (Roth and Morrissey, 1952).

B. Prevalence of Multi-infarct Dementia

Turning from how to when, if these stringent diagnostic criteria are applied we find that arteriopathic dementia accounts for no more than about a quarter of the total of demented patients. Primary neuronal dementia accounts for more than half and the remainder is made up by a large number of other types of encephalopathy, such as tumours, effects of trauma, and alcoholism (Marsden and Harrison, 1972).

II. CHARACTERISTICS OF THE CEREBRAL CIRCULATION

Before going on to describe the results of cerebral blood flow (CBF) studies of the patients with dementia, it is necessary to make some general comments about the cerebral circulation. The brain has a large but fairly stable blood supply and, although there are regional variations in response to metabolic demand, the overall cerebral blood flow remains fairly constant. There is also an exceptionally favourable arterial system with four large arteries connected at the base of the brain, each capable of accommodating a greatly increased flow and offering considerable protection against the effects of occlusion or narrowing. We know from experimental studies and from angiography on patients with advanced arteriosclerosis that any one of these vessels may be capable of supplying sufficient blood for the entire brain. As a further safeguard, the brain has an efficient homeostatic system whereby flow is maintained independent of blood pressure (Lassen, 1959). This means that the mean blood pressure perfusing the brain can fall to 50 mmHg or rise to 180 mmHg without disturbing the blood flow. Although there are many vascular nerves in the walls of cerebral arteries, neurogenic control appears to be of secondary importance in the small intracerebral resistance vessels, although it may possibly influence the calibre of larger basal arteries and may modify the effects of vasodilator agents, such as carbon dioxide (Harper, 1965).

A. Methods of Measurement of CBF

There are a number of methods of assessing the brain's blood supply—the flow may be measured in an individual major artery, usually employing an electromagnetic flow meter or thermistor. This is of limited value since the blood flow through other arteries is unknown. A second method is to introduce a radioactive indicator into the circulation to measure the circulation time or the rate of turnover of the intravascular compartment of the brain. If the volume of blood in the brain is known, then the total cerebral blood flow in millimetres per minute can be calculated. This method suffers from the disadvantage that it is difficult to calculate the volume of the intravascular compartment because of the proximity of other large vascular beds in the skull and scalp. In addition, it makes no allowances for brain size and this may vary widely in different subjects.

The third and most widely used method derives from the classical studies of Kety and Schmidt (Kety, 1956) and uses a diffusible indicator, such as the gas 133-xenon. This is breathed through a face-mask or injected in solution into a vein or into the carotid artery. The resulting radioactive bolus travels to the brain where its arrival and diffusion into cerebral tissue, and its eventual wash-out, are monitored by externally placed counters. From the rate of elution of indicator from the brain can be calculated the cerebral perfusion rate in millilitres of blood per 100 g of brain per minute; the method can be adapted to measure regional or total values (Lassen and coworkers, 1963).

It is important to realize that perfusion rate per unit mass, and not blood flow, is being measured so that a brain may be reduced in size but still have a normal perfusion rate. The main disadvantages of the diffusible indicator method are that in its more reliable form it involves a carotid puncture, and that other techniques using inhalation or intravenous injection are subject to inaccuracies due to slow arrival of the indicator and its presence in extracerebral tissues as well as brain. Correction factors have to be made for this. The method also makes a number of assumptions about the physical distribution of xenon according to its solubility in various compartments of the brain. When brain is diseased, this may be altered and distort the result.

Some workers have used large numbers of detectors enabling regional flow to be measured. In the normal brain there are small differences between various regions, the anterior temporal lobe showing the highest flow. States of heightened physiological activity, such as that produced by hand clenching, stimulation of a limb, or flashing lights, have been shown to produce increases in flow in the appropriate region, (Roland and Larsen, 1976).

III. CBF IN DEMENTIAS: THE RESULT NOT THE CAUSE

Many of the earlier papers on blood flow in dementia are characterized by a poverty of clinical information because few workers attempted to separate the different aetiological types.

In elderly healthy subjects there is a slight reduction in perfusion rate, amounting to 10–20 % of that found in young subjects (O'Brien and Mallett, 1970). In primary neuronal dementia most workers have found that there is a slight reduction of about the same magnitude, but in arteriopathic dementia of similar degree the reduction in flow is more marked and more regional (Hagberg and Ingvar, 1976). The severity of dementia shows a rough correlation with the reduction of blood flow, the fast clearing fraction or flow in grey matter showing the best correlation. With the intra-arterial technique it is possible to resolve the elution curve into fast and slow clearing compartments, thought to correspond to grey and white matter. In some patients with severe dementia the weight of grey matter (calculated by extrapolation of the wash-out curves) has been found to be reduced relative to the weight of white matter (Gustavson and Risberg, 1974).

Where the rate of oxygen consumption has been measured, it has been normal or has shown a mild reduction comparable to that in the cerebral blood flow. Some workers have found a disproportionate fall in cerebral metabolic rate for glucose in elderly patients and in those with arteriopathic dementia, suggesting that alternative energy pathways are being used (Sokoloff, 1975). A further important point is that vascular reactivity to CO_2 is preserved, indicating that flow could increase if it were necessary (Hachinski, Marshall, and Lassen, 1974). When blood flow is deliberately increased by CO_2 breathing there is no change in oxygen or glucose utilization.

How are the results to be interpreted? Is the reduction in blood flow primary or secondary? It seems that in primary neuronal dementia the problem is one of diminished requirements, not diminished supply; there is a reduction in total brain weight and the remaining brain tissue contains fewer cells; metabolism is reduced, possibly due to neurotransmitter failure, and less blood is required. A similar situation obtains in toxic encephalopathy where metabolism is again depressed, this time by the effect of raised intracranial pressure or by barbiturates; brain size is unaltered but blood flow and metabolism are reduced concurrently.

In arteriopathic dementia the situation is slightly different. In most instances small infarcts have already occurred due to occlusion of a number of vessels, producing regions of infarcted brain tissue requiring virtually no circulation and adjacent regions where metabolism is severely depressed. Focally reduced cerebral blood flow values are again usually the consequence, and not the cause, of brain damage.

A. Primary Reduction in CBF

Included in the large number of patients with arteriopathic dementia there is, however, a small group who appear to have a chronic primary reduction in blood flow. Some of these suffer from severe multiple extracranial arterial occlusions, resulting in a reduction in perfusion pressure to the brain. These patients are in a continuous state of borderline cerebral insufficiency and any further reduction in perfusion pressure leads to a fall in blood flow. They are thus extremely sensitive to postural change, minor variations in blood pressure, or to manoeuvres such as neck rotation or extension which cause slight restriction in the calibre of cervical arteries. These patients tend to develop ischaemia and infarction in the border zones between the major arterial territories in the brain, especially those between the middle and posterior cerebral arteries (Russell and Bharucha, 1978). The symptomatology of these patients has been recognized only in recent years.

A further group of patients in whom the reduction in blood flow is the primary event, are those with hyperviscosity states produced, for instance, by poly-cythaemia vera or by disorders of the plasma proteins. These patients, who are known to have a high risk of cerebral and systematic thrombosis, have recently been shown to have substantial generalized reduction in cerebral blood flow which can be reversed in many instances by venesection, a measure which rapidly reduces both the haematocrit and the viscosity (Thomas and coworkers, 1977). Some of these patients also show a state of retardation of mental processes which can be reversed by increasing blood flow.

IV. PRINCIPLES OF TREATMENT: MEDICAL AND SURGICAL

Having considered the question of the pathogenesis of vascular dementia, what rational therapy can be recommended? Those patients in whom multiple infarcts are produced by embolism may benefit from surgical removal of the source of thrombus in the heart or major blood vessels. Ulcerated areas on the arterial wall which do not necessarily cause restriction of the lumen, but which discharge atheromatous debris, may also be appropriately treated by endarterectomy. Patients in whom multiple cerebral infarcts are secondary to hypertensive microvascular disease may show an improved prognosis when the blood pressure is treated, although the neurological deficit usually remains and in this group prevention is better than cure. Patients with very severe extracranial arterial disease and primary reduction in blood flow may be suitable for disobliteration of the extracranial arteries or, alternatively, for a transcranial bypass operation linking the superficial temporal and the middle cerebral arteries. Indications for this operation, which is being done in increasing numbers in the United States, are distal carotid occlusion or proximal middle cerebral occlusion with continuing attacks of ischaemia in the same territory but without a disabling deficit. The number of patients in this group is small.

Finally, we come to the question of vasodilator treatment. Vasodilator drugs are frequently prescribed for demented patients, especially on the Continent but also in the United States. Drugs are of theoretical value only in those patients where the brain is receiving insufficient blood for its metabolic requirements and where this rate can be increased by vasodilation. As we have seen, this state of affairs very rarely occurs and, when it does, the brain is critically dependent on perfusion pressure. It is difficult to find a drug which will produce a selective vasodilatation in the brain and have no effect on systemic blood pressure. Although a number of drugs produce a short-term increase in cerebral perfusion, those trials showing a beneficial effect from vasodilators have not shown an accompanying improvement in cerebral blood flow (McHenry, 1972). It may be that the beneficial effect was due to non-specific altering or antidepressant action.

V. SUMMARY

Although dementia occurs in many patients with cerebral vascular disease, it is seldom caused by a state of chronic underperfusion. Overall cerebral blood flow, measured by diffusible indicator methods, is slightly reduced in primary dementia; in arteriopathic dementia the reduction is more marked and more focal.

These changes in cerebral blood flow are due to reduced metabolic activity of brain or to the presence of infarcted and damaged tissue. Multiple cerebral infarcts in demented patients result from acute occlusion of intracerebral arteries by lipohyaline degeneration or embolism. They are not due to progressive atherosclerosis.

Only in exceptional instances is there evidence of a chronic reduction in cerebral blood flow, secondary to vascular disease of extracranial vessels.

Reconstructive arterial surgery and vasodilator drugs play little part in the treatment of arteriopathic dementia.

REFERENCES

Cole, F. M. and P. O. Yates (1967). The occurrence and significance of intracerebral microaneurysms. *J. Path. Bacter.*, **93**, 393.

Corsellis, J. A. N. and P. H. Evans (1965). *Proceedings of 5th International Congress of Neuropathology.* p. 546.

Fisher, C. M. (1968). Cerebral vascular disease. In J. Toole, R. Siekert, and J. Whisnant (Eds) *South Princeton Conference*, Grune and Stratton, New York and London.

Fisher, C. M. (1969). The arterial lesions underlying lacunes. *Acta Neuropath. (Berl.)*, **12**, 1.

Gustavson, L. and J. Risberg (1974). Cerebral blood flow related to psychiatric symptoms in presenile dementia. *Acta Psychiat. Scand.*, **50**, 516.

Hachinski, V. C., J. Marshall and N. A. Lassen (1974). Multiinfarct dementia. *Lancet*, **2**, 207.

Hagberg, B. and D. Ingvar (1976). Cognitive reduction in presenile dementia related to regional abnormalities of the cerebral blood flow. *Brit. J. Psychiat.*, **128**, 209.

Harper, A. M. (1965). The inter-relationship between $Pa CO_2$ and blood pressure in the regulation of blood flow through the cerebral cortex. *J. Neurol. Neurosurg. Psychiat.*, **28**, 449.

Jorgensen, L. and A. Torvig (1966). Ischaemic cerebrovascular disease in an autopsy series. *J. Neurol. Sci.*, **3**, 490.

Kety, S. S. (1956). *Human Cerebral Blood Flow and Oxygen Consumption as Related to Aging.* Research Publication of Association into Research on Nervous and Mental Diseases. pp. 35, 31.

Lassen, N. A. (1959). Cerebral blood flow and oxygen consumption in man. *Physiol. Rev.*, **39**, 183.

Lassen, N. A., K. Hoedt Rasmussen, S. C. Sorensen, E. Skinhoj, S. Cronquist, B. Bodforss, and D. H. Ingvar (1963). Regional cerebral blood flow in man determined by krypton 85. *Neurology*, **13**, 719.

Marsden, C. D. and M. J. G. Harrison (1972). Outcome of investigations of patients with presenile dementia. *Brit. Med. J.*, **2**, 249.

McHenry, L. (1972). Cerebral vasodilator therapy in stroke. *Stroke*, **3**, 686.

O'Brien, M.D. and B. L. Mallett (1970). Cerebral cortex perfusion rates in dementia. *J. Neurol., Neurosurg. Neuropath.*, **33**, 497–500.

Roland, P. E. and B. Larsen (1976). Focal increase of cerebral blood flow during stereognostic testing in man. *Arch. Neurol.*, **33**, 551–58.

Roth, M. and J. D. Morrissey (1952). Problems in the diagnosis and classification of mental disorder in old age. *J. Mental Sci.*, **98**, 66.

Russell, R. W. R. and N. Bharucha (1978). Recognition and prevention of cerebral border-zone infarctions. *Quart. J. Med., N.S.*, **47**, 303.

Sokoloff, L. (1975). In S. Gershon and A. Raskin. (Eds) Cerebral circulation and metabolism in the aged. (*Aging*, Vol. 2), Raven Press, New York.

Thomas, D. J., G. H. du Boulay, J. Marshall, T. C. Pearson, R. W. Ross Russell, L. Symon, G. Wetherley-Mein, and E. Zilkha (1977). Cerebral blood flow in polycythaemia. *Lancet*, **2**, 161.

Biochemistry of Dementia
Edited by P. J. Roberts
© 1980, John Wiley & Sons Ltd.

Chapter 5

Biochemical Evidence for Selective Vulnerability in Alzheimer's Disease

DAVID M. BOWEN

Institute of Neurology, Queen Square, London, WC1N 2NS, U.K.

I. INTRODUCTION

There are many causes of the clinical state of dementia. Excluding those patients with tumours, infectious or vascular disease, there remains a large group (Corsellis, 1962) whose brains are atrophied and contain an excess of senile degenerative changes (senile plaques and neurofibrillary degeneration) in the neocortex and hippocampus. Altered pre-synaptic axon terminals, pre-synaptic neurites associated with senile plaques, and a decrease in the density of dendritic spines have also been described (for references see Bowen and coworkers, 1976b, 1977a). When this condition occurs before the age of 65 years it is known as 'pre-senile dementia' or 'Alzheimer's disease'; after this age it has been called 'senile dementia' or 'senile dementia of Alzheimer's type'. Since there is no good reason on neuropathological grounds (Corsellis, 1976) to maintain this distinction for all but possibly the rare familial cases (Scheibel and Tomiyasu, 1978), the term Alzheimer's disease is used irrespective of the patient's age.

II. ROLE OF CEREBRAL BIOPSY

Table 1 outlines the usual means of investigating dementia in a neurological unit, psychiatric methods of investigation being reviewed by Blessed (Chapter 1). The tests listed in the right-hand column of Table 1, with the exception, perhaps, of the electroencephalogram, would not be used in an elderly population. The ultimate procedure in the investigation of cerebral disease is that of biopsy. This may be of value in demented patients in whom the tests listed have probably advanced the diagnosis to 'cerebral atrophy of unknown cause'. The procedure is limited to the pre-senile age group. For obvious ethical reasons, biopsy has not been used in the diagnosis of elderly dementia cases. Biopsies, taken by some

Biochemistry of Dementia

Table 1. Investigation of dementia

Full blood count	Cerebrospinal fluid
Erythrocyte sedimentation rate	Chest and skull X-rays
Plasma urea, electrolytes and glucose	Electroencephalography
Liver function tests	Air encephalography
Thyroid function tests	Computerized tomography
Vitamin B_{12}	Isotope cisternography
Serology	? Biopsy ?

Table 2. Some effects of physostigmine on test performance of biopsy-confirmed Alzheimer patient with low choline acetyltransferase activity (modified from Smith and Swash, 1979)

Test	Score (mean $\pm$S.E.M, $n = 6$)		Mann–Whitney U test
	After placebo	After physostigmine	
Ravens I.Q.	11.0 ± 0.63	11.67 ± 0.56	N.S.
Word lists:			
Free recall			
Correct	$8.0 \quad 1.26$	7.67 ± 0.80	N.S.
Intrusions	5.0 ± 1.26	1.38 ± 0.45	$p < 0.052$
Category-cued intrusions	10.0 ± 1.34	4.0 ± 1.56	$p < 0.026$
Memory for names:			
Intrusions	$2.83 - 0.31$	1.33 ± 0.42	$p < 0.034$

physicians either merely to provide a histological diagnosis, genetic advice, or to allow correlation between diagnosis and another variable (Letemendia and Pampiglione, 1958), have only infrequently led to attempts at therapy (Sim and Smith, 1955) (Table 2). Based on biopsy studies, Sim and coworkers conclude that Alzheimer's disease has a discernible clinical pattern and predictable natural history (Sim, Turner, and Smith, 1966; Smith, Turner, and Sim, 1966). The clinical features held to be characteristic of Alzheimer's disease are given in Table 3.

The findings of Sim and coworkers are notable, as 17 of the 59 demented persons by biopsy were found to have non-specific histological changes (Table 3). Spillane (1978) examined cerebral biopsies from 11 patients with dementia due to cerebral atrophy of unknown aetiology. Six were found to have histological evidence of Alzheimer's disease and three had non-specific changes. Thus, both studies, while identifying Alzheimer's disease as the major cause of dementia, are tantalizing also, for they suggest that a cause(s) of at least pre-senile dementia, associated with atrophy, remains unidentified. The other possibility, that the examination of a very small piece of frontal cortex may be misleading, is not the

Table 3. Clinical features in biopsied demented patients
(modified from Sim, Turner, and Smith, 1966)

Clinical features	Dementia due to Alzheimer's disease (34 cases*)	Dementia not due to Alzheimer's disease (25 cases†)
Memory loss	Early	Late
EEG changes	Early	Late
Apraxia	Early	Late
Fits	Late	Early
Incontinence	Late	Early
Neurological signs	Late	Early
Confabulation	Late	Early
Personality changes	Late	Early
Psychotic symptoms	Late	Early

* All had histological evidence of Alzheimer's disease.
† 17 had non-specific histological changes.

opinion of those experienced in the use of biopsy in Alzheimer's disease (McMenemy, 1940; Green and coworkers, 1952; Sim, Turner, and Smith, 1966).

A. Approaches to Study

There have been several approaches to the study of the chemical pathology of the organic dementias. This includes the biochemical examination of the well-defined histological lesions through the use of histochemistry and biochemical separation techniques, e.g. see Shelanski (1978) and Grundke-Iqbal and coworkers (1979) on the origin of abnormal proteins in tangle-bearing neurons.

Subcellular fractionation of post-mortem brain tissue, pioneered by Stahl, Sumi, and Swanson (1971), is another approach. Although the total protein (per gram wet weight) in one fraction (the interphase between 0. 32 mol l^{-1} and 0.8 mol l^{-1} sucrose solution) may be selectively abnormal in Alzheimer brain, the results are remarkable for they fail to demonstrate extensive differences between normal and diseased tissues (White, Bowen, and Davison, 1978).

The nature of a possible metabolic disturbance, indicated by the findings of reduced cerebral oxygen uptake and cerebral blood flow (CBF) (Raiche and coworkers, 1978) might be investigated further, using cortical biopsies. This approach has already provided preliminary data on glucose utilization (Suzuki, Katzman, and Korey, 1965) and energy-dependent high-affinity uptake of transmitters (Spillane and coworkers, 1977a, 1977b). Cerebral oxygen uptake but not CBF is reduced in other neurological disorders (Lenzi and coworkers, 1979). Thus, the blood flow deficit in Alzheimer cases, although controversial (Hachinski and coworkers, 1975), may be a key change.

Biochemical analyses of unfractionated brain tissue, useful in elucidating neurotransmitter changes in Parkinson's disease and Huntington's chorea, have now been carried out on brain samples of Alzheimer's disease. These data provide information about the possible extent and selectivity of cellular changes, such as neuronal loss.

B. Difficulties of Interpreting Autopsy Data

Polyacrylamide electrophoretic profiles of soluble acidic proteins from neocortex show that one such protein, NS6, clearly occurs in normal human brain. This protein is of interest because it is sensitive to conditions that might be expected to cause 'oxygen deprivation' (Bowen and coworkers, 1976a, 1976b; Smith and Bowen, 1976). For example, the concentration of the protein is markedly reduced in caudate nucleus from non-demented patients dying of severe respiratory disease, and is reduced in cortex from baboons made ischaemic, in acute experiments, by occlusion of the middle cerebral artery. In cases of Alzheimer's disease dying of bronchopneumonia, the protein is reduced not only in frontal cortex but more markedly so in brain regions in which senile degeneration is infrequent. We believe that this phenomenon is due to a combination of the terminal state and reduced CBF. Glutamate decarboxylase (GAD), a marker of γ-aminobutyric acid (GABA)-containing neurons, appears to be similarly affected. For example, in cortex from ischaemic baboon the activity decreases as the intensity of terminal ischaemia increases. The threshold flow taken for the calculation of degree of ischaemia or flow deficit was low (22 ml per 100 g per min). Since most Alzheimer cases die of respiratory disease, and presumably have reduced CBF, these and other data indicate that in this disease GAD activity is not a reliable index of the pre-terminal state of GABA-containing neurons. The marker of cholinergic neurons, choline acetyltransferase (CAT) activity, appears to be relatively unaffected by the terminal state. Other factors that have been considered in post-mortem studies are age, clinical history, drug treatment, time of day of death, place of death, sampling delay, interval between death and refrigeration of corpse, and intensity of cerebral pathology (including possible histological changes in controls).

1. Reduction in CAT Activity

When the factors described above are taken into account, there appears to be a disease-related reduction in CAT activity in Alzheimer's disease (Table 4). Note that the control autopsy specimens and normal-appearing tissues removed at craniotomy for tumour (biopsy controls) have similar CAT activities; furthermore, that the CAT activity in Alzheimer's disease is reduced at both biopsy and autopsy. Other data obtained with post-mortem specimens suggest that there is a correlation between CAT activity and the intensity of senile degeneration. GAD activity appears to correspond to neuronal loss which itself may be

Table 4. Neocortical CAT activities measured pre- and post-mortem

Tissue and reference	CAT activity	
	Control (nmol per min per 100 mg protein)	Alzheimer's disease (% control)
Biopsy		
Bowen and coworkers (1979)	6.5	46†
Autopsy		
Bowen and coworkers (1976b)*	7.2	51†
Davies and Maloney (1976)*	15.6	35
Perry and coworkers (1977a)	3.9	31†
Reisine and coworkers (1978a)	8.3	40†
White and coworkers (1977)	5.4	50†

* Calculated from data expressed per g fresh weight.
† p at least < 0.05, usually < 0.01.

reflected in CBF changes (Bowen and coworkers, 1976b). In an elegant study, Perry and coworkers (1978) have extended this work with respect to senile plaque formation and mental test score.

2. Cholinoreceptive Cells

Muscarinic cholinergic receptor binding, measured using atropine (White and coworkers, 1977; Bowen and coworkers, 1979), scopolamine (Perry and coworkers, 1977a), or quinuclidinyl benzilate (QNB) (Davies and Verth, 1978; Bowen and coworkers, 1979), appears to be normal in Alzheimer's disease.

C. Extent of Neocortical Neuronal Loss

The neurochemical changes in the Parkinsonian and choreic brain are accompanied by demonstrable neuronal loss from discrete regions of the brain. Ball (1977) has shown that neuronal loss occurs from the hippocampus in normal ageing and is more marked in age-matched Alzheimer cases.

The narrowing of the cortical ribbon, loss in brain weight, and shrinkage that occur in Alzheimer's disease have been ascribed to neuronal fall-out. As neocortical cell counts yield no information about *total* cell numbers, there are limitations in current morphological methods to test such a hypothesis. Therefore, we have used biochemical methods in an attempt to assess *overall* cellular and subcellular changes in the brain. The analyses were carried out on aliquots of whole temporal lobe and the results were expressed per lobe. It was anticipated that this procedure would reduce any errors due to oedema, water loss or differences in tissue sampling. The temporal lobe was chosen for study because it is particularly affected in Alzheimer's disease and may show changes in control subjects that reflect the functional deficits that are associated with normal ageing.

The content of DNA, ganglioside NANA, myelin protein, and NS5 (also called the 14.3.2. protein), ratio of DNA to RNA, and activities of β-galactosidase and adenosine 2, 3-cyclic nucleotide 3-phosphohydrolase (phosphohydrolase) were measured as potential indices of nerve cell number. None of these markers alters significantly with age in temporal lobe from non-demented subjects aged 50–100 years, living normal lives appropriate to their age, from whom histologically normal brains were obtained.

Due to secondary glial reactions (Bowen and coworkers, 1977a), or post-mortem artefact (Smith and Bowen, 1976), or terminal changes (Bowen and coworkers, 1977b), only ganglioside NANA and phosphohydrolase activities appear to be relatively reliable as quantitative markers in the temporal lobe. Twenty Alzheimer brains have so far been examined, and both constituents are significantly reduced to 57–70 % of control, compared with controls matched with respect to post-mortem handling, or terminal status, or age (Bowen and coworkers 1977b, 1979).

It can be concluded that neocortical neurons of the temporal lobe, representing much of the massive neocortical development in man, are able to be maintained into normal old age, but that in Alzheimer's disease there is significant shrinkage and probably loss of these neurons. This suggests that Alzheimer's disease, like Huntington's chorea, is a primary degenerative nerve cell disorder. Thus, until some way to prevent cell death and other structural biochemical changes is found, it can be anticipated that it will be difficult to alter the course of such diseases (Bird, 1978).

1. CAT Activity and Markers of Nerve Cells

Of the 43 biochemical constituents measured in the temporal lobe (Table 5) CAT activity was the most depleted component, being reduced twice as much as the indices of nerve cells and the serotonin system (Table 6). Note that the high-affinity binding of LSD was taken as an index of serotonin or 5HT receptors. The ratio of 5HIAA/5HT was calculated as an index of 5HT turnover. Further work is needed here, for we cannot rule out the possibility that this ratio is affected by the terminal state. The high-affinity binding of other ligands (QNB, atropine, dihydroalprenolol, or DHA and naloxone) was not significantly reduced, suggesting that muscarinic cholinergic, β-adrenergic, and opiate receptors are not depleted. There was no evidence of significant change in the whole caudate nucleus (Bowen and coworkers, 1979). Thus, the reduction in neocortical CAT activity appears to be a key change in Alzheimer's disease.

Table 5. Biochemical constituents measured in temporal lobe

Potential indices	Biochemical constituents
Specific transmitter pathways	High-affinity binding of: atropine and quinuclidinyl benzilate (muscarinic receptors); dihydroaloprenolol (β-adrenergic receptors); naloxone (opiate receptors); muscimol (GABA receptors); LSD (serotonin receptors)
Transmitters, their metabolites and modulators	Serotonin; 5-hydroxyindoleacetate; angiotensin-converting enzyme; acetylcholinesterase; CAT
Nerve cells	Ganglioside NANA; phosphohydrolase; NS5; β-galactosidase; galactolipid; myelin protein; DNA; DNA/RNA
Glial cells	Carbonic anhydrase; β-glucuronidase
Atrophy	Lobe weight; total protein
Subcellular structures	ATPases (Mg^{2+}, Na^+/K^+ and total); protein kinases; (cyclic-AMP, independent and dependent); succinate dehydrogenase
Pentose phosphate cycle	Glucose 6-phosphate dehydrogenase; 6-phosphogluconate dehydrogenase
Glycolysis	
Initial reactions	Hexokinase; aldolase; phosphohexoisomerase; phosphofructokinase
Intermediate reactions	Phosphoglycerate mutase; triosephosphate isomerase; glyceraldehyde 3-phosphate dehydrogenase; glycerate phosphokinase; enolase
Terminal reactions	Pyruvate kinase; lactate dehydrogenase
?	Alcohol dehydrogenase

For details see Bowen and coworkers (1977a, 1977b, 1979).

Table 6. Selected changes in whole temporal lobe (modified from Bowen and coworkers, 1979)

Potential indices	Significant ($p < 0.01$) changes in Alzheimer's disease* (content % control[†])
Cholinergic neurons (CAT)	35
Number of nerve cells (ganglioside NANA; phosphohydrolase) Serotinergic system (5HIAA/5HT; high-affinity LSD binding)	60–70
Atrophy (lobe weight; total protein)	77–81

* $N = 17$; † $N = 16$.

Abbreviations: 5HIAA, 5-hydroxyindoleacetate; 5HT, serotonin; LSD, lysergic acid diethylamide.

2. Accelerated Ageing

Perry and coworkers (1977b) found that CAT activity is age-dependent in hippocampus from control brain, while in age-matched Alzheimer cases the activity is reduced further. Our biochemical results on temporal lobe suggest that there is no significant loss of neocortical neurons in histologically normal brain from non-demented elderly people. Furthermore, the CAT activities per lobe and per gram of neocortex (obtained at either biopsy or autopsy) are independent of age in controls, yet are nevertheless markedly decreased in Alzheimer's disease (for references see Bowen and coworkers, 1979).

Due to the difficulty of obtaining specimens from psychometrically proven mentally normal elderly subjects, the analysis of animal brain should provide supportive data about possible age-related changes in human brain. Thus, Meek and coworkers (1978) found that neocortical CAT activity is not reduced in elderly rats. The activity was significantly reduced in the caudate nucleus (Table 7), which is in agreement with data obtained for human specimens (McGeer and McGeer, 1976).

Table 7. CAT activity in aged rat (modified from Meek and coworkers, 1977)

Region	CAT (nmol, per 100 mg protein per min $\pm$ S.E.M.)	
	Control	Aged
Caudate nucleus	550 ± 50	400 ± 25*
Neocortex	90 ± 10	103 ± 13
Hippocampus	150 ± 14	167 ± 9

* $p < 0.05$ (N for both groups = 24).
Control and aged animals were 35–45 days and 24 months old, respectively.

Two studies provide evidence that muscarinic cholinergic receptors decline in normal old age. Firstly, blockade of central muscarinic receptors converts the pattern of intellectual performance of young adults to that of elderly subjects (Table 8). Secondly, a significant age-related decline of 32 % in muscarinic receptor binding occurs in the neocortex, with little or no histological evidence of senile degeneration from subjects aged 65–92 years (White and coworkers, 1977).

D. Significance and Selectivity of the Reduction in CAT Activity

CAT activity may not be the rate-limiting factor in acetylcholine (ACh) synthesis (Tucek, 1978); thus ACh content may *not* be reduced in Alzheimer's disease (Bowen, 1978). However, studies on rate-limiting factors have been

Table 8. Comparison of the effect of normal ageing and
scopolamine on test performance (modified from Drachman and
Leavitt, 1974)

Function tested	Loss of performance (%) due to:	
	(a) Normal ageing	(b) Inactivated central ACh receptors
Memory storage	42	45
I.Q. test: 1	19	17
2	17	16
3	12	11
4	3	0
Immediate memory	0	0
Memory retrieval	0	0

(a) Performance of medical students compared with that of elderly subjects.
(b) Performance of medical students without medication compared with that of the same students treated with scopolamine.

limited to rodent brain, where CAT specific activity is at least ten times higher than in human brain (see Tables 7 and 9). Furthermore, there may be a limiting pool of CAT, preferentially localized at the nerve terminal plasma membrane (Burgess, Atterwill, and Prince, 1978).

CAT activity may depend upon neuronal activity, which may itself be reduced in dementia patients (Bowen, 1979). Disuse of cholinergic motor neurons, produced by blockade of nerve conduction by repeated subperineural injection of tetrodotoxin, had no effect on CAT activity of sciatic nerve (Butler, Drachman, and Goldberg, 1978). Nevertheless, the relationship between cortical CAT activity and neuronal activity in animals with chronic CBF changes should be investigated.

Although CAT activity of grey matter obtained at biopsy is significantly reduced, GAD activity has not been so extensively measured, but preliminary data indicate that the enzyme is spared (Table 9). However, apart from CAT activity no other reliable and specific enzymatic marker of nerve terminals has been measured in *autopsy* samples. As judged by a histochemical technique, as well as by chemical analyses, noradrenergic neurons (Berger, Escourolle, and Moyne, 1976; Gottfries, Chapter 10) may also be affected in Alzheimer's disease. Receptor binding data suggest that GABA, as well as serotonin receptor pathways, may deteriorate (Reisine and coworkers, 1978a, 1978b; Bowen and coworkers, 1979), indicating that there are changes in several transmitter systems, as has now been found in Parkinson's and Huntington's diseases. Table 9 is a summary of some of the data which provide direct biochemical evidence of

Table 9. Summary of changes in markers of specific neocortical transmitter pathways

Variable	Specific activity or high-affinity binding			Specimen and reference
	Control	Dementia due to Alzheimer's disease	Dementia not due to Alzheimer's disease	
CAT (nmol per 100 mg protein per min ± S.D.)	6.73 ± 2.23 (10)	3.22 ± 1.58* (6)	5.66 ± 1.90 (5)	Biopsy Spillane (1978)
GAD (mol per 100 mg protein per min ± S.D.)	7.86 ± 2.68 (9)	8.99, 7.85	6.53, 7.43	Biopsy Spillane (1978)
5HT binding (fmol per mg protein ± S.D.)	218 ± 42 (5)	109	139, 196	Biopsy Goodhardt (1979)
DHA binding (fmol per mg protein ± S.D.)	56 ± 20 (12)	46 ± 11 (8)	N.D.	Autopsy Goodhardt (1979)
Atropine binding (nmol per g protein ± S.D.)	0.660 ± 0.156 (14)	0.597 ± 0.071 (8)	N.D.	Autopsy White and coworkers (1977)
GABA binding (mmol per mg protein ± S.E.M.)	1800 ± 79 (3)	913 ± 86† (4)	N.D.	Autopsy Reisine and coworkers (1978b)
Spiroperidol binding (mmol per mg protein ± S.E.M.)	24 ± 5 (3)	17 ± 4 (4)	N.D.	Autopsy Reisine and coworkers (1978b)

* Significantly lower than either control ($p < 0.01$) or non-Alzheimer dementias ($p < 0.05$).
† Significantly lower than control ($p < 0.05$).

selectivity. Clinicopathological studies suggest that neuropeptides, such as vasoactive intestinal peptide, vasopressin, and angiotensin should be examined in Alzheimer's disease (Fahrenkrug and coworkers, 1977; Bowen and Davison, 1978; Legros and coworkers, 1978; Bowen and coworkers, 1979). Dopamine has also been implicated (Lewis, Ballinger, and Presly, 1978; Gottfries, Chapter 10), but the beneficial effects of L-dopa therapy is controversial, particularly in the pre-senile age group (Kristensen, Olsen, and Theilgaard, 1977).

III. SUMMARY AND CONCLUSIONS

Extensive biochemical analysis of autopsy brain specimens indicates that CAT activity is selectively reduced in Alzheimer's disease. Further work is needed to establish, for example, if this phenomena reflects selective loss of either cholinergic neurons or cholinergic nerve endings (with sparing of the perikarya). It is essential to establish whether or not ACh synthesis is reduced. Further work may provide the foundation for rational therapy. At present the best existing treatment is, unfortunately, the positive diagnosis of some other more treatment-responsive condition which masquerades as Alzheimer's disease (Cole and Branconnier, 1978).

ACKNOWLEDGEMENTS

The close collaboration of Professor A. N. Davison, Drs C. B. Smith, J. A. Spillane and P. White and Ms. M. J. Goodhardt is greatly valued.

REFERENCES

Adolfsson, R.,C. G. Gottfries, L. Oreland, B. E. Roos, and B. Winblad (1978). Reduced levels of catecholamines in the brain and increased activity of monoamine oxidase in platelets in Alzheimer's disease: therapeutic implications. In R. Katzman, R. D. Terry, and K. L. Bick (Eds) *Alzheimer's Disease: Sensile Dementia and Related Disorders* (*Aging*, Vol. 7) Raven Press, New York, pp. 441–51.
Ball, M. J. (1977). Neuronal loss, neurofibrillary tangles and granulovacuolar degeneration in the hippocampus with aging and dementia. A quantitative study. *Acta Neuropath. (Berl.)*, **37**, 111–8.
Berger, B., R. Escourolle, and M. A. Moyne (1976). Axones, caticholaminerques du cortex cerebral humain. *Rev. Neurol. (Paris)*, **136**, 183.
Bird, E. D. (1978). Huntington's chorea. In N. J. Legg (Ed.) *Neurotransmitter Systems and their Clinical Disorders*, Academic Press, London. pp.142–50.
Bowen, D. M. (1978). Vulnerability of cholinergic neurones in Alzheimer's disease. *Brit. J. Clin. Practice*, **32** (Suppl. 2), 19–21.
Bowen, D. M. (1979) Biochemistry of Alzheimer's disease. In G. Curzon (Ed.) *The Biochemistry of Psychiatric Disturbances*. John Wiley, London. In Press.
Bowen, D. M. and A. N. Davison (1978). Biochemical changes in the normal aging brain and in dementia. In B. Isaacs (Ed.) *Recent Advances in Geriatric Medicine,*Vol. I, Livingstone, Edinburgh. pp.41–60.

Bowen, D. M., M. J. Goodhardt, A. J. Strong, C. B. Smith, P. White, N. M. Branston, L. Symon and A. N. Davison (1976a). Biochemical indices of brain structure, function and 'hypoxia' in cortex from baboons with middle cerebral artery occlusion. *Brain Res.*, **117**, 503–7.

Bowen, D. M., C. B. Smith, P. White, and A. N. Davison (1976b). Neurotransmitter-related enzymes and indices of hypoxia in senile dementia and other abiotrophies. *Brain*, **99**, 459–96.

Bowen, D. M.,C. B. Smith, P. White, M. J. Goodhardt, J. A. Spillane, R. H. A. Flack, and A. N. Davison (1977a). Chemical pathology of the organic dementias. I. Validity of biochemical measurements on human post-mortem brain specimens. *Brain*, **100**, 397–426.

Bowen, D. M., C. B. Smith, P. White, R. H. A. Flack, L. H. Carrasco, J. L. Gedye, and A. N. Davison (1977b). Chemical pathology of the organic dementias. II. Quantitative estimation of cellular changes in post-mortem brains. *Brain*, **100**, 427–53.

Bowen, D. M., P. White, J. A. Spillane, M. J. Goodhardt, G. Curzon, P. Iwangoff, W. Meier-Ruge, and A. N. Davison (1979). Accelerated aging or elective neuronal loss as an important cause of dementia? *Lancet*, **i**, 11–14.

Burgess, E. J., C. K. Atterwill, and A. K. Prince (1978). Choline acetyl transferase and the high-affinity uptake of choline in corpus striatum of reserpinised rats. *J. Neurochem.*, **31**, 1027–33.

Butler, I. J., D. B. Drachman, and A. M. Goldberg (1978). The effect of disease on cholinergic enzymes. *J. Physiol.*, **274**, 593–600.

Cole, J. O. and R. Branconnier (1978). The therapeutic efficacy of psychopharmacologic agents in senile organic brain syndrome. In K. Nandy (Ed.) *Senile Dementia: A Biomedical Approach*. Elsevier/North Holland, New York. pp. 271–86.

Corsellis, J. A. N. (1962). *Mental Illness and the Aging Brain*, Maudsley Monograph No. 9, Oxford University Press, Oxford.

Corsellis, J. A. N. (1976). Aging and the dementias. In W. Blackwood and J. A. N. Corsellis (Eds) *Greenfield's Neuropathology*, Edward Arnold, London. pp. 796–849.

Davies, P. and A. J. F. Maloney (1976). Selective loss of central cholinergic neurones in Alzheimer's disease. *Lancet*, **ii**, 1403.

Davies, P. and A. H. Verth (1978). Regional distribution of muscarinic acetylcholine receptor in normal and Alzheimer-type dementia brains. *Brains Res.*, **138**, 385–92.

Drachman, D. A. and J. Leavitt (1974). Human memory and the cholinergic system. *Arch. Neurol.*, **30**, 113–21.

Fahrenkrug, J., O. B. Schaffalitzky de Muckadell, and A. Fahrenkrug (1977). Vasoactive intestinal polypeptide (V. I. P.) in human cerebrospinal fluid. *Brain Res.*,**124**, 581–4.

Goodhardt, M. J. (in prep.) *Neurotransmitter Uptake and Binding in Ischaemia and Senile Dementia*. Ph.D. Thesis. University of London.

Green, M. A., L. D. Stevenson, J. E. Fonseca, and S. B. Wortis (1952). Cerebral biopsy in patients with presenile dementia. *Dis. Nerv. Syst.*, **13**, 303–7.

Grundke-Iqbal, I., A. Johnson, H. M. Wisniewski, R. D. Terry, and K. Iqbal (1979). Evidence that Alzheimer-neurofibrillary tangles originate from neurotubules. *Lancet*, **i**, 578–9.

Hachinski, V. C., L. D. Iliff, E. Zilkha, G. H. du Boulay, V. L. McAllister, J. Marshall, R. W. Ross Russell, and L. Symon (1975). Cerebral blood flow in dementia. *Arch. Neurol.*, **32**, 632.

Kristensen, V., M. Olsen, and A. Theilgaard (1977). Levodopa treatment of presenile dementia. *Acta Psychiat. Scand.*, **55**, 41–51.

Legros, J. J., P. Gilot, X. Seron, J. Claessens, A. Adam, J. M. Moeglen, A. Audibert, and P. Berchier (1978). Influence of vasopressin on learning and memory. *Lancet*, **i**, 41–2.

Lenzi, G. L., T. Jones, J. L. Reid, and S. Moss (1979). Regional impairment of cerebral oxidative metabolism in Parkinson's disease. *J. Neurol., Neurosurg. Psychiat.,* **42,** 59–62.

Lewis, C., B. R. Ballinger, and A. S. Presly (1978). Trial of levodopa in senile dementia. *Brit. Med. J.,* **1,** 550.

Letemendia, F. and G. Pampiglione (1958). Clinical and electroencephalographic observations in Alzheimer's disease. *J. Neurol., Neurosurg. Psychiat.,* **21,** 167–72.

McGeer, P. L. and E. G. McGeer (1976). Enzymes associated with the metabolism of catecholamines, acetylcholine and GABA in human controls and patients with Parkinson's disease and Huntington's chorea. *J. Neurochem.,* **26,** 331–5.

McMenemey, W. H. (1940). Alzheimer's disease: a report of six cases. *J. Neurol. Psychiat.,* **3,** 211–40.

Meek, J. L., L. Bertilsson, D. L. Cheyney, G. Zsilla, and E. Costa (1978). Aging-induced changes in acetylcholine and serotonin content of discrete brain nuclei. *J. Gerontol.,* **12,** 129–31.

Perry, E. K., R. H. Perry, G. Blessed, and B. E. Tomlinson (1977a). Necropsy evidence of central cholinergic deficits in senile dementia. *Lancet,* **i,** 189.

Perry, E. K., R. H. Perry, P. H. Gibson, G. Blessed, and B. E. Tomlinson (1977b). A cholinergic connection between normal aging and senile dementia in the human hippocampus. *Neurosci. Lett.,* **6,** 85–9.

Perry, E. K., B. E. Tomlinson, G. Blessed, K. Bergmann, P. H. Gibson, and R. H. Perry (1978). Correlation of cholinergic abnormalities with senile plaques and mental test scores in senile dementia. *Brit. Med. J.,* **2,** 1457–9.

Raiche, M. E., R. L. Grubb, M. H. Gado, J. O. Eichling, and C. P. Hughes (1978). Cerebral hemodynamics and metabolism in dementia: Features distinguishing normal pressure hydrocephalus from atrophy. In K. Nandy (Ed.) *Senile Dementia: A Biomedical Approach.* Elsevier/North Holland, New York. pp. 131–8.

Reisine, T. D., E. D. Bird, E. Spokes, S. J. Enna, and H. I. Yamamura (1978a). Pre- and post-synaptic neurochemical alterations in Alzheimer's disease, *Trans. Amer. Soc. Neurochem.,* **9,** 203.

Reisine, T. D., H. I. Yamamura, E. D. Bird, E. Spokes, and S. J. Enna (1978b). Pre- and post-synaptic neurochemical alterations in Alzheimer's disease. *Brain Res.,* **159,** 477–82.

Scheibel, S. B. and U. Tomiyasu (1978). Dendritic sprouting in Alzheimer's pre-senile dementia. *Exp. Neurol.,* **60,** 1–8.

Shelanski, M. L. (1978). Discussion. In R. Katzman, R. D. Terry, and K. L. Bick (Eds) *Alzheimer's Disease, Senile Dementia and Related Disorders* (*Aging,* Vol. 7), Raven Press, New York. p. 429.

Sim, M. and W. T. Smith (1955). Alzheimer's disease confirmed by biopsy: A therapeutic trial with cortisone and ACTH. *J. Mental Sci.,* **101,** 604–12.

Sim, M., S. Turner, and W. T. Smith (1966). Cerebral biopsy in the investigation of pre-senile dementia, I. Clinical aspects. *Brit. J. Psychiat.,* **112,** 119–25.

Smith, C. B. and D. M. Bowen (1976). Soluble proteins in normal and diseased human brain. *J. Neurochem.,* **27,** 1521–8.

Smith, C. M. and M. Swash (1979). Physostigmine in Alzheimer's disease. *Lancet,* **i,** 42.

Smith, W. T., E. Turner, and M. Sim (1966). Cerebral biopsy in the investigation of pre-senile dementia. *Brit. J. Psychiat.,* **112,** 127–33.

Spillane, J. A. (1978). *Alzheimer's Disease: A State of Cholinergic Deficiency?* M. D. Thesis, University of London.

Spillane, J. A., M. J. Goodhardt, P. White, D. M. Bowen, and A. N. Davison (1977a). Choline in Alzheimer's disease. *Lancet,* **ii,** 826.

Spillane, J. A., P. White, M. J. Goodhardt, R. H. A. Flack, D. M. Bowen, and A. N. Davison (1977b). Selective vulnerability of neurones in organic dementia. *Nature* (*London*), **266**, 558–9.

Stahl, W. L., S. M. Sumi, and P. D. Swanson (1971). Subcellular distribution of cerebral cholesterol in cerebrotendinous xanthomatosis. *J. Neurochem.*, **18**, 403–4.

Suzuki, K., R. Katzman, and S. R. Korey (1965). Chemical studies on Alzheimer's disease. *J. Neuropath. Exp. Neurol.*, **24**, 211–21.

Tucek, S. (1978). *Acetylcholine Synthesis in Neurons*. Chapman and Hall, London.

White, P., D. M. Bowen, and A. N. Davison (1978). Alzheimer's disease: distribution of protein on sucrose density gradient centrifugation. *Acta Neuropath.* (*Berl.*), **41**, 253–6.

White, P., C. R. Hiley, M. J. Goodhardt, L. H. Carrasco, J. P. Keet, I. E. I. Williams, and D. M. Bowen (1977). Neocortical cholinergic neurones in elderly people. *Lancet*, **i**, 668–70.

Biochemistry of Dementia
Edited by P. J. Roberts
© 1980, John Wiley & Sons Ltd.

Chapter 6

Adverse Factors Affecting Neuronal Metabolism: Relevance to the Dementias

BO K. SIESJÖ and STIG REHNCRONA

Laboratory of Experimental Brain Research, E-Blocket,
University of Lund, Lund, Sweden

Histopathological changes in the brains of patients with various forms of dementias include not only vacuolation and loss of neurons with hypertrophy of glial elements, but also more characteristic changes such as accumulation of neuritic plaques, neurofibrillary tangles, and lipofuscin granulae, as well as congophilic angiopathy (Tomlinson, Blessed, and Roth, 1970; Terry, 1976, 1978a, 1978b). In some of the dementias, cerebral atrophy with loss of neurons is mainly observed in the neocortex, hippocampus, and cerebellar cortex, i.e. in the classical 'selectively vulnerable areas', while neuritic plaques and neurofibrillary tangles tend to be concentrated to the neocortex and to sectors h_1 and h_2 of the hippocampus. Undoubtedly, the widespread disappearance of neurons and the associated loss of dendritic arborization (Scheibel, 1978) must be responsible for the deterioration of mental functions observed in the dementias. However, it should be emphasized that neither the loss of neurons or dendritic arbor, nor the more characteristic plaques, tangles, lipofuscin granulae, or congophilic vascular changes occur exclusively in the dementias, since all have been observed in the brains of non-demented elderly individuals. Thus, the differences between dementia and normal ageing are quantitative rather than qualitative (Terry, 1978b).

Studies of cerebral blood flow (CBF) and cerebral metabolic rate for oxygen ($CMRo_2$) and glucose ($CMRGL$) have given three main results. Firstly, although some optimally healthy individuals, with remarkably well-preserved brain function, have normal CBF and $CMRo_2$ at a mean age of 71 years (Dastur and coworkers, 1963; Sokoloff, 1966), studies of mixed populations of elderly individuals show an age-related reduction in cerebral blood flow and metabolic rate, and these reductions are more pronounced in patients with arteriosclerotic disease and/or dementia (Scheinberg, 1950; Freyhan, Woodford, and Kety, 1951; Kety, 1956; Lassen, Feinberg, and Lane, 1960; Hachinski and coworkers, 1975). Secondly, the reduction in regional CBF is not homogeneous but is accentuated in certain regions, e.g. temporal and temporal-parietal-occipital areas, demonstrating a correlation between loss of function, reduction in CBF, and histopathological alterations (Gustafson and Risberg, 1974; Brun and Gustafson, 1976; Hagberg and Ingvar, 1976; Ingvar and coworkers, 1978). Thirdly, at least in some of the demented patients the reduction in CBF is associated with a moderately reduced cerebral venous Po_2, suggesting the presence of some degree of cerebral hypoxia (Dastur and coworkers, 1963; Sokoloff, 1966). It has also been proposed that patients with cerebral arteriosclerosis demonstrate a larger reduction in CMR GL than in $CMRo_2$ (Dastur and coworkers, 1963; Gottstein, Bernsmeier, and Sedlmeyer, 1964; Hoyer, 1978). Although this finding could be compatible with a block in glucose utilization, and with oxidation of endogenous substrates, it is perhaps more likely that a ketoacidosis triggered cerebral oxidation of acetoacetate and β-hydroxybutyrate.

At present, little is known about the mechanisms that lead to cell loss in the dementias, or to the more characteristic neuronal alterations. Thus, apart from multi-infarct dementia, which should have a vascular basis, the evidence that cerebral hypoxia underlies the neuronal damage is inconclusive. Probably, many of the neuronal alterations observed in dementia have another aetiology. It has been shown, for example, that aluminium can give rise to neurofibrillary tangles (Klatzo, Wisnieski, and Streicher, 1965), and demented patients appear to have high brain aluminium concentrations (Crapper, Karlik, and De Boni, 1978). Furthermore, both autoimmunization and transmissible agents ('slow virus') have been implicated in the pathogenesis of neuronal alterations in dementia (see review by Tower, 1978).

Although all neuronal (and glial) alterations in dementia must be caused by a deranged cellular metabolism, neither the nature of this derangement nor its causes are known. For that reason we will focus the present discussion on pathophysiological factors and biochemical mechanisms contributing to cell damage in acute disease, and consider their possible involvement in pathological ageing.

I. BRAIN METABOLISM AND NEURONAL VULNERABILITY

It has been well-documented that brain tissues have a high metabolic rate and hence require a constant and plentiful supply of oxygen and substrate to provide the necessary energy for cellular work. Since the tissues have virtually no oxygen stores and contain slender amounts of their principal fuel (glucose), curtailment of the oxygen or substrate supply quickly leads to neuronal dysfunction and, provided the conditions are sufficiently pronounced, to reversible or irreversible cell damage. When this damage is slight or moderate it is virtually confined to neurons and often shows a selective localization to certain regions, affecting mainly small pyramidal cells in the neocortex and hippocampus, and Purkinje cells in the cerebellum (Schadé and McMenemey, 1963; Brierley, 1976). A preferential localization of cell injury to these regions has been observed not only in hypoxia and hypoglycaemia but also in some models of ischaemia and, with a notable sparing of the Purkinje cells in paralysed animals, also in status epilepticus (Table 1).

Table 1. Selective vulnerability of cerebral neurons—localization and occurrence

Localization:	1. Neocortex (layers 3, 5, and 6)
	2. Hippocampus (h_1 and h_5)
	3. Cerebellum (Purkinje cells)
Occurrence:	1. Hypoxia
	2. Complete ischaemia
	3. Hypoglycaemia
	4. Status epilepticus

It is not known why neurons are particularly vulnerable in a variety of adverse conditions but, most probably, the vulnerability reflects their large energy requirements. Thus, despite suggestions to the contrary (Hertz, 1978) several facts indicate that neurons have a metabolic rate appreciably higher than that of glial cells (see Siesjö, 1978). Firstly, measurements of respiratory activity of microdissected neurons and lumps of glia indicate that neurons have an appreciably higher oxygen consumption than glial cells (Epstein and O'Connor, 1965; Hydén and Lange, 1965). Secondly, indirect calculations based on the *in vitro* oxygen consumption of glial preparations and tissue slices or homogenates, and on estimates of the number of neurons and glial cells, suggest that in the cerebral cortex neurons account for at least 75 % of the total oxygen consumption (Elliott and Heller, 1957; Korey and Orchen, 1959; Hess, 1961). Thirdly, both *in vitro* and *in vivo* data demonstrate that oxygen consumption of cerebral cortex or whole brain varies inversely with body (or brain) weight (Fig. 1). Since there is a corresponding, inverse relationship between brain weight and neuron packing density (Tower and Young, 1973), the data support the view that neurons account for the major share of the oxygen consumed.

It would seem that the loss of neurons in elderly and/or demented patients could adequately account for the decrease in $CMRo_2$ (and CBF). However, several facts indicate that a quantitative relationship cannot be expected. For example, if neuronal loss is largely confined to circumscript regions, e.g. to the hippocampus and related structures, a correlation between cell loss and metabolic rate can be expected only if the latter is measured with truly local methods. Furthermore, there are results suggesting that the high metabolic rate

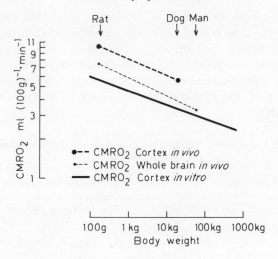

Figure 1. Cerebral metabolic rate related to the body weight in different species. Uninterrupted line: relationship between body weight and cerebral metabolic rate *in vitro*, as reported by Elliott and Henderson (1948). Thick stippled line: corresponding relationship for 'cortical' CMR_{O_2} *in vivo*, as obtained by joining the points for rat and dog. Thin interrupted line: corresponding relationship for 'whole brain' CMR_{O_2} in rat and man. (Reproduced with permission from Nilsson and Siesjö, 1976)

in grey matter structures are mainly dendritic (Lowry, 1957), a suggestion which has been corroborated by results obtained with the autoradiographic ^{14}C-deoxyglucose (DOG) technique for measuring local glucose consumption (Sokoloff and coworkers, 1977). Thus, it could be expected that loss of dendritic arbor should decrease metabolic rate even if the neuronal cell density is not appreciably reduced.

Accepting that the vulnerability of neurons is at least partly due to their high metabolic rate and energy requirements, we must consider the basic functions which deteriorate when oxygen or substrate supply fails. Probably, a major share of the energy consumed is spent in recharging the ionic batteries following the activity-coupled fluxes of Na^+, K^+, and other ions along their thermodynamic gradients. However, a substantial part of the energy may be spent in maintaining the internal household of the neuron, i.e. in synthesizing enzymes and organelles required centrally or peripherally, and in transporting these essential cell components to distant axonal and dendrite arborizations (see Barondes, 1969; Droz and Koenig, 1970; Jeffrey and Austin, 1973). It follows from this that energy failure will not only dissipate the ionic gradients, reduce or abolish the transmembrane potential, and upset osmotic regulation, but also that it will deplete the periphery of enzymes and organelles required for cell-to-cell communication. It is also clear that depletion of cellular energy stores upsets the balance between degradation and resynthesis of cellular constituents and, when degradation reaches a certain point, the cell is damaged beyond repair.

When sufficiently severe, both cellular hypoxia and hypoglycaemia give rise to extensive deterioration of cerebral energy state (see below). In view of what was discussed above, such deterioration provides a logical explanation for both cell dysfunction and reversible or irreversible cell injury. However, two important facts should be recalled. Firstly, as will be discussed in more detail below, cell dysfunction occurs at degrees of hypoxia or hypoglycaemia that do not measurably alter cerebral energy state. By itself, this fact suggests that metabolic alterations other than energy failure underlie the derangement of cell-to-cell communication. Secondly, it now seems established that prolonged epileptic seizures irreversibly damage cerebral neurons, even though tissue oxygenation is upheld and cerebral energy state is only marginally affected (see below). We then arrive at the conclusion that neither extensive energy depletion nor hypoxia or tissue acidosis provide common mechanisms of cell damage, and tissue blood flow can vary from zero to several hundred per cent of control (Table 2). Clearly, these facts must be taken into account when discussing mechanisms of cell damage. We also recognize the need to consider the possibility of oxidative damage. In the following we shall discuss the factors which adversely affect neuronal metabolism (and brain circulation) in hypoxia, ischaemia, hypoglycaemia, and status epilepticus, before considering possible mechanisms of cell damage.

Table 2. Pathophysiological conditions in hypoxia, ischaemia, hypoglycaemia, and status epilepticus

Condition	Blood flow	Metabolic rate	P_{O_2}	Acidosis	Energy state
Hypoxia	Increased	Normal → low	Decreased	Marked	Decreased
Ischaemia	Low	Normal → low	Decreased	Marked	Decreased
Hypoglycaemia	Increased	Normal	Increased	Absent	Decreased
Status epilepticus	Increased	Increased	Normal or increased	Moderate	Close to normal

II. CEREBRAL HYPOXIA

The two most common causes of cellular hypoxia are a reduction in arterial P_{O_2} and oxygen saturation (arterial hypoxia), and a reduction in cerebral blood flow (ischaemia). Although they often occur in combination, we shall discuss them separately.

A. Arterial Hypoxia

1. Clinical Effects

It is now well-established that even relatively mild hypoxia leads to signs and symptoms of neuronal dysfunction, despite the fact that the phosphorylation state of the adenine nucleotide system is not measurably altered (see Siesjö, 1978, Ch. 14). For obvious reasons, most data on functional effects of hypoxia have been collected in man (see Luft, 1965; Ernsting, 1966). Such results show that mild degrees of hypoxia (the equivalent of 14–16 % O_2 in inspired air) affect some brain functions, e.g. the acuity of the dark-adapted eye, and the learning of complex tasks (Fig. 2). At somewhat more severe degrees (12–13 %O_2) short-term memory fails and, at about 10 %O_2, subjects often lose their ability of critical judgment; consciousness, though, is usually retained until severe degrees of hypoxia are reached (6–7 % O_2). It should be clearly emphasized that such signs and symptoms poorly correlate to arterial Po_2. This is mainly due to the fact that hypoxia is accompanied by overventilation and that the ensuing fall in

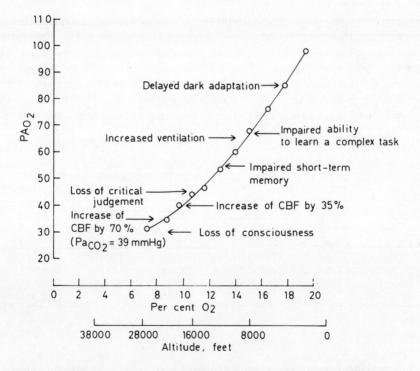

Figure 2. Some symptoms and physiological responses in man to hypoxia. The alveolar Po_2 is plotted against the inspired oxygen concentration. Equivalent altitudes are indicated at the bottom. (Modified from Siesjö and coworkers, 1974)

P_{CO_2} reduces CBF or, more to the point, abolishes or curtails the rise in CBF which would otherwise occur. Supportive evidence is the fact that when CO_2 is added to a hypoxic gas mixture, both the EEG changes and the symptoms are ameliorated (Gibbs, Gibbs, and Lennow, 1943; Otis and coworkers, 1946).

Extensive data exist for chronic hypoxia, particularly since it occurs at high altitude in the form of mountain sickness (Carson and Evans, 1969; Singh, 1969; Hackett and Rennie, 1976). The cardinal symptoms are headache, insomnia, anorexia, lassitude, and ataxia. Such symptoms may progress to a life-threatening condition with signs of cerebral (and pulmonary) oedema, even though the hypoxia is seemingly mild. Possibly, this may be related to a jeopardized circulatory adaptation to hypoxia, secondary to such factors as hyperventilation and polycythaemia.

We recognize that at least some of the symptoms of acute and more sustained hypoxia show a resemblance to those encountered in the dementias. Quite naturally, this does not demonstrate that clinical symptoms in the dementias are due to tissue hypoxia but it could mean that the same neuronal circuits are affected due to reversible dysfunction (hypoxia) or cellular degeneration (dementia).

2. *Metabolic Sequelae*

If the arterial P_{O_2} is progressively lowered in acute animal experiments, one observes metabolic alterations at a P_{O_2} of about 50 mmHg and, when the P_{O_2} is reduced further, these alterations become more pronounced. In summary, these alterations involve increases in the lactate concentration and the lactate/pyruvate ratio, reductions in cellular redox systems, a perturbation of the concentrations of citric acid cycle intermediates which seem secondary to the redox changes and the rise in pyruvate concentration, and changes in tissue concentrations of amino acids such as alanine, aspartate, and GABA (for results and further references, see Norberg and Siesjö 1975a, 1975b; Berntman and Siesjö, 1978; Siesjö, 1978, ch. 14). However, if the perfusion pressure is upheld, the energy charge of the adenine nucleotide pool is not measurably affected at P_{O_2} values exceeding 20 mmHg, despite the fact that the EEG shows clear signs of tissue hypoxia (see Bachelard and coworkers, 1974; Siesjö and coworkers, 1975).

The discrepancy between symptomatology and changes in energy state warrants a search for biochemical mechanisms underlying the disordered function. Presumably, the symptoms are more related to 'transmission failure' than to 'energy failure' (e.g. Siesjö and Plum, 1973). This assumption receives some support from the fact that the concentrations of established or putative amino acid transmitters are perturbed (see above). However, more conclusive are the results pertaining to the effect of hypoxia on the synthesis rates of biogenic amines and acetylcholine.

It was observed by Davis and Carlsson (1973) that in unanaesthetized rats breathing gas mixtures with low oxygen content, the synthesis rates of catechol and indole amines in the brain declined. Later results (Davis, 1976) showed that if the animals were paralysed and ventilated to constant CO_2 tension, the synthesis rate of serotine, but not that of catecholamines, was reduced. Although Davis (1976) postulated that this was due to the influence of stress on the affinity of tyrosine hydroxylase for oxygen, the results could well reflect an influence of intracellular acidosis (see Brown, Snider, and Carlsson, 1974; Carlsson and coworkers, 1977). We have recently observed that, although hypoxia in paralysed rats does not influence tyrosine hydroxylation in the cerebral cortex, it *raises* the rate of synthesis in striatum, indicating acceleration of dopamine synthesis (Sakabe and coworkers, in preparation). Thus, the effect of hypoxia on amine synthesis is complex.

Comparable results exist for acetylcholine, synthesis of which is reduced in even relatively moderate hypoxia (Gibson and Blass, 1976). Recently, Gibson, Shimada, and Blass (1978) have reported that such degrees of hypoxia are accompanied by reduced tissue concentrations of cyclic-GMP. Taken together with those pertaining to biogenic amines and amino acids, these results provide some support to the postulate that the signs and symptoms of mild to moderate hypoxia are related to 'transmission failure'.

3. Histopathology

It has been well established that arterial hypoxia (i.e. a reduction in tissue Po_2 in the absence of a fall in CBF below normal) can give rise to irreversible cell damage in the brain. However, in acute conditions, such a pronounced tissue hypoxia, it is required that, at arterial Po_2 values of 20 mmHg or higher, a complicating fall in perfusion pressure must occur. This condition of hypoxia with *relative* ischaemia can be experimentally induced by combining a lowering of arterial Po_2 with unilateral clamping of a carotid artery. Using this model, Salford, Plum, and Siesjö (1973) and Salford, Plum, and Brierley (1973) showed that there was extensive deterioration of cerebral energy state on the clamped side with cell damage occurring in the neocortex, hippocampus, and cerebellum after a 30-minute period of hypoxia-related ischaemia (Fig. 3). With short recovery periods, this damage is in the form of microvacuolation due to swollen mitochondria and 'ischaemic cell change', while the later result is necrosis and loss of neurons with glial hypertrophy. Subsequent results suggest that some damage is observed after similar insults of only 5–10 minutes' duration (Levy and coworkers, 1975). It should be clearly stated, though, that cell damage was evaluated after a 30-minute period of reoxygenation/recirculation. Thus, it cannot be excluded that the damage occurred or 'matured' in this period.

Regrettably, there is little precise information on histopathological sequelae of mild, chronic hypoxia. In healthy, experimental animals (or individuals) there is a brisk circulatory adaptation to hypoxia, ensuring increased supply of oxygen.

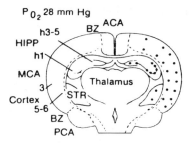

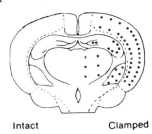

Intact   Clamped

Figure 3. Distribution and relative
density of neuronal lesions 30 min
after unilateral carotid artery clamping and hypoxia. ACA, MCA, PCA:
anterior, medial, and posterior cerebral arteries, respectively; BZ: boundary zone between cerebral arteries;
HIPP: hippocampus, with subdivisions of pyramidal layers (h_1 to h_5);
STR: striatum. (Reproduced with permission from Salford, Plum, and
Brierley, 1973)

This adaptation may well deteriorate in old age, augmenting the cellular impact
of hypoxia. In addition, if mild hypoxia occurs in conjunction with mild
hypotension, the added impacts could be harmful.

B. Ischaemia

Since ischaemia is just another cause of cellular hypoxia, it leads to changes in
cellular metabolism similar to those encountered in severe arterial hypoxia. The
main difference between the conditions is the state of the circulation which, to
some extent, determines the localization of ischaemic cell damage (e.g. Brierley,
1973, 1976). Details of metabolic and circulatory effects of ischaemia are outside
the scope of the present communication (see Siesjö, 1978, ch. 15) and we shall

confine ourselves to emphasizing that in many elderly patients the cerebral circulation shows a decreased capacity to compensate for variations in blood pressure. In normal individuals (and experimental animals) the cerebral circulation shows autoregulation in the sense that CBF is upheld even if the perfusion pressure is appreciably reduced (e.g. Lassen, 1959). This autoregulatory ability is decreased in elderly individuals, especially in those with hypertensive and arteriosclerotic disease. For example, although normal individuals may tolerate a decrease in blood pressure to 50mmHg without signs of cerebral hypoxia, those with hypertensive disease can develop such signs when blood pressure falls to normotensive levels (Kety and coworkers, 1950; see also Finnerty, Witkin, and Fazekas, 1954). It follows from this that, in patients with arteriosclerotic and hypertensive disease, relatively moderate reductions in blood pressure can jeopardize cellular oxygen supply.

III. HYPOGLYCAEMIA

Like hypoxia, hypoglycaemia can give rise to signs and symptoms of brain dysfunction and, when sufficiently severe and prolonged, it causes irreversible cell damage. There is evidence that many of the signs and symptoms represent a 'transmission failure'. Thus, whereas a reduction of blood glucose concentrations to 3 μmol g^{-1} or lower, gives objective evidence of cerebral dysfunction in man and in experimental animals, experiments show that cerebral cortex concentrations of ATP, ADP, or AMP remain unaltered until blood glucose concentrations fall to 1 μmol g^{-1} or lower, and spontaneous EEG activity ceases (Hinzen and Müller, 1971; Lewis and coworkers, 1974b; Norberg and Siesjö, 1976). There is also ample evidence of a deranged metabolism of cerebral transmitters. For example, even relatively moderate hypoglycaemia depresses cerebral acetylcholine synthesis (Gibson and Blass, 1976). Furthermore, recent data demonstrate that in animals with an EEG pattern of slow waves-polyspikes, brain concentrations of noradrenaline and dopamine are reduced despite an enhanced rate of catecholamine synthesis (Agardh, and coworkers, 1979).

In severe hypoglycaemia, endogenous carbohydrate and amino acid substrates are oxidized with a resulting gross perturbation of concentrations of citric acid cycle intermediates and associated amino acids (Lewis and coworkers, 1974a; Norberg and Siesjö, 1976; Agardh, Folbergrová, and Siesjö, 1978). Although mobilization of endogenous substrates from intracellular sites carries the risk of structural damage, such damage seems to occur first when the hypoglycaemia is sufficiently severe to disrupt cerebral energy state. As mentioned, lesions tend to be localized mainly to the selectively vulnerable areas, i.e. to the neocortex, hippocampus, and cerebellum (Brierley, Brown, and Meldrum, 1971). It now seems established that hypoglycaemia alone, i.e. substrate deficiency in the absence of oxygen deficiency, is the cause of the cell damage. Thus, even when hypoglycaemia extinguishes EEG activity for 30 min, CBF is increased above normal (Siesjö and Abdul-Rahman, 1979a). Furthermore, in this condition of cerebral energy failure, calculations from substrate couples indicate oxidation of cellular redox systems (Lewis and coworkers, 1974a; Norberg and Siesjö, 1976). In this sense then, the cellular lesions in severe hypoglycaemia are truly 'oxidative'.

The facts discussed should not be taken to indicate that circulatory factors do not contribute to the final cell lesions incurred after severe hypoglycaemia. In the clinical setting an embarrassed lung ventilation and/or arterial hypotension may well add a hypoxic insult to that caused by substrate deficiency. Recent results have also shown that, following prolonged hypoglycaemic coma, a delayed hypoperfusion of cortical and subcortical structures develops (Fig. 4) that could well contribute to the final cell damage (Siesjö and Abdul-Rahman, 1979a).

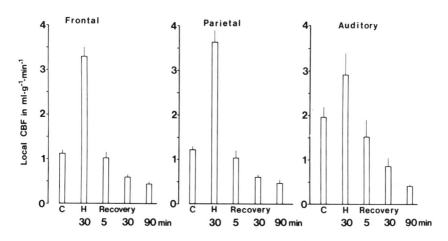

Figure 4. Local cerebral blood flow (CBF) in different cortical regions of the rat at 30 min of severe hypoglycaemia (H) and during recovery (glucose administration). C: control values

IV. EPILEPTIC SEIZURES

Cerebral metabolic and circulatory changes in experimentally induced seizures have been intensely explored (for literature, see Siesjö, 1978, ch. 12). In the present context, our main concern is the influence of seizures on cerebral metabolic rate, and the possibility that systemic factors modifying oxygen and substrate supply influence the lesions that occur after repeated or sustained seizures.

All types of seizure lead to an increased cerebral metabolic rate, either globally or locally (see Plum, Posner, and Troy, 1968; Plum and Duffy, 1975; Meldrum and Nilsson, 1976; Sokoloff, 1978). In most models studied, overall metabolic rate increases 1.5- to 2.5-fold. The most extensive data exist for bicuculline-induced status epilepticus in rats which increases oxygen and glucose consumption about 2.5-fold (Borgström, Chapman, and Siesjö, 1976; Meldrum and Nilsson, 1976). However, if blood pressure is upheld or increased, there is an even more pronounced rise in CBF. Under conditions in which the arterial oxygenation is also maintained, tissue Po_2 does not fall (e.g. Caspers and Speckmann, 1972) and, despite an accumulation of lactate and an elevation of the lactate/pyruvate ratio, mitochondrial redox systems may become oxidized (Jöbsis and coworkers, 1971; Duffy, Howse, and Plum, 1975; Howse and Duffy, 1975; Chapman, Meldrum, and Siesjö, 1977).

Repeated seizures, or those maintained for at least two hours (status epilepticus) have been shown to give rise to neuronal cell damage, mainly localized to the selectively vulnerable areas (Meldrum and Brierley 1973; Wasterlain, 1974; Brierley, 1976). In paralysed and ventilated baboons, in which systemic factors such as hypoxia, hypotension, hypoglycaemia, and hyperthermia could be largely avoided, the lesions were more moderate and were absent in the cerebellum (Meldrum, Vigouroux, and Brierley, 1973). However, the fact that cell damage did occur hints at the possibility of 'oxidative' damage. This assumption was corroborated by recent results on bicuculline-induced seizures in paralysed rats (Blennow and coworkers, 1978). Thus, in normoxic rats with 2 hours of bicuculline-induced status epilepticus, neuronal damage occurred in the neocortex and hippocampus, to some extent also in the thalamus and striatum, but lesions were not observed in the cerebellum and brain stem. Most interestingly, a restriction of cerebral oxygen supply by induced, moderate hypoxia or hypotension virtually prevented the cell damage from occurring, despite uninterrupted seizure activity (Table 3). The results obviously corroborate the hypothesis that oxygen deficiency does not contribute to the lesions, and suggest the occurrence of 'oxidative' damage.

Table 3. Number of animals showing microvacuolation and/or ischaemic cell change in the brain after 2-hour seizure activity under various physiological conditions (modified from Blennow and coworkers, 1978)

| | No. in group | Region | | | | | |
| | | Cortex | Hippocampus | | | Striatum | |
			h_1	h_{3-5}	Total		Total
Standard	13	11	9	3	9	3	11
Moderate hypotension (MABP = 70–75 mmHg)	12	1	0	0	0	0	1*
Hypoxia (Pao_2 45–51 mmHg)	7	0	0	0	0	0	0*

*Significantly different from the *standard* group at 1 % level (Fisher's exact probability test).

Recent results demonstrate a correlation between local metabolic rate and localization of neuronal injury. Thus, local glucose consumption, as measured with the autoradiographic ^{14}C-deoxyglucose technique of Sokoloff and co-workers (1977) showed greatly enhanced values in cortex, hippocampus, thalamus, and amygdala, and low values in cerebellar cortex and brain stem (Siesjö and Abdul-Rahman, 1979b). The results strongly indicate that the cell damage occurring may be related to excessive neuronal activity and greatly enhanced metabolic rate.

V. OXIDATIVE CELL DAMAGE—A SPECULATIVE HYPOTHESIS

Obviously, in two of the conditions discussed (hypoglycaemia and status epilepticus) the cell damage is oxidative in the sense that it occurs at unchanged or increased tissue oxygen tensions, and in only one of these (hypoglycaemia) is cell injury related to extensive energy failure. There is now a growing suspicion that oxygen-dependent mechanisms may contribute to the final damage also in cerebral hypoxia and ischaemia. For example, some results hint at the possibility that an incomplete interruption of oxygen (and substrate) supply, as occurs in pronounced cerebral hypoxia and in incomplete ischaemia, leads to more severe injury than complete ischaemia (see Hossmann and Kleihues, 1973; Nordström, Rehncrona, and Siesjö, 1978; Rehncrona, Mela, and Siesjö, 1979). Further-more, some reactions of a degradative nature are observed first when oxygen supply is restored after ischaemia (Cooper and coworkers, 1977). Finally, it cannot be excluded that the secondary hypoperfusion following ischaemia (see Hossmann, 1977) has a metabolic basis. If one assumes that part of the final damage.after hypoxia and ischaemia is incurred in the reoxygenation/recirculation period, it is possible to formulate a tentative hypothesis which predicts that some mechanisms of damage are common to hypoxia, ischaemia, hypoglycaemia, and status epilepticus, and involve oxygen-dependent degradation of cell structure.

Some of the hydrolytic enzymes that degrade macromolecular cell complexes, e.g. proteins, are oxygen- and energy-dependent (e.g. Marks and Lajtha, 1971). Theoretically, it is therefore possible that a trickling oxygen supply to the tissue, in conditions in which the energy production is insufficient for a corresponding resynthesis, can hasten the damage to the cells. The significance of such mechanisms is, however, poorly known and, at present, interest is focussed on another oxygen-dependent mechanism of potentially injurious nature, namely that which, via production and release of free radicals, leads to lipid peroxidation and other deleterious effects.

A. Free Radicals—Formation and Cellular Effects

It now appears clear that free radicals, i.e. molecules with an unpaired electron in an outer shell, are formed in the normal metabolism of all aerobic cells, mainly in the respiratory chain, e.g. in the flavin- and ubiquinone-dependent steps, and in certain cytoplasmic reactions, e.g. those that lead to oxidation of xanthine and certain amino acids (see Demopoulos and coworkers, 1973; and reviews by Slater, 1972; Fridovich, 1976; Mead, 1976; Pryor, 1976; Dormandy, 1978). It is also known that free radicals are an integral part of the normal intermediates in prostaglandin synthesis (Samuelsson, 1972, 1976). The majority of the radicals that are formed are probably oxygen radicals that occur because, in the respiratory metabolism, a univalent reduction of oxygen is preferred. Thus, the combination of oxygen with one, two, and three electrons leads to the development of superoxide anions ($^{\bullet}O_2{}^-$), hydrogen peroxide (H_2O_2), and hydroxyl radicals ($OH^{\bullet}$). Furthermore, there occurs in the reaction described by Harber and Weiss (1934) another radical, namely singlet oxygen (O_2^*):

$$H_2O_2 + O_2{}^- \longrightarrow OH^- + OH^{\bullet} + O_2^* \qquad (1)$$

The radical-dependent reactions do not normally lead to a net production of radicals, as those that (transiently) develop are quenched when the reaction sequences are completed. If free radicals are formed in an increasing number and/or are dislocated from the sites of production, there is a risk of harmful side-effects that are often of an autocatalytic chain-reaction character. This is because of the fact that most free radicals are highly reactive and can abstract hydrogen from, or add themselves to, surrounding macromolecules. The best-studied of these reactions is that which, via a radical attack on α-methylene carbon atoms in unsaturated fatty acids, leads to the development of peroxides and hydroperoxides, and to a final fragmentation of the fatty acids (lipid peroxidation). Other harmful effects are due to radicals adding themselves to nucleic acids and proteins, thus causing abnormal links between macromolecules (cross-linking). The final result on the part of the cell can mean an irreversible breakdown of intracellular membranes (e.g. in mitochondria and endoplasmatic reticulum), DNA damage, inactivation of enzymes, and autolysis. It must be pointed out that most of these reactions are non-enzymatic. Some cellular reactions of a degrading radical nature are, however, enzymatically catalysed, e.g. those that, via a NADPH-ADP-Fe^{2+}-mediated reaction sequence lead to peroxidation of microsomal lipids in the liver, kidney, and brain (Hochstein and Ernster, 1963; Hochstein, Nordenbrand, and Ernster, 1964).

B. Cellular Defence against Radical Damage

It is obvious that the potential danger of free-radical reactions for the cellular function and integrity demands an effective antioxidative defence. This defence appears to be based on (a) spatial separation of radical reactions and vulnerable biomolecules; (b) enzymatic quenching of free radicals; and (c) the presence of antioxidants and non-enzymatic 'scavengers'.

1. Spatial Separation

If certain tissues (e.g. liver, kidney, brain) are homogenized in the presence of oxygen, a pronounced lipid peroxidation occurs that is accelerated by the addition of certain initiators (particularly Fe^{2+} and ascorbic acid). The reason appears to be that by the disintegration of the tissue, a disruption is achieved of the spatial separation that normally prevents the interaction between free radicals and vulnerable biomolecules, and that metal ions (Fe^{2+}, Cu^{2+}) are released from their binding sites. A corresponding lipid peroxidation is also seen if the structure of isolated mitochondria is disrupted by means of the addition of chaotropic substances (Hanstein and Hatefi, 1970). Theoretically one can, therefore, postulate that radical impairment can occur *in vivo* if the cell structure is damaged (e.g. by the effect of phospholipases and other destructive enzymes), or if initiators such as Fe^{2+} are released (e.g. through bleeding or trauma).

2. Enzymatic Defence

Three enzymes dominate the enzymatic defence of the cell against free radicals: superoxide dismutase, catalase, and glutathione peroxidase. Superoxide dismutase, an enzyme found in all aerobic cells, catalyses the reaction:

$$\overset{\bullet}{O}_2{}^- + \underset{\bullet}{O}_2{}^- + 2H^+ \longrightarrow H_2O_2 + O_2 \tag{2}$$

Together with catalase, superoxide dismutase can therefore keep the concentrations of $\overset{\bullet}{O}_2{}^-$ and H_2O_2 low, and thereby minimize the formation of hydroxyl radicals and singlet oxygen, i.e. those radicals that are probably chiefly responsible for oxidative damage (see Kellogg and Fridovich, 1975; Fridovich, 1976). Glutathione peroxidase appears to have partly the same effect as catalase, but the glutathione system plays a more complex role (see below).

3. Substances with an Antioxidative Effect

The most important 'scavengers' in the cell are probably vitamin E, vitamin C, and thioles, such as glutathione. The effect of vitamin E (here denoted as ArOH) appears to depend on the ability of the molecule to 'donate' hydrogen to free radicals ($Q^{\bullet}$)

$$Q^{\bullet} + ArOH \longrightarrow QH + ArO^{\bullet} \tag{3}$$

and on the fact that the newly-formed radical ($ArO^{\bullet}$) has only a slight tendency to propagate chain-reactions (see Slater, 1972; Pryor, 1976). The effect of ascorbic acid and of glutathione is more complex, particularly as these substances in certain concentrations (and under special conditions) can *initiate* the formation of free radicals.

4. Glutathione: a Special case

During recent years great attention has been paid to glutathione, a thiol-containing amino acid compound that occurs in high concentrations in many organs. It is considered by many today that the most important function of the glutathione system, which consists of reduced (GSH) and oxidized (GSSG) tripeptide, is antioxidative (Flohé and coworkers, 1974; Orlowski and Karkowsky, 1976). The following functions of the system can be defined:

(i) GSH works as a direct scavenger in reactions such as:

$$Q^{\bullet} + GSH \longrightarrow QH + GS^{\bullet} \tag{4}$$

$$GS^{\bullet} + GS^{\bullet} \longrightarrow GSSG \tag{5}$$

(ii) GSH regenerates other scavengers such as vitamin E and ubiquinone (cf. reaction 3):

$$ArO^{\bullet} + GSH \longrightarrow ArOH + GS^{\bullet} \tag{6}$$

$$GS^{\bullet} + GS^{\bullet} \longrightarrow GSSG \tag{5}$$

(iii) The GSH–GSSG system takes part in thiol-disulphide reactions that prevent (and reverse) oxidation of thiol groups in enzymes and other proteins, an oxidation that could otherwise, for instance, lead to enzyme inactivation:

$$R_1SSR_2 + 2GSH \longrightarrow R_1SH + R_2SH + GSSG \tag{7}$$

(iv) The enzyme glutathione peroxidase causes a reduction of hydrogen peroxide and other hydroperoxides, including those that occur in lipid peroxidation:

$$2ROOH + 2GSH \longrightarrow 2ROH + H_2O + GSSG \tag{8}$$

It is of interest that the cell catalyses a rapid regeneration of the GSSG formed in reactions 5, 7, and 8. Thus, the enzyme glutathione reductase catalyses the reaction

$$GSSG + 2NADPH + 2H^+ \longrightarrow 2GSH + 2NADP^+ \tag{9}$$

while the phosphogluconate sequence (hexose monophosphate shunt) regenerates NADPH from the $NADP^+$ that is formed.

C. Is Free-radical Damage Occurring *in vivo*?

It has proved to be difficult to show convincingly that a free radical-mediated lipid peroxidation constitutes an important mechanism for cell damage. A direct measurement of free radicals is extremely difficult because of the lability and short life of these substances, and suitable techniques (for example electron spin reasonance measurements) can only be used successfully on relatively homogeneous *in vitro* systems. The available techniques are therefore those that measure the *effects* of radical reactions, especially lipid peroxidation. *In vitro* this can be carried out with a number of techniques such as the thiobarbituric acid (TBA) method which quantifies malondialdehyde and similar substances, i.e. substances that are formed when lipid peroxides are broken down (Barber and Bernheim, 1967; Slater, 1972). Further techniques measure other effects of lipid peroxidation, e.g. diene conjugation or an increase in 'peroxide number' (see Slater, 1972). Unfortunately, these are hardly suitable *in vivo*, partly because malondialdehyde and different lipid peroxides can be metabolized (Recknagel and Ghoshal, 1966; Little and O'Brien, 1968). Of greater interest, therefore, are those results which show that lipid peroxidation in liver microsomes leads to relatively typical changes in the phospholipid pattern of the tissue, with a preferential loss of unsaturated fatty acids, especially 20:4 and 22:6 (see Table 5) (May, Poyer, and McCay, 1965; Recknagel and Ghoshal, 1966; May and McCay, 1968; Flohé and Zimmerman, 1974). Another potentially valuable technique has been reported by Tappel and coworkers (see Tappel, 1975) who reported that lipid peroxidation *in vitro* (and *in vivo*) leads to the formation of fluorescent products that appear to be identical with those that accumulate in the lipofuscin granulae of the cell with ageing.

Normally, the production (in *in vitro* systems) of free radicals is proportional to the oxygen pressure, and anoxia excludes, of course, peroxidative changes. It can therefore appear to be paradoxical to suggest that the damage that occurs in tissue hypoxia is partly caused by free radicals. As long as there is a certain supply of oxygen this possibility cannot be ignored, however, particularly as continued electron transport in the respiratory chain, when there is a lack of oxygen (the terminal free radical quencher), can possibly lead to accelerated dislocation of radicals. Two research groups have reported results that hint at tissue hypoxia giving oxidative damage. Widemann and Domańska-Janik (1974) found that hypoxia (arterial Po_2 about 30 mmHg) reduced the content (indirectly measured) of GSH in the brain, and these authors postulated that a corresponding increase of GSSG occurred (this was not measured). The authors concluded that oxidative mechanisms contribute to tissue damage in hypoxia. Results from Demopoulos' groups in New York have more directly implicated free radicals and lipid peroxidation. These authors ligated the middle cerebral artery in the cat and observed a continuous reduction of the concentration of a natural scavenger (ascorbic acid) in the affected area (Demopoulos and coworkers, 1977a; Flamm and coworkers, 1978). They have subsequently, in abstract form, reported that typical changes in phospholipid and fatty acid patterns occur in the ischaemic tissues (Flamm and coworkers, 1977). As it has previously been shown that barbiturates have a pronounced protective effect in this form of ischaemia (Smith and coworkers, 1974; Hoff and coworkers, 1975; Michenfelder and Milde, 1975), it is interesting to note that the Demopoulos group, in model experiments, has found that such substances act as scavengers of free radicals (Demopoulos and coworkers 1977b).

The reports mentioned above are not entirely convincing in their arguments that tissue hypoxia can lead to oxidative damage. The hypothesis can, however, hardly be ignored in a thorough analysis of the pathogenesis of hypoxic-ischaemic brain damage, particularly if one supposes that this develops partly during the reoxygenation/recirculation period. Thus, an alternative working hypothesis can be proposed that postulates the possibility of oxidative damage in a phase when reactive hyperaemia increases the oxygen pressure to above normal in tissues whose structure could have been partially degraded by hydrolytic enzymes (Siesjö, 1978).

Three recent series of experiments cast further light on the mechanisms discussed. They will be considered under the headings (1) glutathione metabolism in hypoxia and ischaemia; (2) changes in phospholipids and fatty acids; and (3) mechanisms of action of barbiturates.

1. Glutathione Metabolism in Hypoxia and Ischaemia

We tested the proposition that hypoxia leads to a change in the ratio of reduced (GSH) to oxidized (GSSG) glutathione in the brain, using newly-developed enzymatic, fluorometric techniques for measuring GSH and GSSG in tissue (Folbergrová, Rehncrona, and Siesjö, 1979). When precautions were taken to avoid artefactual oxidation of GSH during sample preparation, GSSG concentrations were about 0.7 % of GSH concentrations. Moderate or marked hypoxia failed to alter GSH concentrations or GSSG/GSH ratios, nor did it affect CSF concentrations of GSSG (Table 4). Obviously, the results failed to corroborate the hypothesis of Widemann and Domańska-Janik (1974).

Table 4. The influence of 60 minutes of moderate hypoxia on GSH and GSSG concentrations in cerebral cortex and cisternal CSF (modified from Folbergrová, Rehnorona, and Siesjö, 1979)

Sample	Arterial P_{O_2}	GSH	GSSG
Cortex	105–135 mmHg	2.04 ±0.04	0.014 ±0.002
	28–35 mmHg	2.02 ±0.04	0.008 ±0.001*
CSF	105–135 mmHg	0.04 ±0.01	0.010 ±0.002
	28–35 mmHg	0.02 ±0.01	0.006 ±0.001

The values are means ± S.E.M. for groups of four animals.
*$P < 0.05$

Other results have shown that although complete and pronounced incomplete ischaemia give rise to a decrease in tissue GSH concentration, there is no change in GSSG/GSH ratio during or after the ischaemia, and no rise in CSF GSSG concentration (Rehncrona, and coworkers, 1980a). Thus, rather than demonstrating a conversion of GSH to GSSG, the results show that energy failure due to ischaemia leads to a reduction in the size of the glutathione pool, probably because degradation of the tripeptide is unmatched by a corresponding resynthesis.

Clearly, the results fail to support the hypothesis of oxidative damage during or following hypoxia or ischaemia. However, the results cannot exclude that such damage occurs, since the glutathione reductase reaction and the phosphogluconate pathway could well have regenerated any GSSG formed.

2. Changes in Phospholipids and Fatty Acids in vitro and in vivo

An *in vitro* system was set up in which brain tissue is homogenized in phosphate buffer (0.05 mol l^{-1}, pH 7) and equilibrated with 5 % O_2 in the presence of free-radical initiators (0.01 mmol l^{-1} Fe^{2+} and 0.25 mmol l^{-1} ascorbic acid). In this system lipid peroxidation, as measured with the TBA test for MDA and related cleavage products, proceeds at an approximately linear rate for at least 60 min (Smith and coworkers, 1979; Westerberg and coworkers, 1979). Subsequent results have shown that parallel increases occur in diene conjugation and in concentrations of fluorescent products (Rehncrona, and coworkers 1980b). As Table 5 shows, lipid peroxidation is accompanied by typical changes in concentrations of phosphoglyceride ethanolamine and of the polyunsaturated arachidonic and docosahexanoic acids.

Table 5. Effects of *in vitro* induced lipid peroxidation on fatty acids and phospholipids in cortical tissue from the rat brain (from Westerberg and coworkers, 1979)

	5 % O_2	100 % N_2	Probability (p)
Total fatty acids	113 ±4	122 ±3	$p < 0.01$
20:4	10.8 ±0.4	12.3 ±0.4	$p < 0.01$
22:6	14.8 ±0.7	18.7 ±0.4	$p < 0.001$
Ethanolamine phosphoglyceride	22.5 ±0.6	26.5 ±0.5	$p < 0.001$
Choline phosphoglyceride	25.1 ±0.7	25.0 ±0.3	N.S.

*No. of carbon atoms: no. of double bonds.
Homogenates of rat cerebral cortex were incubated in the presence of Fe^{2+} and ascorbic acid for 45 minutes with 5 % O_2 or 100 % N_2. In O_2-incubated samples an appreciable amount of malondialdehyde (MDA) was formed, indicating peroxidative processes, while the MDA formed in N_2-incubated samples was negligible.

Of the *in vitro* methods used for estimating lipid peroxidation, that quantitating changes in phospholipids and fatty acids is applicable to *in vivo* conditions. So far, we have failed to obtain evidence that changes in these parameters occur in the recirculation period following complete or incomplete ischaemia (Rehncrona, and coworkers in preparation).

3. Mechanisms of Action of Barbiturates

In other experiments it could be demonstrated that thiopental, in a concentration of 1 mmol l^{-1}, efficiently prevents lipid peroxidation *in vitro* (Fig. 5) and the associated changes in phospholipids and fatty acids (Smith and coworkers, 1979). These results are seemingly in line with the assumption that barbiturates protect the tissue in ischaemia by acting as a free-radical scavenger. However, under similar conditions, methohexital had a very small effect, and neither pentobarbital nor phenobarbital had any influence. Since all these barbiturates have been shown to protect in conditions of ischaemia (Smith and coworkers, 1974; Hoff and coworkers, 1975; Michenfelder and Milde, 1975), the results lend little support to the view that they act by scavenging free radicals.

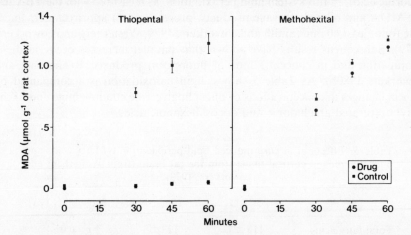

Figure 5. Effects of thiopental and methohexital on Fe^{2+}-induced lipid peroxidation (formation of malondialdehyde (MDA)) in brain cortical homogenates incubated for different periods in 5% O$_2$. (From Smith and coworkers, 1979)

Clearly, the results quoted fail to corroborate the hypothesis that free-radical damage is an important mechanism for cell injury, at least in hypoxia and ischaemia. It remains to be studied whether or not free-radical damage occurs in subcellular fractions, and to explore the potential importance of radical pathology in hypoglycaemia and in status epilepticus. In general, it seems warranted to explore in further detail the possibility of free-radical damage in the brain, especially since the mechanism has been implicated as a cause of nerve cell degeneration in ageing (Barber and Bernheim 1967; Tappel, 1968).

VI. THE IMPORTANCE OF TISSUE ACIDOSIS

If lipid peroxidation does not provide an important damaging mechanism in hypoxia and ischaemia, the question remains what mechanisms are involved. The problem may seem academic since both conditions, by causing energy failure, upset the balance between degradation and resynthesis of cell structures. However, it remains to be explained why hypoxia and incomplete ischaemia seem more harmful than complete ischaemia. Or, posed in another way, why does clinical ischaemia, of only 4–5-minutes' duration, often lead to gross brain damage (e.g. Cole and Corday, 1956), when experimentally induced complete ischaemia of 20–25-minutes' duration sometimes does not (see Neely and Youmans, 1963; Miller and Myers, 1970)? One clue to this problem is offered by recent results on the influence of the dietary status of experimental animals subjected to ischaemia, and on the effects of excessive cellular acidosis.

The potentially deleterious effect of acidosis has usually been attributed to the fact that a lowered pH is one of the factors that activate or release those hydrolytic enzymes which are normally sequestered in lysosomes (De Duve and Wattieaux, 1966; Koenig, 1969). Since excessive acidosis also alters the activity of many enzymes modulating anabolic and catabolic sequences in the energy metabolism in the cell, it has been postulated that a marked lowering of intracellular pH predisposes to metabolic damage and autolysis (e.g. Friede and van Houten, 1961; Swanson, 1969; Wasterlain, 1974).

In experiments with arterial hypoxia combined with unilateral carotid artery ligation, we found that the energy charge of the adenine nucleotide pool of cortical tissue on the ligated side fell continuously with increasing lactic acid concentrations (Salford and Siesjö, 1974). It was speculated that excessive lactic acidosis was responsible for the irreversible metabolic damage that appeared in about 50 % of the animals during the reoxygenation/recirculation period. An attempt was made to demonstrate a correlation between acidosis and tissue damage by inducing hyper- and hypoglycaemia before complete ischaemia was induced (Ljunggren, Norberg, and Siesjö, 1974). The results showed that the resulting tissue lactic acidosis varied with the pre-ischaemic tissue concentrations of glucose plus glycogen (hypoglycaemia: 5 μmol g^{-1}; hyperglycaemia: 21 μmol g^{-1}). However, these alterations did not influence recovery of cerebral energy state. Probably, the results are inconclusive since the duration of the ischaemia was limited to 5 minutes. Furthermore, even in hyperglycaemic animals the resulting lactic acidosis is less marked than that observed in severe hypoxia and in incomplete ischaemia, conditions that allow a continued supply of substrate for anaerobic glycolysis. Thus, in the latter conditions tissue lactate concentrations may rise to 30–50 μmol g^{-1}.

Recently, Myers and collaborators have reported results suggesting that accumulation of lactic acid in brain tissues to levels exceeding 25 μmol g^{-1} predisposes to massive cellular oedema and irreversible brain damage (Myers and Yamaguchi, 1976; Myers, 1977). An adverse effect of acidosis has also been observed by others (Ginsberg, Welsh, and Budd, 1978; Welsh and coworkers, 1978; Rehncrona, Rosén and Siesjö, in preparation). It is worth noting that starved animals tolerate ischaemia better than those that are first starved and then given glucose by infusion. Presumably, the deleterious effects of glucose administration is related to the magnitude of the resulting tissue acidosis. However, it has not yet been possible to exclude other mechanisms, nor is it known whether the primary event is vascular (with secondary metabolic damage) or metabolic (with subsequent reduction in blood flow due to cell oedema).

VII. CELL DAMAGE IN ACUTE DISEASE: RELEVANCE TO THE DEMENTIAS

When considering the possibility that some of the factors and mechanisms contributing to neuronal cell damage in acute disease are instrumental in causing cell degeneration and cell loss in the dementias, the histopathological characteristics must be kept in mind. Thus, although cell death and necrosis are common to both classes of disease, the dementias involve alterations not observed in acute disease, e.g. neurofibrillary tangles and neuritic plaques. At first sight, therefore, only multi-infarct dementia would seem to provide a link to the mechanisms discussed, since the focal areas of tissue necrosis should have a vascular basis in the form of local reductions in blood flow due to thrombosis or arteriosclerotic narrowing of resistance vessels. Conceivably, one pathophysiological factor of importance is the reduced ability of the microcirculation to autoregulate in patients with a relative fall in perfusion pressure, and one possible contributing mechanism of damage is cellular acidosis.

However, it seems that also the more characteristic alterations observed in the dementias show some relationship to the acute conditions discussed, especially to ischaemia. Thus, neurofibrillary tangles have been observed in dementia pugilistica (Corsellis, 1978), a condition which presumably results from repeated trauma and its pathophysiological consequences (intraparenchymal bleeding and/or vascular spasm). In this particular condition, it cannot be excluded that post-traumatic paroxysmal neuronal activity is contributory.

A special interest has been focussed on lipid peroxidation as a cause of neuronal cell death in elderly patients. Theoretically, one may assume that peroxidative damage to intracellular membranes, to DNA molecules, and even to vascular endothelium represents cumulative events reflecting a less than complete cellular defence against free-radical formation, possibly accelerated by an age-related decline in enzymatic and non-enzymatic scavenging ability. One may also speculate that intracerebral bleeding, due to vascular rupture or trauma, accelerates free-radical formation by providing initiators such as Fe^{2+}. At present, the evidence that lipid peroxidation occurs is circumstantial and resides mainly in the belief that lipofuscin granulae represent partly peroxidized intracellular membranes that have been engulfed by lysosomes. It is also of interest the the fluorescence characteristic of lipofuscin granulae seems identical with that obtained when tissues are peroxidized *in vitro* (Tappel, 1975).

The problem with the free radical hypothesis of ageing is that it is not known whether lipofuscin accumulation is a parallel phenomenon of marginal pathogenetic importance, or if it represents one mechanism by which cells are punched out of the neuronal population in normal or pathological ageing. Current information seems to favour the first alternative (Terry, 1976), but it seems warranted to obtain further data in models of 'oxidative' damage, particularly hypoglycaemia and epileptic seizures.

In summary, with the notable exception of multi-infarct dementia and dementia pugilistica, there is at present no proof that neuronal cell death in the dementias is related to a reduced supply of oxygen or substrate, or to paroxysmal neuronal activity, nor has it been shown that lipid peroxidation is an important mechanism of cell damage. However, although emphasis is at present laid on other mechanisms (autoimmunization, slow virus disease, or aluminium intoxication) much more work is required on age-related changes in neuronal energy metabolism.

ACKNOWLEDGEMENTS

Research from the authors' own laboratory was supported by funds from the Swedish Medical Research Council (project No. B79-14X-263), and from U.S. PHS Grant No. 2 RO1 NS-07838.

REFERENCES

Agardh, C.-D., A. Carlsson, M. Lindquist, and B. K. Siesjö (1979). The effect of pronounced hypoglycemia on monoamine metabolism in rat brain. *Diabetes.* **28**, 804–809.

Agardh, C.-D., J. Folbergrová, and B. K. Siesjö (1978). Cerebral metabolic changes in profound, insulin-induced hypoglycemia, and in the recovery period following glucose administration. *J. Neurochem.*, **31**, 1135–42.

Bachelard, H. S., L. D. Lewis, U. Pontén, and B. K. Siesjö (1974). Mechanisms activating glycolysis in the brain in arterial hypoxia. *J. Neurochem.*, **22**, 395–401.

Barber, A. A. and F. Bernheim (1967). Lipid peroxidation: its measurement, occurrence, and significance in animal tissues. *Advan. Gerontol. Res.*, **2**, 355–403.

Barondes, S. H. (1969). Axoplasmic transport. In A. Lajtha (Ed.) *Handbook of Neurochemistry*, Vol. II, Plenum Press, New York. pp. 435–46.

Berntman, L. and B. K. Siesjö (1978). Cerebral metabolic and circulatory changes induced by hypoxia in starved rats. *J. Neurochem.*, **31**, 1265–7.

Borgström, L., A. G. Chapman, and B. K. Siesjö (1976). Glucose consumption in the cerebral cortex of rat during bicuculline-induced status epilepticus. *J. Neurochem.*, **27**, 971–3.

Blennow, G., J. B. Brierley, B. S. Meldrum, and B. K. Siesjö (1978). Epileptic brain damage: The role of systemic factors that modify cerebral energy metabolism. *Brain.*, **101**, 687–700.

Brierley, J. B. (1973). Pathology of cerebral ischemia. In F. H. McDowell and R. W. Brennan (Eds) *Cerebral Vascular Diseases*, Grune and Stratton, New York, pp. 59–75.

Brierley, J. B. (1976). Cerebral hypoxia. In W. Blackwood and J. A. N. Corsellis (Eds) *Greenfield's Neuropathology* Edward Arnold, London. pp. 43–85.

Brierley, J. B., A. W. Brown, and B. S. Meldrum (1971). The nature and time course of the neuronal alterations resulting from oligaemia and hypoglycaemia in the brain of *Macaca Mulatta*. *Brain Res.*, **25**, 483–99.

Brown, R. M., S. R. Snider, and A. Carlsson (1974). Changes in biogenic amine synthesis and turnover induced by hypoxia and/or foot shock stress. II. The central nervous system. *J. Neurol. Transmission*, **35**, 293–305.

Brun, A. and L. Gustafson (1976). Distribution of cerebral degeneration in Alzheimer's disease. A clinico-pathological study. *Arch. Psychiat. Nervenkr.*, **223**, 15–33.

Carlsson, A., T. Holmin, M. Lindqvist, and B. K. Siesjö (1977). Effect of hypercapnia and hypocapnia on tryptophan and tyrosine hydroxylation in rat brain. *Acta physiol. scand.*, **99**, 503–9.

Carson, R. and W. Evans (1969). Symptomatology, pathophysiology, and treatment of acute mountain sickness. *Fed. Proc.*, **28**, 1085–91.

Caspers, H., and E.-H. Speckmann (1972). Cerebral Po_2, Pco_2, and pH changes during convulsive activity and their significance for spontaneous arrest of seizures. *Epilepsia*, **13**, 699–725.

Chapman, A. G., B. S. Meldrum, and B. K. Siesjö (1977). Cerebral metabolic changes during prolonged epileptic seizures in rats. *J. Neurochem.*, **28**, 1025–35.

Cole, S. L. and E. Corday (1956). Four-minute limit for cardiac resuscitation. *J. Amer. Med. Assoc.*, **161**, 1454–8.

Cooper, H. K., T. Zalewska, S. Kawakami, K.-A. Hossmann, and P. Kleihues (1977). The effect of ischemia and recirculation on protein synthesis in the rat brain. *J. Neurochem*, **28**, 929–34.

Corsellis, J. A. N. (1978). Post-traumatic dementia. In R. Katzman, R. D. Terry, and K. L. Bick (Eds) *Alzheimer's Disease: Senile Dementia and Related Disorders* (Aging, Vol. 7), Raven Press, New York. pp. 125–33.

Crapper, D. R., S. Karlik, and U. De Boni (1978). Aluminum and other metals in senile (Alzheimer) dementia. In R. Katzman, R. D. Terry, and K. L. Bick (Eds) *Alzheimer's Disease: Senile Dementia and Related Disorders* (Aging, Vol. 7), Raven Press, New York. pp. 471–85.

Dastur, D. K., M. H. Lane, D. B. Hansen, S. S. Kety, R. N. Butler, S. Perlin, and L. Sokoloff (1963). Effects of aging on cerebral circulation and metabolism in man. In J. E. Birren, R. N. Butler, S. W. Greenhouse, L. Sokoloff, and M. R. Yarrow (Eds) *Human Aging*, Publ. Health Service Publ. No. 986. pp. 59–76.

Davis, J. N. (1976). Brain tyrosine hydroxylation: alteration of oxygen affinity *in vivo* by immobilization or electroshock in the rat. *J. Neurochem.*, **27**, 211–5.

Davis, J. N. and A. Carlsson (1973). The effect of hypoxia on monoamine synthesis, levels and metabolism in rat brain. *J. Neurochem.*, **21**, 783–90.

De Duve, C. and R. Wattieaux (1966). Functions of lysosomes. *Ann. Rev. Physiol.*, **28**, 435–92.

Demopoulos, H. B. (1973). Free radical pathology. *Fed. Proc.*, **32**, 1859–908.

Demopoulos, H., E. Flamm, M. Seligman, R. Power, D. Pietronigro, and J. Ransohoff (1977a). Molecular Pathology of lipids in CNS membranes. In F F. Jöbsis (Ed.) *Oxygen and Physiological Function*, Professional Information Library, Dallas, Texas. pp. 491–508.

Demopoulos, H. B., E. S. Flamm, M. L. Seligman, E. Jorgensen, and J. Ransohoff (1977b). Antioxidant effects of barbiturates in model membranes undergoing free radical damage. *Acta Neurol. Scand.*, 56 (Suppl. 64), 152–3.

Dormandy, T. L. (1978). Free-radical oxidation and antioxidants. *Lancet*, I, 647–50.

Droz, B. and H. L. Koenig (1970). Localization of protein metabolism in neurons. In A. Lajtha (Ed.) *Protein Metabolism of the Nervous System*, Plenum Press, New York. pp. 93–106.

Duffy, T. E., D. C. Howse, and F. Plum (1975). Cerebral energy metabolism during experimental status epilepticus. *J. Neurochem.*, 24, 925–34.

Elliott, K. A. C. and I. H. Heller (1957). Metabolism of neurons and glia. In D. Richter (Ed.) *Metabolism of the Nervous System*, Pergamon Press, Oxford. pp. 286–90.

Elliott, K. A. C. and N. Henderson (1948). Metabolism of brain tissue slices and suspensions from various mammals. *J. Neurophysiol.*, 11, 473–84.

Epstein, M. H. and J. S. O'Connor (1965). Respiration of single cortical neurons and of surrounding neuropil. *J. Neurochem.*, 12, 385–95.

Ernsting, J. (1966). The effects of hypoxia upon human performance and the electroencephalogram. In J. P. Payne and D. W. Hill (Eds.) *Oxygen Measurements in Blood and Tissues and their Significance*, J. & A. Churchill, London. pp. 245–59.

Finnerty, F. A. Jr, L. Witkin, and J. F. Fazekas (1954). Cerebral hemodynamics during cerebral ischemia induced by acute hypotension. *J. Clin. Invest.*, 33, 1227–32.

Flamm, E. S., H. B. Demopoulos, M. L. Seligman, R. G. Poser, and J. Ransohoff (1978). Free radicals in cerebral ischemia. *Stroke*, 9, 445–7.

Flamm, E. S., H. B. Demopoulos, M. L. Seligman, and J. Ransohoff (1977). Possible molecular mechanisms of barbiturate-mediated protection in regional cerebral ischemia. *Acta Neurol. Scand.*, 56 (Suppl. 64), 150–1.

Flohé, L., H. Ch. Benöhr, H. Sies, H. D. Waller, and A. Wendel (Eds) (1974). *Glutathione*. Georg Thieme Publishers, Stuttgart.

Flohé, L. and R. Zimmermann (1974). G-SH-induced high-amplitude swelling of mitochondria. In L. Flohé, H. Ch. Benöhr, H. Sies, H. D. Waller, and A. Wendel (Eds) *Glutathione*, Georg Thieme, Stuttgart. pp. 245–59.

Folbergrová, J., S. Rehncrona, and B. K. Siesjö (1979). Oxidized and reduced glutathione in the rat brain under normoxic and hypoxic conditions. *J. Neurochem.* 32, 1621–1627.

Freyhan, F. A., R. B. Woodford, and S. S. Kety (1951). Cerebral blood flow and metabolism in psychoses of senility. *J. Nerv. Mental Dis.*, 113, 449–56.

Fridovich, I. (1976). Oxygen radicals, hydrogen peroxide and oxygen toxicity. In W. A. Pryor (Ed.) *Free Radicals in Biology*, Academic Press, New York. pp. 239–77.

Friede, R. L. and W. H. van Houten (1961). Relations between post-mortem alterations and glycolytic metabolism in the brain. *Exp. Neurol.*, 4, 197–204.

Gibbs, F. A., E. L. Gibbs, and W. G. Lennow (1943). The value of carbon dioxide in counteracting the effects of low oxygen. *J. Aviat. Med.*, 14, 250–61.

Gibson, G. E. and J. P. Blass (1976). Impaired synthesis of acetylcholine in brain accompanying mild hypoxia and hypoglycemia. *J. Neurochem.*, 27, 37–42.

Gibson, G. E., M. Shimada, and J. P. Blass (1978). Alterations in acetylcholine synthesis and in cyclic nucleotides in mild cerebral hypoxia. *J. Neurochem.*, 31, 757–60.

Ginsberg, M. D., F. A. Welsh, and W. W. Budd (1978). Accentuation of post-ischemic cerebral perfusion impairment by pre-ischemic glucose administration. *Fed. Proc. Abstracts*, 37, 873.

Gottstein, U., A. Bernsmeier, and I. Sedlmeyer (1964). Der Kohlenhydratstoffwechsel des menschlichen Gehirns. II. Untersuchungen mit Substratspezifischen enzymatischen Methoden bei Kranken mit verminderter Hirndurchblutung auf dem Boden einer Arteriosklerose der Hirngefässe. *Klin. Wochenschr.*, **42**, 310–3.

Gustafson, L. and J. Risberg (1974). Regional cerebral blood flow related to psychiatric symptoms in dementia with onset in the presenile period. *Acta Psychiat. Scand.*, **50**, 516–38.

Hachinski, V. C., L. D. Iliff, E. Zilhka, G. H. Du Boulay, V. L. McAllister, J. Marshall, R. W. R. Russel, and L. Symon (1975). Cerebral blood flow in dementia. *Arch. Neurol.*, **32**, 632–7.

Hackett, P. and D. Rennie (1976). The incidence, importance, and prophylaxis of acute mountain sickness. *Lancet*, **2**, 1150.

Hagberg, B. and D. H. Ingvar (1976). Cognitive reduction in presenile dementia related to regional abnormalities of the cerebral blood flow. *Brit. J. Psychiat.*, **128**, 209–22.

Hanstein, W. G. and Y. Hatefi (1970). Lipid oxidation in biological membranes. II. Kinetics and mechanism of lipid oxidation in submitochondrial particles. *Arch. Biochem. Biophys.*, **38**, 87–95.

Harber, F. and J. Weiss (1934). The catalytic decomposition of hydrogen peroxide by iron salts. *J. Proc. Roy. Soc. Lond.* **A 147**, 332–51.

Hertz, L. (1978). Energy metabolism of glial cells. In E. Schoffeniels, G. Franck, D. B. Towers, and L. Hertz (Eds) *Dynamic Properties of Glia Cells*, Pergamon Press, Oxford. pp. 121–32.

Hess, H. (1961). The rates of respiration of neurons and neuroglia in human cerebrum. In S. S. Kety and J. Eldes (Eds) *Regional Neurochemistry*, Pergamon Press, Oxford. pp. 200–2.

Hinzen, D. H. and U. Müller (1971). Energiestoffwechsel und Funktion des Kaninchengehirns während Insulinhypoglykämie. *Pflügers Arch. ges. Physiol.*, **322**, 47–59.

Hochstein, P. and L. Ernster (1963). ADP-activated lipid peroxidation coupled to the TPNH oxidase system of microsomes. *Biochem. Biophys. Res. Com.*, **12**, 388–94.

Hochstein, P., K. Nordenbrand, and K. Ernster (1964). Evidence for the involvement of iron in the ADP-activated peroxidation of lipids in microsomes and mitochondria. *Biochem. Biophys. Res. Com.*, **14**, 323–8.

Hoff, J. T., L. Smith, H. L. Hankinson, and S. L. Nielsen (1975). Barbiturate protection from cerebral infarction in primates. *Stroke*, **6**, 28–33.

Hossmann, K.-A. (1977). Total ischaemia of the brain. In K. J. Zülch, W. Kaufmann, K.-A. Hossmann, and V. Hossmann (Eds), *Brain and Heart Infarct*, Springer Verlag, Berlin. pp. 107–22.

Hossmann, K.-A. and P. Kleihues (1973). Reversibility of ischemic brain damage. *Arch Neurol. (Chicago)*, **29**, 375–82.

Howse, D. C. and T. E. Duffy (1975). Control of the redox state of the pyridine nucleotides in the rat cerebral cortex. Effect of electroshock-induced seizures. *J. Neurochem.*, **24**, 935–40.

Hoyer, S. (1978). Blood flow and oxidative metabolism of the brain in different phases of dementia. In R. Katzman, R. D. Terry, and K. L. Bich (Eds) *Alzheimer's Disease: Senile Dementia and Related Disorders (Aging, Vol. 7)*, Raven Press, New York. pp. 219–26.

Hydén, H. and P. W. Lange (1965). The steady state and endogenous respiration in neurons and glia. *Acta Physiol. Scand.*, **64**, 6–14.

Ingvar, D. H., A. Brun, B. Hagberg, and L. Gustafson (1978). Regional cerebral blood flow in the dominant hemisphere in confirmed cases of Alzheimer's disease, Pick's disease, and multi-infarct dementia: Relationship to clinical symptomatology and neuropathological findings. In R. Katzman, R. D. Terry, and K. L. Bick (Eds) *Alzheimer's Disease: Senile Dementia and Related Disorders* (*Aging*, Vol. 7), Raven Press, New York. pp. 203–11.

Jeffrey, P. L. and L. Austin (1973). Axoplasmic transport. *Progr. Neurobiol.*, **2** (part 3), 205–55.

Jöbsis, F. F., M. O'Connor, A. Vitale, and H. Wreman (1971). Intracellular redox changes in functioning cerebral cortex. I. Metabolic effects of epileptiform activity. *J. Neurophysiol.*, **5**, 735–49.

Kellogg, E. W. III and I. Fridovich (1975). Superoxide, hydrogen peroxide and singlet oxygen in lipid peroxidation by a xanthine oxidase system. *J. Biol. Chem.*, **250**, 8812–7.

Kety, S. S. (1956). Human cerebral blood flow and oxygen consumption as related to aging. *J. Chron. Dis.*, **3**, 478–86.

Kety, S. S., B. D. King, S. M. Horvath, W. A. Feffers, and J. H. Hafhenschiel (1950). The effects of an acute reduction in blood pressure by means of differential spinal sympathetic block on the cerebral circulation of hypertensive patients. *J. Clin. Invest.*, **29**, 402–7.

Klatzo, I., H. Wisnieski, and F. Streicher (1965). Experimental production of neurofibrillary degeneration. 1. Light microscope observations. *J. Neuropathol. Exp. Neurol.*, **24**, 187–99.

Koenig, H. (1969). Lysosomes. In A. Lajtha (Ed.) *Handbook of Neurochemistry*, Vol. II, Plenum Press, New York. pp. 255–301.

Korey, S. R. and M. Orchen (1959). Relative respiration of neuronal and glial cells. *J. Neurochem.*, **3**, 277–85.

Lassen, N. A. (1959). Cerebral blood flow and oxygen consumption in man. *Physiol. Rev.*, **39**, 183–238.

Lassen, N. A., I Feinberg, and M. H. Lane (1960). Bilateral studies of cerebral oxygen uptake in young and aged normal subjects and in patients with organic dementia. *J. Clin. Invest.*, **39**, 491–500.

Levy, D. E., J. B. Brierley, D. G. Silverman, and F. Plum (1975). Brain hypoxia initially damages cerebral neurons. *Arch. Neurol. (Chicago)*, **32**, 450–5.

Lewis, L. D., B. Ljunggren, K. Norberg, and B. K. Siesjö (1974a). Changes in carbohydrate substrates, amino acids and ammonia in the brain during insulin-induced hypoglycemia. *J. Neurochem.*, **23**, 659–71.

Lewis, L. D., B. Ljunggren, R. A. Ratcheson, and B. K. Siesjö (1974b). Cerebral energy state in insulin-induced hypoglycemia, related to blood glucose and to EEG. *J. Neurochem.*, **23**, 673–9.

Little, C. and P. J. O'Brien (1968). An intracellular GSH-peroxidase with a lipid peroxide substrate. *Biochem. Biophys. Res. Commun.*, **31**, 145–50.

Ljunggren, B., K. Norberg, and B. K. Siesjö (1974). Influence of tissue acidosis upon restitution of brain energy metabolism following total ischemia. *Brain Res.*, **77**, 173–86.

Lowry, O. H. (1957). Enzyme concentrations in individual nerve cell bodies. In D. Richter (Ed.) *Metabolism of the Nervous System*, Pergamon Press, London. pp. 323–8.

Luft, U. C. (1965). Aviation physiology—the effects of altitude. In W. O. Fenn and H. Rahn (Eds) *Handbook of Physiology*, Vol. II, American Physiological Society, Washington. pp. 1099–145.

Marks, N. and A. Lajtha (1971). Protein and polypeptide breakdown. In A. Lajtha (Ed.) *Handbook of Neurochemistry*, Vol. V, Part A, Plenum Press, New York. pp. 49–139.

May, H. E. and P. B. McCay (1968). Reduced triphosphopyridine nucleotide oxidase-catalyzed alterations of membrane phospholipids. II. Enzymic properties and stoichiometry. *J. Biol. Chem.*, **243**, 2296–305.

May, H. E., J. L. Poyer, and P. B. McCay (1965). Lipid alterations occurring in microsomes during the enzymic oxidation of TPNH. *Biochem. Biophys. Res. Commun.*, **19**, 166–70.

Mead, J. F. (1976). Free radical mechanisms of lipid damage and consequences for cellular membranes. In W. A. Pryor (Ed.) *Free Radicals in Biology*, Academic Press, New York. pp. 51–68.

Meldrum, B. S. and J. B. Brierley (1973). Prolonged epileptic seizures in primates: ischemic cell change and its relation to ictal physiological events. *Arch. Neurol. (Chicago)*, **28**, 10–7.

Meldrum, B. S. and B. Nilsson (1976). Cerebral blood flow and metabolic rate early and late in prolonged seizures induced in rats by bicuculline. *Brain*, **99**, 523–42.

Meldrum, B. S., R. A. Vigouroux, and J. B. Brierley (1973). Systemic factors and epileptic brain damage. Prolonged seizures in paralyzed, artificially ventilated baboons. *Arch. Neurol. (Chicago)*, **29**, 82–7.

Michenfelder, J. D. and J. H. Milde (1975). Influence of anesthetics on metabolic, functional and pathological responses to regional cerebral ischemia. *Stroke*, **6**, 405–10.

Miller, J. R. and R. E. Myers (1970). Neurological effects of systemic circulatory arrest in the monkey. *Neurology (Minneap.)*, **20**, 715–24.

Myers, R. E. (1977). Experimental models of perinatal brain damage: relevance to human pathology. In L. Gluck (Ed.) *Intrauterine Asphyxia and the Developing Fetal Brain*, Year Book Medical Publishers, New York. pp. 37–97.

Myers, R. E. and M. Yamaguchi (1976). Effects of serum glucose concentration on brain response to circulatory arrest. *J. Neuropath. Exp. Neurol.*, **35**, 301.

Neely, W. A. and J. R. Youmans (1963). Anoxia of canine brain without damage. *J.A.M.A*, **183**, 1085–7.

Nilsson, B. and B. K. Siesjö (1976). A method for determining blood flow and oxygen consumption in the rat brain. *Acta Physiol. Scand.*, **96**, 72–82.

Norberg, K. and B. K. Siesjö (1975a). Cerebral metabolism in hypoxic hypoxia. I. Pattern of activation of glycolysis; a re-evaluation. *Brain Res.*, **86**, 31–44.

Norberg, K. and B. K. Siesjö (1975b). Cerebral metabolism in hypoxic hypoxia. II. Citric acid cycle intermediates and associated amino acids. *Brain Res.*, **86**, 45–54.

Norberg, K. and B. K. Siesjö (1976). Oxidative metabolism of the cerebral cortex of the rat in insulin-induced hypoglycemia. *J. Neurochem.*, **26**, 345–52.

Nordström, C.-H., S. Rehncrona, and B. K. Siesjö (1978). Effects of phenobarbital in cerebral ischemia. II. Restitution of cerebral energy state, as well as of glycolytic metabolites, citric acid cycle intermediates and associated amino acids after pronounced incomplete ischemia. *Stroke*, **9**, 335–43.

Orlowski, M. and A. Karkowsky (1976). Glutathione metabolism and some possible functions of glutathione in the nervous system. *Int. Rev. Neurobiol. (New York)*, **19**, 75–121.

Otis, A. B., H. Rahn, M. A. Epstein, and W. O. Fenn (1946). Performance as related to composition of alveolar air. *Amer. J. Physiol.*, **146**, 207–21.

Plum, F. and T. E. Duffy (1975). The couple between cerebral metabolism and blood flow during seizures. In D. H. Ingvar and N. A. Lassen (Eds) *Brain Work, Alfred Benzon Symposium VIII*, Munksgaard, Copenhagen. pp. 197–214.

Plum, F., J. B. Posner, and B. Troy (1968). Cerebral metabolic and circulatory responses to induced convulsions in animals. *Arch. Neurol. (Chicago)*, **18**, 1–13.

Pryor, W. A. (1976). The role of free radical reactions in biological systems. In W. A. Pryor (Ed.) *Free Radicals in Biology*, Academic Press, New York. pp. 1–49.

Recknagel, R. O. and A. K. Ghoshal (1966). Lipoperoxidation as a vector in carbon tetrachloride hepatotoxicity. *Lab. Invest.*, **15**, 132–45.

Rehncrona, S., J. Folbergrova, D. S. Smith and B. K. Siesjö (1980a). Influence of complete and pronounced incomplete cerebral ischemia and subsequent recirculation on cortical concentrations of oxidized and reduced glutathione in the rat. *J. Neurochem.*, **34** (4).

Rehncrona, S., L. Mela, and B. K. Siesjö (1979). Recovery of brain mitochondrial function in the rat after complete and incomplete cerebral ischemia. *Stroke.* **10**, 437–446.

Rehncrona, S., D. S. Smith, B. Åkesson, E. Westerberg and B. K. Siesjö (1980b). Peroxidative changes in brain cortical fatty acids and phospholipids, as characterized during Fe^{++} – and ascorbic acid-stimulated lipid peroxidation *in vitro. J. Neurochem.*, (In Press).

Salford, L. G., F. Plum, and J. B. Brierley (1973). Graded hypoxia-oligemia in rat brain. II. Neuropathological alterations and their implications. *Arch. Neurol.*, **29**, 234–8.

Salford, L. G., F. Plum, and B. K. Siesjö (1973). Graded hypoxia-oligemia in rat brain. I. Biochemical alterations and their implications. *Arch. Neurol.*, **29**, 227–33.

Salford, L. G. and B. K. Siesjö (1974). The influence of arterial hypoxia and unilateral carotid artery occlusion upon regional blood flow and metabolism in the rat brain. *Acta Physiol. Scand.*, **92**, 130–41.

Samuelsson, B. (1972). Biosynthesis of prostaglandins. *Fed. Proc.*, **31**, 1442–50.

Samuelsson, B. (1976). Introduction: New trends in prostaglandin research. In B. Samuelsson and R. Paoletti (Eds) *Advances in Prostaglandin and Thromboxane Research*, Vol. I, Raven Press, New York.

Schadé, J. P. and W. H. McMenemey (Eds) (1963). *Selective Vulnerability of the Brain in Hypoxaemia*, Blackwell, Oxford.

Scheibel, A. B. (1978). Structural aspects of the aging brain: Spine systems and the dendritic arbor. In R. Katzman, R. D. Terry and K. L. Bick (Eds) *Alzheimers's Disease: Senile Dementia and Related Disorders (Aging*, Vol. 7), Raven Press, New York. pp. 353–73.

Scheinberg, P. (1950). Cerebral blood flow in vascular disease of the brain. *Amer. J. Med.*, **8**, 139–47.

Siesjö, B. K. (Ed.) (1978). *Brain Energy Metabolism*, John Wiley, London.

Siesjö B. K. and A. Abdul-Rahman (1979a). Delayed hypoperfusion in the cerebral cortex of the rat in the recovery period following severe hypoglycemia. *Acta Physiol. Scand.* **106**, 375–376.

Siesjö, B. K. and A. Abdul-Rahman (1979b). A metabolic basis for the selective vulnerability of neurons in status epilepticus. *Acta Physiol. Scand.* **106**, 377–378.

Siesjö, B. K., H. Jóhansson, B. Ljunggren, and K. Norberg (1974). Brain dysfunction in cerebral hypoxia and ischemia. In F. Plum (Ed.) *Brain Dysfunction in Metabolic Disorders*, Res. Publ. Assoc. Nerv. Ment. Dis., Vol. 53, Raven Press, New York. pp. 75–112.

Siesjö, B. K., H. Jóhansson, K. Norberg, and L. G. Salford (1975). Brain function, metabolism and blood flow in moderate and severe arterial hypoxia. In D. H. Ingvar and N. A. Lassen (Eds) *Brain Work, Alfred Benzon Symposium VIII*, Munksgaard, Copenhagen. pp. 101–5.

Siesjö, B. K. and F. Plum (1973). Pathophysiology of anoxic brain damage. In G. E. Gaull (Ed.) Biology of Cerebral Dysfunction, Vol. I, Plenum Press, New York. pp. 319–72.

Singh, A. (1969). Acute mountain sickness. *New Engl. J. Med.*, **280**, 175–84.

Slater, T. F. (1972). *Free Radical Mechanisms in Tissue Injury*, Pion, London.

Smith, A. L., J. T. Hoff, S. L. Nielsen, and C. P. Larson (1974). Barbiturate protection in acute focal cerebral ischemia. *Stroke*, **5**, 1–7.

Smith, D. S., S. Rehncrona, E. Westerberg, B. Åkesson, and B. K. Siesjö (1979). Lipid peroxidation in brain tissue *in vitro*: antioxidant effects of barbiturates. *Acta Physiol. Scand.* **105**, 527–529.

Sokoloff, L. (1966). Cerebral circulatory and metabolic changes associated with aging. *Res. Publ. Assoc. Res. Nerv. Mental Dis.*, **41**, 237–54.

Sokoloff, L. (1978). Mapping cerebral functional activity with radioactive deoxyglucose. *T.I.N.S.*, **Sept.**, 75–9.

Sokoloff, L., M. Reivich, C. Kennedy, M. H. Des Rosiers, C. S. Patlak, K. D. Pettigrew, D. Sakurada, and M. Shinohara (1977). The [^{14}C]deoxyglucose method for the measurement of local cerebral glucose utilization: theory, procedure, and normal values in the conscious and anesthetized albino rat. *J. Neurochem.*, **28**, 879–916.

Swanson, P. D. (1969). Acidosis and some metabolic properties of isolated cerebral tissues. *Arch. Neurol. (Chicago)*, **20**, 653–63.

Tappel, A. L. (1968). Will antioxidant nutrients slow aging processes? *Geriatrics.*, **Oct.**, 97–105.

Tappel, A. L. (1975). Lipid peroxidation and fluorescent molecular damage to membranes. In B. F. Trump and A. V. Arstila (Eds) *Pathobiology of Cell Membranes*, Vol. I, Academic Press, New York. pp. 145–70.

Terry, R. D. (1976). Morphology of the aging brain. In P. Scheinberg (Ed.) *Cerebrovascular Diseases. Tenth Princeton Conference*, Raven Press, New York. pp. 351–6.

Terry, R. D. (1978a). Ultrastructural alterations in senile dementia. In R. Katzman, R. D. Terry, and K. L. Dick (Eds) *Alzheimer's Disease: Senile Dementia and Related Disorders (Aging*, Vol. 7), Raven Press, New York. pp. 375–82.

Terry, R. D. (1978b). Aging, senile dementia, and Alzheimer's disease. In R. Katzman, R. D. Terry, and K. L. Bick (Eds) *Alzheimer's Disease: Senile Dementia and Related Disorders (Aging*, Vol. 7), Raven Press, New York. pp. 11–4.

Tomlinson, B. E., G. Blessed, and M. Roth (1970). Observations on the brains of demented old people. *J. Neurol. Sci.*, **11**, 205–42.

Tower, D. B. (1978). Alzheimer's disease—senile dementia and related disorders: neurobiological status. In R. Katzman, R. D. Terry, and K. L. Bick (Eds) *Alzheimer's Disease: Senile Dementia and Related Disorders (Aging*, Vol. 7), Raven Press, New York. pp. 1–4.

Tower, D. B. and O. M. Young (1973). Interspecies correlations of cerebral cortical oxygen consumption, acetylcholinesterase activity and chloride content: studies on the brains of the fin whale (*Balaenophera physalus*) and the sperm whale (*Physeter catodon*). *J. Neurochem.*, **20**, 253–67.

Wasterlain, C. G. (1974). Mortality and morbidity from serial seizures: an experimental study. *Epilepsia*, **15**, 155–76.

Welsh, F. A., M. D. Ginsberg, W. Rieder, and W. W. Budd (1978). Impairment of metabolic recovery from cerebral ischemia by prior administration of glucose. *Fed. Proc.* (Abstr.), **37**, 873.

Westerberg, E., B. Åkesson, S. Rehncrona, D. S. Smith, and B. K. Siesjö (1979). Lipid peroxidation in brain tissue *in vitro*: effects on phospholipids and fatty acids. *Acta Physiol. Scand.* **105**, 524–526.

Widemann, J. and K. Domańska-Janik (1974). Regulations of thiols in the brain. I. Concentrations of thiols and glutathione reductase activity in different parts of the rat brain during hypoxia. *Resuscitation*, **3**, 27–36.

Biochemistry of Dementia
Edited by P. J. Roberts
© 1980, John Wiley & Sons Ltd.

Chapter 7

Brain Carbohydrate Metabolism and Dementias

J. P. BLASS, G. E. GIBSON,

*The Dementia Research Service, Department of Neurology,
Cornell University Medical College, at The Burke Rehabilitation Center,
785 Mamaroneck Avenue, White Plains, N.Y. 10605, U.S.A.*

M. SHIMADA, T. KIHARA, M. WATANABE, and K. KURINÏOTO

*Department of Anatomy, Osaka Medical College, 2–7 Daigakumachi, Takatuski
City, Osaka 569, Japan*

A variety of biochemical and anatomical abnormalities of the brain can impair memory and other higher integrative functions, and lead to the abnormal behaviour we label 'demented' (Wells, 1977). Decreases of cerebral carbohydrate oxidation have been among the earliest, most characteristic, and best-documented metabolic alterations in dementia (Sokoloff, 1966).

Several lines of evidence can be brought together to support the significance of these abnormalities in carbohydrate oxidation. Firstly, they occur. In dementias, and specifically in senile dementia of the Alzheimer type, there are typically falls in cerebral blood flow (CBF), oxygen uptake (CMR_{O_2}), and glucose utilization (CMR_{GL}). Secondly, cerebral hypoxia—even mild cerebral hypoxia—characteristically impairs higher integrative functions including memory, learning, and judgment. Other conditions which reduce cerebral carbohydrate utilization have similar effects. Thirdly, impairing cerebral carbohydrate oxidation impairs the synthesis of a number of putative neurotransmitters, notably of acetylcholine. Finally, abnormalities of cholinergic and other neurotransmitter systems appear to be common in, and perhaps characteristic of, certain types of dementias. However, which of these changes are cause and which are effect remains to be clarified.

121

I. CEREBRAL CARBOHYDRATE OXIDATION IN DEMENTIAS

Shortly after they introduced techniques to measure CBF, CMR_{O_2} and CMR_{GL} in living humans, Kety and Sokoloff and their coworkers reported decreases in these activities in older patients with dementias (Freyhan, Woodford, and Kety, 1951). These decreases occurred in both senile dementia of the Alzheimer type (SDAT) and in what would now be called multi-infarct dementias (Sokoloff, 1966). While there were discrepancies in individual patients, overall there was a good correlation between the fall in CMR_{O_2} and clinical state (Table 1).

Table 1. CMR_{O_2} in Dementias

	CMR_{O_2} (ml per 100 g per min)
Normal young	3.5
Paranoid, chronic brain syndrome	3.4
Aged, non-senile quality	3.3
Normal aged	3.3
Aged, senile quality	3.0
Aged, extreme senile quality	2.7
Chronic brain syndrome with psychosis and arteriosclerosis	2.7
Chronic brain syndrome	2.4
Pre-senile dementia	2.4

Data are from Butler (1966), which gives the clinical and experimental details.

These results have been extensively confirmed (Sokoloff, 1966). Lassen, Feinberg, and Lane (1960) reported that performance correlated better with metabolic rate in the dominant than in the non-dominant hemisphere. Ingvar, Risberg, Gustafson and their coworkers have even attempted to use regional decrements in blood flow in the diagnosis of different types of dementia (Ingvar and Gustafson, 1970; Obrist and coworkers, 1970; Risberg, 1979). The current state of CBF and CMR_{O_2} measurements in evaluating dementias is reviewed elsewhere in this volume (Chapters 4 and 6).

II. MENTAL FUNCTION IN HYPOXIA

The profound dependence of the brain on a continuous supply of oxygen has been recognized at least since the days of Lavoisier and Priestly. Furthermore, since the 1930s it has been widely appreciated that even mild hypoxia can profoundly impair memory and other higher integrative functions. Detailed observations were supported by the military of many countries, who realized that the performance of warplanes in the Second World War would otherwise be limited not by the hardware but by the supply of oxygen and blood to the brains of the pilots (Luft, 1965). Reduction of the percentage of O_2 in inspired air to 12–15 % impairs critical judgment, short-term memory and the ability to learn a complex task (Luft, 1965; Siesjö and coworkers, 1974). Other conditions which can impair cerebral oxidative metabolism in a graded fashion have similar effects; these include, among many other conditions, hypoglycaemia and thiamine deficiency (Williams and coworkers, (1940); Blass and Gibson, 1976a, 1976b, 1976c). The neurochemistry of graded hypoxia and related conditions is discussed in detail by Siesjö and Rehncrona in Chapter 6. Two essential points need to be repeated here. The major substrate of cerebral oxidation under normal circumstances is glucose, which is converted to pyruvate by glycolysis and oxidized in the Krebs tricarboxylic acid cycle, and normally accounts for virtually all of the oxygen taken up by the brain. Milder impairments of cerebral oxidative metabolism, which profoundly impair higher integrative functions, do not impair the supply of energy in the brain, as measured by the levels of ATP and other 'high-energy compounds' or by the ability of the tissue to maintain osmotic gradients for Na^+ (Ingvar and Lassen, 1975; Yatsu, Lee and Liao, 1975). Thus, the confusion and loss of judgment which accompany milder impairments of cerebral oxidative metabolism cannot be explained as a 'power failure' (Blass and Gibson, 1976a, 1976b).

III. NEUROTRANSMITTERS AND CARBOHYDRATE METABOLISM

A number of studies have appeared within the last decade which indicate that graded impairments of cerebral carbohydrate catabolism impair the synthesis of a number of neurotransmitters including, particularly, acetylcholine (Blass and Gibson, 1979a, 1979b, 1979c). These studies support the proposal that synapses are often more sensitive to metabolic insults than are other parts of the brain (Kety, 1974). This proposal implies that the *functional* abnormalities associated with mild hypoxia result from 'neurotransmitter failure', at least in part.

Acetylcholine synthesis has been demonstrated to be tightly linked to carbohydrate utilization *in vitro*, *in vivo*, and in physiological studies. The mechanism of the linkage involves compartmentation of glucose and pyruvate catabolism with respect to acetylcholine metabolism.

In vitro, Quastel and coworkers (Quastel, Tennenbaum, and Wheatley, 1936; Mann and Quastel, 1940) reported that acetylcholine synthesis is impaired in conditions which impair respiration, and related the deficit to impaired pyruvate catabolism. The significance of that observation has only recently been generally recognized (Blass and Gibson, 1979a). It was soon established that the normal physiological source of the acetyl moiety of cerebral acetylcholine is acetyl-coenzyme A, produced by oxidation of pyruvate, but less than 1 % of the pyruvate oxidized is incorporated into acetylcholine. It was therefore widely assumed that only the most profound impairments of cerebral carbohydrate oxidation—impairments profound enough to stop almost everything—would impair the synthesis of acetylcholine.

However, Gibson, Jope, and Blass (1975) demonstrated in brain slices that impairment of pyruvate oxidation lead to proportional impairment of acetylcholine synthesis, even if the impairment is less than 10 % (Fig. 1). This proportionality held whether pyruvate oxidation was inhibited by 3-bromopyruvate, a non-competitive inhibitor of the pyruvate dehydrogenase complex (PDHC), which oxidizes pyruvate to acetyl-coenzyme A; by 2-oxobutyrate, a

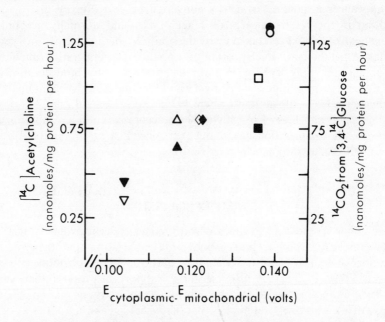

Figure 1. Proportionality between oxidation and acetylcholine synthesis in rat brain slices. Rat brain slices were incubated with $[U-{}^{14}C]$glucose and the production of ${}^{14}CO_2$ and acetylcholine measured. Note that both the production of acetylcholine (left vertical axis and open symbols) and of ${}^{14}CO_2$ (right vertical axis and closed symbols) were proportional to transmitochondrial potentials, and therefore also proportional to each other. Transmitochondrial potentials were calculated from the lactate dehydrogenase (LDH) and glutamate dehydrogenase (GDH) potentials. For experimental details and explicit statements of the assumptions involved, see Gibson and Blass (1976c). For discussion of the difficulties in using GDH potentials in brain, see Berntman and Siesjö (1978) and Dennis and Clark (1978). o, Control; $\triangle$, flasks flushed with N_2; ∇, cyanide; $\Diamond$, low glucose; $\square$, amobarbital. Open symbols, acetylcholine; solid symbols, ${}^{14}CO_2$

competitive inhibitor and alternate substrate of PDHC; by barbiturates or cyanide, which presumably act on the electron transport system (Gibson, Jope, and Blass, 1975); by the branched-chain 2-oxoacids, which inhibit the tricarboxylic acid cycle probably primarily by competitive inhibition of the 2-oxoglutarate dehydrogenase complex (Gibson and Blass, 1976a); or by reducing the glucose or oxygen in the media (Gibson and Blass, 1976c). Ketone bodies, which are alternate substrates for brain, reduced the synthesis of acetylcholine from glucose to the extent that they reduced the utilization of glucose in other processes (Gibson and Blass, 1979). The proportionality held whether the substrate was glucose or pyruvate, and whether the synthesis of acetylcholine was measured by following the incorporation of labelled precursors of the accumulation of total acetylcholine, determined by gas–liquid chromatography–mass spectrometry.

The tight linkage between acetylcholine synthesis and carbohydrate oxidation has also been found in synaptosomes by several groups (Barker, Mittag, and Krespan, 1977; Jope, Weiler, and Jenden, 1978; Lefresne, Beaujouan, and Glowinski, 1978a, 1978b).

In vivo, impairment of cerebral carbohydrate oxidation also lead to proportional decreases in the synthesis of acetylcholine from either radioactive glucose or deuterated choline (Gibson and Blass, 1976c; Gibson, Shimada and Blass, 1979). This proportionality held whether cerebral carbohydrate metabolism was impaired by reducing the oxygen-carrying capacity of the blood with $NaNO_2$ (anaemic hypoxia), by inhibiting cytochrome-c oxidase with cyanide (histotoxic hypoxia), by reducing the oxygen content of inspired air (hypoxic hypoxia), or by hypoglycaemia induced by large doses of insulin. It held whether acetylcholine synthesis was followed from glucose or from choline, and in both rats and mice.

Furthermore, the depression in acetylcholine synthesis occurred with mild

Table 2. Acetylcholine synthesis in hypoxic hypoxia

	Control	15 % O_2	12 % O_2
Neocortex	7.8 ±0.05	8.6 ±0.09	2.7 ±0.04*
Hippocampus	5.7 ±0.8	4.5 ±0.7	0.35 ±0.07*
Striatum	14 ±1	15 ±1	13 ±1
Septum	13 ±1	10 ±2	5.5 ±0.6*

Adult mice were exposed to various concentrations of O_2 in N_2 at sea level; controls breathed room air (21 % O_2). Animals were injected with [U-^{14}C]glucose and sacrificed by microwave irradiation, and acetylcholine metabolism studied using gas–liquid chromatography–mass spectrometry and radiochemical methods, as described previously (Gibson, Blass, and Jenden, 1978). Original data and methods are in Shimada and coworkers (1979).
Values are dpm/mg protein ±S.E.M.
* $p < 0.01$.

hypoxia. Reducing the oxygen content of inspired air (Shimada and coworkers, 1979) to 12 % reduced acetylcholine synthesis in mouse hippocampus to less than 10 % of normal (Table 2). As noted, this level of hypoxia impairs performance but not consciousness or gross motor behaviour. The changes in acetylcholine synthesis occur with hypoxia so mild that there are no significant changes in the levels of ATP, ADP, AMP, cyclic-AMP, or lactate (Gibson, Shimada, and Blass, 1978), all of which have been used as indicators of cerebral hypoxia. The only neurochemical change other than that in acetylcholine, which has been identified in these animals, is a doubling of the concentration of cyclic-GMP (Fig. 2). The significance of that alteration is not clear, since the $NaNO_2$ or KCN used to induce hypoxia in those animals can stimulate guanylate cyclase directly (Kimura, Mittal, and Murad, 1975; Gibson, Blass, and Jenden, 1978). Another possibility is that there is a slight rise in free fatty acids under these conditions, and that they stimulate cyclic-GMP formation (Asakawa and coworkers, 1978).

Physiological and pharmacological experiments support the significance of the impairment of acetylcholine synthesis which accompanies impaired carbohydrate oxidation. In extensive studies of superior cervical ganglia from rats,

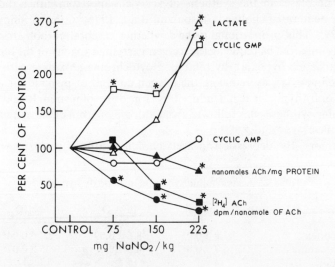

Figure 2. Sensitivity of Acetylcholine synthesis to mild anaemic hypoxia in mouse brain *in vivo*. Adult mice were injected with [U-^{14}C]glucose and [$^2H_4$]choline intravenously, after the induction of anaemic hypoxia by s.c. injection of $NaNO_2$. The synthesis of acetylcholine and the levels of a number of other metabolites were measured. Note that the *levels* of total brain acetylcholine remained normal under conditions where the incorporation of precursors fell. Experimental details and complete data are in Gibson, Blass, and Jenden (1978)

Dolivo (1974) demonstrated that removing glucose or oxygen from the incubation media severely impaired transmission across the cholinergic synapse, while axonal conduction remained intact. The transmission failure was associated with the loss of pre-synaptic vesicles known to contain acetylcholine. The response of the post-synaptic membrane to added acetylcholine remained intact. In analogous studies, Perri, Sacchi, and Casella (1970) demonstrated that ganglia from thiamine-deficient rats lost the ability to transmit impulses across the cholinergic synapse in response to rapid stimulation (20 Hz) while the response to slow stimulation (2 Hz) remained intact, as did axonal conduction. They attributed the deficit in rapid transmission to deficient acetylcholine synthesis and subsequently confirmed that suggestion by direct measurement (Sacchi and coworkers, 1978).

Pharmacological experiments have shown that pre-treatment with appropriate doses of the cholinesterase inhibitor, physostigmine, could delay seizures or death in hypoxia and prevent death from hypoglycaemia (Gibson and Blass, 1976c). The protective effect was not due to slower absorption of the agents used to induce hypoxia or hypoglycaemia since brain glucose and methaemoglobin concentrations were not altered by physostigmine. Interpreting the protective effect in detail is difficult. Physostigmine has peripheral as well as central effects, and a host of agents of many pharmacological types ameliorate the effects of hypoxia (Cohen, 1973; Berlet, 1974). Furthermore, the levels of acetylcholine can remain constant under conditions where the incorporation of precursors falls markedly. The change in synthetic rate may, therefore, reflect a decrease in utilization secondary to a decrease in firing rate, rather than a direct limitation of the capacity of the cells to synthesize this transmitter.

Mechanisms linking acetylcholine synthesis to carbohydrate oxidation have been studied.

Compartmentation of glucose and pyruvate metabolism with respect to acetylcholine synthesis has been shown directly (Gibson, Blass, and Jenden, 1978). The pathway is known to be, in outline:

$$\text{glucose} \longrightarrow \text{pyruvate} \longrightarrow \text{acetylcholine}$$

When mice were injected i.v. with [U-^{14}C]glucose and the specific activity of glucose, pyruvate, and acetylcholine in the brain followed, there was a typical precursor–product relationship between glucose and acetylcholine, but the specific activity of pyruvate never reached that of acetylcholine (Fig. 3). This observation (higher specific activity in a product than in its precursor) is the conventional criterion for demonstration of metabolic compartmentation. This result agrees with extensive studies by Tucek and Cheng (1974), indicating compartmentation of pyruvate metabolism in the brain (Cheng, Kumar, and Casella, 1972; Cheng and Brunner, 1978). It also agrees with experiments with synaptosomes by Lefresne, Beaujouan, and Glowinski (1978a, 1978b), indicating that pyruvate or glucose can be preferentially used for acetylcholine synthesis

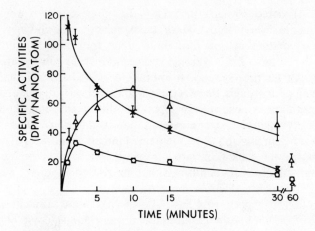

Figure 3. Compartmentation of glucose and pyruvate metabolism with respect to acetylcholine synthesis. Adult mice were injected with [*U*-¹⁴C]glucose intravenously, and the specific activities of glucose (×), pyruvate (O), and acetylcholine (△) were measured as described in detail in Gibson Blass, and Jenden (1978). (Reprinted by permission of the Editor of the *Journal of Neurochemistry*)

or for oxidation, depending on the exact experimental conditions chosen.

The cellular mechanisms responsible for this compartmentation are not known in detail. Lefresne, Beaujouan, and Glowinski (1978a, 1978b) have proposed that there is a PDHC located extramitochondrially which is specifically involved in acetylcholine synthesis. However, the kinetic data cited to support this attractive hypothesis can also be interpreted in other ways. Nestorescu, Siess, and Wieland (1973) have proposed that there is a proportion of PDHC in the outer mitochondrial space, on the basis of electron microscopic evidence of pyruvate-dependent $Fe(CN)_3{}^{6+}$ reduction there. A correlation has been reported between changes in NAD/NADH ratios and acetylcholine synthesis (Gibson and Blass, 1976b, 1976c; Blass and Gibson, 1979c). Although there was a relatively high correlation with cytoplasmic $NADH/NAD^+$ potentials (calculated from the lactate dehydrogenase equilibrium), the closest correlation was with transmitochondrial potentials (Figure 1). Indeed, impaired neurological function in a variety of neurometabolic disorders could be correlated with falls in transmitochondrial potentials (Blass and Gibson, 1979c). However, this calculation requires the use of the glutamate dehydrogenase potential to calculate mitochondrial NADH/NAD potentials. That calculation is questionable (Berntman & Siesjö, 1978; Dennis and Clark, 1978). Furthermore, the mechanism by which the acetylcoenzyme A, produced from pyruvate oxidation, reaches the cytoplasmic enzyme which synthesizes acetylcholine has not been established unequivocally. Current proposals include, among others, that the carrier from mitochondria to cytoplasm is citrate (Sollenberg and Sorbö, 1970; Sterling and O'Neill, 1978), something else (Gibson and Shimada, 1977; Pollack, Molenaar, and Braggar-Schaap, 1977), or that no carrier is needed (Lefresne, Beaujouan, and Glowinski, 1978a, 1978b). Once this neurochemical problem is solved, it should be possible to propose and test discrete mechanisms which might link oxidation and acetylcholine synthesis. For instance, PDHC is known to be inhibited by NADH, so increases in the cytoplasmic NADH/NAD ratio could be invoked to inhibit a cytoplasmic PDHC, if that were proven to exist. Until the intermediate(s) are identified, proposals about control mechanisms are likely to remain conjectural.

Amino acids, which are putative neurotransmitters, have not been studied in graded hypoxia in as much detail as acetylcholine has, but their synthesis does appear to be impaired when carbohydrate catabolism is impaired. This result is expected, since they are typically derived metabolically from tricarboxylic acid cycle intermediates. Indeed, glucose can preferentially label the neurotransmitter pool of amino acids (Berl, Clarke, and Schneider, 1974). Yoshino and Elliot (1970) demonstrated that the synthesis of glutamate, aspartate, and γ-aminobutyric acid (GABA) from [U-^{14}C]glucose was reduced when rats were exposed to 5 % O_2 (Table 3).

Table 3. Hypoxia and amino acids
(from Yoshino and Elliot, 1970)

Amino acid	Specific activity (dpm μg^{-1})	
	Normal	Hypoxic
Alanine	872	483*
Glutamate	479	173†
Aspartate	552	254†
GABA	432	155†

Adult rats were exposed to 5 % O_2 in N_2 and the incorporation of [U-^{14}C]glucose into amino acids was measured.
* $p < 0.01$; † $p < 0.001$.

Fluorocitrate, which inhibits the tricarboxylic acid cycle by its action on citrate synthase, impairs the synthesis of amino acids in the brain (Clarke, Nicklas, and Berl, 1970; Patel and Koenig, 1971; Cheng, Kumar, and Casella, 1972). Thiamine deficiency also alters amino acid metabolism (Gaitonde and Nixey, 1974; Gaitonde, Fayein, and Johnson, 1975). The metabolism of amino acids in the brain is complex and compartmentalized (Berl, Clarke, and Schneider, 1974), and the effects of graded hypoxia on the putative transmitter amino acids deserves further detailed and direct studies.

Catecholamine and 5-hydroxytryptamine (5HT) synthesis is impaired by mild hypoxia under some but not all experimental conditions (Davis and Carlsson, 1973; Brown, Kehr, and Carlsson, 1975; Carlsson, 1978). The hydroxylases involved in the biosyntheses of these compounds utilize molecular oxygen, and their K_m for O_2 is close to the physiological Po_2 of brain. However, thiamine deficiency, which does not alter the Po_2 of brain, does impair metabolism of catecholamines (Iwata, 1976) and 5HT (Pliatakis, Nicklas, and Berl, 1978). Furthermore, catechols can alter cerebral carbohydrate metabolism. For instance, stimulation of the nigra can activate phosphorylase specifically in the ipsilateral striatum (Anchors and Garcia-Rill, 1977). The interactions between cerebral carbohydrate and catechol and 5HT metabolism are complex, and deserve further investigation.

IV. NEUROTRANSMITTERS IN DEMENTIA

Demonstrations of abnormalities in cholinergic and other neurotransmitter systems in dementias are discussed in detail by Perry and Gottfries in Chapters 8 and 10, respectively. However, it is worth stressing here that in human dementias, as in experimental studies, correlations can be drawn between impairments of cerebral oxidative metabolism and impairments of neurotransmitter systems.

V. IMPLICATIONS

In analysing the relations between brain metabolism and neurotransmitters, a major problem lies in separating primary from secondary events. A variety of insults have been demonstrated to alter brain metabolism or neurotransmitter function, or both (Plum, 1974; Ingvar and Lassen, 1975). There is even a report that slow virus infection damages cholinergic systems (McDermott, Fraser, and Dickinson, 1978). As indicated above, impairing carbohydrate catabolism impairs the synthesis of acetylcholine and other putative neurotransmitters. On the other hand, it is known that the metabolic rate of neurons depends in part on their rate of firing, so that impairments of neurotransmitter function might be expected to alter overall brain metabolism. Indeed, from one viewpoint the function of neurons is to manufacture chemicals which alter the firing of other neurons and to excrete them into synaptic clefts. Thus, disorders of brain function, such as dementias, necessarily involve some level of abnormalities in brain metabolism and neurotransmission. The problem is to pin-point which of the changes are critical and so provide a basis for devising better treatments than are now available. Unfortunately, at this point we not only do not know chicken from egg, but also whether or not we are looking at omelettes.

On the other hand, it is encouraging that the changes in brain metabolism and in neurotransmitters which have been reported in dementias can be related to each other. Presumably, the pathophysiological processes involve a chain of related events. If analogies with other areas of medicine hold, breaking one of these links may ameliorate many of the other changes. For instance, it is conceivable that treatment directed to substitution of a deficient neurotransmitter might increase the metabolism of the cells normally stimulated by that transmitter, and be reflected in increases in overall brain metabolism. Similarly, effective treatment of metabolic impairments could be expected to improve the ability of the sick cells to manufacture and secrete neurotransmitters. The little relevant data available support these ideas. If analogies with other areas of medicine again hold, then identification of pathophysiological events and of their inter-relations should increase our understanding of these disorders. That knowledge should increase the precision of diagnosis, make possible more precise counselling, and perhaps even allow more effective treatments, whatever the primary events which lead to these devastating disorders turn out to be.

ACKNOWLEDGMENTS

Supported by grants from the N.I.H. (NS–15125) and from the Winifred Masterton Burke Relief Foundation.

REFERENCES

Anchors, J. M. and E. Garcia-Rill (1977). Dopamine, a modulator of carbohydrate metabolism in the caudate nucleus. *Brain Res.*, **133**, 183–9.

Asakawa, T., M. Takenoshita, S. Uchida, and S. Tanaka (1978). Activation of guanylate cyclase in synaptic plasma membranes of cerebral cortex by free fatty acids. *J. Neurochem.*, **30**, 161–6.

Barker, L. A., T. W. Mittag, and B. Krespan (1977). Studies on substrates, inhibitors and modifiers of the high affinity choline transport–acetylation system present in rat brain synaptosomes. In D. J. Jenden (Ed.) *Cholinergic Mechanisms and Psychopharmacology*, Plenum Press, New York. pp. 465–80.

Berl, S., D. D. Clarke, and D. Schneider (Eds) (1974). *Metabolic Compartmentation and Neurotransmission*, Plenum Press, New York.

Berlet, H. H. (1974). Effect of 6-aminonicotinamide on the tolerance of mice to hypoxic hypoxia. *Experientia*, **30**, 1065–7.

Berntman, L. and B. K. Siesjö (1978). Cerebral metabolic and circulatory changes induced by hypoxia in starved rats. *J. Neurochem.*, **31**, 1265–76.

Blass, J. P. and G. E. Gibson (1979a). Carbohydrates and acetylcholine synthesis: implications for cognitive disorders. In K. L. Davis and P. A. Berger (Eds) *Brain Acetylcholine and Neuropsychiatric Disease*, Plenum Press, New York. pp 215–236.

Blass, J. P. and G. E. Gibson (1979b). Thiamine and the Wernicke–Korsakoff syndrome. In M. H. Briggs (Ed.) *Vitamins in Human Biology and Medicine*, C.R.C. Press, Miami. In press.

Blass, J. P. and G. E. Gibson (1979c). Consequences of mild, graded hypoxia, *Adv. Neurol.* **26**, 229–253.

Brown, R. M., W. Kehr, and A. Carlsson (1975). Functional and biochemical aspects of catecholamine metabolism in brain under hypoxia. *Brain Res.*, **85**, 491–509.

Butler, R. N. (1966). Psychiatric aspects of cerebrovascular disease in the aged. *Proc. Ass. Res. Nerv. Mental Dis.*, **41**, 255–66.

Carlsson, A. (1978). Effects of low oxygen on brain monoamine metabolism. *Proc. Eur. Soc. Neurochem.*, **1**, 266–70.

Cheng, S. C. and E. A. Brunner (1978). Alteration of tricarboxylic acid cycle metabolism in rat brain slices by halothane. *J. Neurochem.*, **30**, 1421–30.

Cheng, S. C., S. Kumar, and G. A. Casella (1972). Effects of fluoroacetate and fluorocitrate on the metabolic compartmentation of tricarboxylic acid cycle in rat brain slices. *Brain Res.*, **42**, 117–28.

Clarke, D. D., W. J. Nicklas, and S. Berl (1970). Tricarboxylic acid cycle metabolism in brain. Effect of fluoroacetate and fluorocitrate on the labelling of glutamate, aspartate, glutamine, and γ -aminobutyrate. *Biochem. J.*, **120**, 345–51.

Cohen, M. M. (1973). Biochemistry of cerebral anoxia, hypoxia and ischemia. *Monagr. Neurol. Sci.*, **1**, 1–49.

Davis, J. N. and A. Carlsson (1973). Effect of hypoxia on tyrosine and tryptophan hydroxylation in unanesthetized rat brain. *J. Neurochem.*, **20**, 913–5.

Dennis, S. G. C. and J. B. Clark (1978). The synthesis of glutamate by rat brain mitochondria, *J. Neurochem.*, **31**, 673–80.

Dolivo, M. (1974). Metabolism of mammalian sympathetic ganglia. *Fed. Proc.*, **33**, 1043–8.

Freyhan, F. A., R. B. Woodford, and S. S. Kety (1951). Cerebral blood flow and metabolism in psychoses of senility. *J. Nerv. Mental Dis.*, **113**, 449–56.

Gaitonde, M. K., N. A. Fayein, and A. L. Johnson (1975). Decreased metabolism *in vivo* of glucose into amino acids of the brain of thiamine-deficient rats after treatment with pyrithiamine. *J. Neurochem.*, **24**, 1215–23.

Gaitonde, M. K. and R. W. K. Nixey (1974). The effect of deficiency of thiamine on the metabolism of [U-^{14}C]glucose and [U-^{14}C]ribose and the levels of amino acids in rat brain. *J. Neurochem.*, **22**, 53–61.

Gibson, G. E. and J. P. Blass (1976a). Inhibition of acetylcholine synthesis and of carbohydrate utilization by metabolites from maple-syrup-urine-disease. *J. Neurochem.*, **26**, 1073–7.

Gibson, G. E. and J. P. Blass (1976b). A relation between NAD$^+$/NADH potentials and glucose utilization in rat brain slices. *J. Biol. Chem.*, **251**, 4127–30.

Gibson, G. E. and J. P. Blass (1976c). Impaired synthesis of acetylcholine in brain accompanying hypoglycemia and mild hypoxia. *J. Neurochem.*, **27**, 37–42.

Gibson, G. E. and J. P. Blass (1979). Proportional inhibition of acetylcholine synthesis accompanying impairment of 3-hydroxybutyrate oxidation in rat brain slices. *Biochem. Pharmacol.*, **28**, 133–9.

Gibson, G. E., J. P. Blass, and D. J. Jenden (1978). Measurement of acetylcholine turnover using glucose as precursor. Evidence for compartmentation of glucose metabolism in brain. *J. Neurochem.*, **30**, 71–6.

Gibson, G. E., R. Jope, and J. P. Blass (1975). Reduced synthesis of acetylcholine accompanying impaired oxidation of pyruvic acid in rat brain minces. *Biochem. J.*, **148**, 17–29.

Gibson, G. E. and M. Shimada (1977). Studies on the origin of the acetyl moiety of acetylcholine. *Trans. Amer. Soc. Neurochem.*, **8**, 127 (abstract); and for *Biochem. Pharmacol.*, (in press).

Gibson, G. E., M. Shimada, and J. P. Blass (1978). Alterations in acetylcholine synthesis and in cyclic nucleotides in mild cereberal hypoxia. *J. Neurochem.*, **31**, 757–60.

Ingvar, D. H. and L. Gustafson (1970). Regional cerebral blood flow in organic dementia with early onset. *Acta Neurol. Scand.*, **46**, (Suppl. 43), 42–73.

Ingvar, D. H. and N. A. Lassen (Eds) (1975). *Brain Work*, Munksgaard, Copenhagen.

Iwata, H. (1976). Catecholamine metabolism in thiamine-deficient rats. *J. Nutr. Sci. Vitaminol.*, **22** (Suppl.), 25–7.

Jope, R. S., M. H. Weiler, and D. J. Jenden (1978). Regulation of acetylcholine synthesis: control of choline transport and acetylation in synaptosomes. *J. Neurochem.*, **30**, 949–54.

Kety, S. S. (1974). Discussion. In F. Plum (Ed.) *Brain Dysfunction in Metabolic Disorders*, Raven Press, New York. p. 111.

Kimura, H., C. Mittal, and F. Murad (1975). Activation of guanylate cyclase from rat liver and other tissues by sodium azide. *J. Biol. Chem.*, **250**, 8016–22.

Lassen, N. A., I. Feinberg, and M. H. Lane (1960). Bilateral studies of cerebral oxygen uptake in young and aged normal subjects and in patients with organic dementias. *J. Clin. Invest.*, **39**, 491–500.

Lefresne, P., J. C. Beaujouan, and J. Glowinski (1978a). Origin of the acetyl moiety of acetylcholine in rat striatal synaptosomes: a specific pyruvate dehydrogenase involved in acetylcholine synthesis. *Biochimie*, **60**, 479–87.

Lefresne, P., J. C. Beaujouan, and J. Glowinski (1978b). Evidence for extramitochondrial pyruvate dehydrogenase involved in acetylcholine synthesis in nerve endings. *Nature (London)*, **274**, 497–500.

Luft, U. C. (1965). Aviation physiology: the effects of altitude. In W. O. Fenn and K. Rhan (Eds) *Handbook of Physiology—Respiration*. American Physiological Society, Washington, D.C. pp. 1099–1145.

Mann, P. J. G. and J. H. Quastel (1940). Vitamin B_1 and acetylcholine formation in isolated brain. *Nature (London)*, **145**, 856–857.

McDermott, J. R., H. Fraser, and A. G. Dickinson (1978). Reduced choline acetyltransferase activity in scrapie mouse brain. *Lancet*, **2**, 318–9.

Nestorescu, M. L., E. A. Siess, and O. H. Wieland (1973). Ultra-structural localization of pyruvate dehydrogenase in rat heart muscle. *Histochemie*, **34**, 355–60.

Obrist, W. D., E. Chivian, S. Cronquist, and D. H. Ingvar (1970). Regional cerebral blood flow in senile and presenile dementia. *Neurology*, **20**, 315–22.

Patel, A. and H. Koenig (1971). Some neurochemical aspects of fluorocitrate intoxication. *J. Neurochem.*, **18**, 621–8.

Perri, V., O. Sacchi, and C. Casella (1970). Nervous transmission in the superior cervical ganglion of the thiamine-deficient rat. *J. Exp. Physiol.*, **55**, 25–35.

Pliatakis, A., W. J. Nicklas and S. Berl (1978). Thiamine deficiency: selective impairment of the cerebellar serotonergic system. *Neurology*, **28**, 691–8.

Plum, F. (Ed.) (1974). *Brain Dysfunction in Metabolic Disorders*, Raven Press, New York.

Pollack, R. L., P. C. Molenaar, and P. Braggar-Schaap (1977). Regulation of acetylcholine synthesis in rat brain. In D. J. Jenden (Ed.) *Cholinergic Mechanisms and Psychopharmacology*, Plenum Press, New York. pp. 511–24.

Quastel, J. H., M. Tennenbaum, and A. H. M. Wheatley (1936). Dependence of acetylcholine synthesis on tissue respiration. *Biochem. J.*, **30**, 1668–79.

Risberg, J. (1979). Regional cerebral blood flow measurements by ^{133}Xe-inhalation: methodology and applications in neuropsychology and psychiatry. *Brain and Language*. In press.

Sacchi, O., H. Ladinsky, I. Prigioni, S. Consolo, G. Peri, and V. Perri (1978). Acetylcholine turnover in the thiamine-depleted superior cervical ganglion of the. rat. *Brain Res.*, **151**, 609–14.

Shimada, M., T. Kihara, M. Watanabe, and K. Kurinioto (1979). Decreased acetylcholine synthesis in mild hypoxic hypoxia. Submitted for publication.

Siesjö, B. K., H. Johannsson, B. Ljunggren, and K. Norberg (1974). Brain dysfunction in cerebral hypoxia and ischemia. In F. Plum (Ed.) *Brain Dysfunction in Metabolic Disorders*, Raven Press, New York. pp. 75–112.

Sokoloff, L. (1966). Cerebral circulatory and metabolic changes associated with aging, *Res. Publ. Assoc. Res. Nerv. Mental Dis.*, **41**, 237–49.

Sollenberg, J. and B. Sorbö (1970). On the origin of the acetyl moiety of acetylcholine in brain studied with a differential labelling technique using [^{3}H-^{14}C]-mixed labelled glucose and acetate. *J. Neurochem.*, **17**, 201–7.

Sterling, G. H. and J. J. O'Neill (1978). Citrate as the precursor of the acetyl moiety of acetylcholine. *J. Neurochem.*, **31**, 525–30.

Tucek, S. and S. C. Cheng (1974). Provenance of the acetyl group of acetylcholine and compartmentation of acetyl-CoA and Krebs cycle intermediates in the brain *in vivo*. *J. Neurochem.*, **22**, 893–914.

Wells, C. E. (Ed.) (1977). *Dementia*, 2nd edn, F. A. Davis, Philadelphia.

Williams, R. D., H. L. Mason, R. M. Wilder, and B. F. Smith (1940). Observations on induced thiamine (vitamin B$_1$) deficiency in man. *Arch. Int. Med.*, **66**, 785–99.

Yatsu, F. M., L. W. Lee, and C. L. Liao (1975). Energy metabolism during brain ischemia. Stability during reversible and irreversible damage. *Stroke*, **6**, 678–83.

Yoshino, Y. and K. A. C. Elliot (1970). Hypoxia and amino acid transmitters, *Biochemistry*, **48**, 228–35.

Biochemistry of Dementia
Edited by P. J. Roberts
© 1980, John Wiley & Sons Ltd.

Chapter 8

The Cholinergic System in Alzheimer's Disease

ELAINE K. PERRY and ROBERT H. PERRY

*Department of Neuropathology, Newcastle General Hospital,
Newcastle upon Tyne, U.K.*

I. INTRODUCTION

'The more pointedly and logically we formulate a thesis, the more irresistibly it cries out for its antithesis'

(Herman Hesse, *The Glass Bead Game*)

Acetylcholine (ACh) was the first neurotransmitter to be demonstrated (Loewi, 1921), and its role in the peripheral nervous system and at the neuromuscular junction is now well established. Cholinergic function in the brain is, by comparison, less well characterized and its role in cerebral disorders has not generally been investigated as extensively as other transmitter systems, such as the catecholamines. This apparent neglect of central cholinergic systems is partly due to the lack of a reliable histochemical method for mapping cholinergic pathways in the brain, and to difficulties in assessing components of cerebral (as opposed to peripheral) acetylcholine metabolism from blood, cerebrospinal fluid, or urine. Despite these limitations, there is now convincing evidence of a role for the cerebral cholinergic system in diverse behavioural patterns such as sleep, arousal, emotion, sensory, motor, and learning activities (reviewed by De Feudis, 1974; Karczmar, 1975), and of a widespread distribution of ACh and its associated enzyme, receptor, and uptake activities in the brain (reviewed by Kuhar and Atweh, 1978). Investigation of cerebral cholinergic activities in mental disorders is thus a fertile area for research which has already produced a number of reports on cholinergic parameters in schizophrenia and Huntington's, Parkinson's, and Alzheimer's diseases.

In this chapter biochemical and histochemical observations in Alzheimer's disease*, particularly those relating to cholinergic activities in necropsy brain, are

---

* Senile dementia of Alzheimer type occurring in people over 60 years.

discussed (Section IV), and relevant aspects of the neuroanatomy, biochemistry, and psychopharmacology of cerebral cortical cholinergic systems are considered (Sections II and V). The evidence in favour of a 'cholinergic hypothesis', which links abnormalities of the cholinergic system to certain functional and pathological changes in Alzheimer's disease, is assessed. In this hypothesis it is suggested that the cortical cholinergic system may play an important role in cognitive functions (including memory) and that there may be a particular association between cortical cholinergic abnormalities and some of the pathological features of Alzheimer's disease. There are obvious pitfalls in attempting to allocate malfunction of a particular transmitter to a specific mental disease, like Alzheimer's disease, but such a concept may provide a useful means of assessing current evidence relating to the cholinergic system.

II. THE CORTICAL CHOLINERGIC NETWORK

A. Biochemical Aspects

The major biochemical pathways of ACh metabolism, including various enzyme, receptor, and uptake systems, are summarized in Fig. 1. Biochemical aspects of the cholinergic system have been extensively reviewed (Silver, 1974; Browning, 1976; Mautner, 1977; Rossier, 1977; Jenden, 1978; Tuček, 1978) and this description is limited to certain components which are reasonably stable in post-mortem tissue and can be routinely investigated in the human brain.

1. Choline Acetyltransferase

Choline acetyltransferase (CAT), discovered in 1943 by Nachmansohn and Michado, catalyses the conversion of the precursors acetyl-coenzyme A and choline to ACh (Fig. 1). One of these precursors, acetyl-coenzyme A, is normally derived from glucose in the brain, although the immediate source of the acetyl group is uncertain (reviewed by Tuček, 1978). Choline, in contrast, is not synthesized in the brain but supplied by the blood as both free choline and phospholipid-bound choline, although the role of the latter in ACh synthesis is not yet clear (Ansell and Spanner, 1978). The enzyme CAT is probably mainly, if not totally, confined to cholinergic neurons in the brain. Its association with both ACh (Hebb, 1963) and high-affinity choline uptake (Kuhar and coworkers, 1973) have led to its use as a biochemical 'marker' for cholinergic neurons. At the subcellular level CAT appears to be concentrated in the nerve terminal cytoplasmic fraction (Fonnum, 1970). The enzyme is synthesized in the nerve cell body (in which at least some portion must obviously be localized) and transported along the axon by the slower component of axonal transport (reviewed by Tuček, 1978).

The extent to which alterations in CAT activities reflect functional activities of

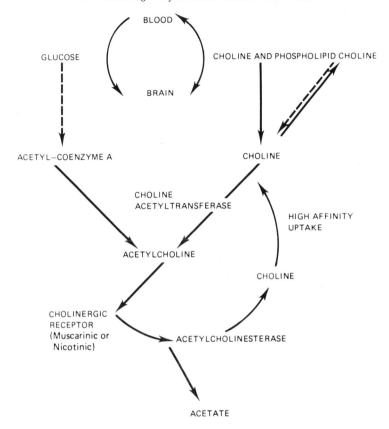

Figure 1. Biochemical pathways involved in acetylcholine metabolism in the brain. Pathways which have not yet been clearly established in connection with acetylcholine synthesis are indicated as broken lines

the cholinergic neuron has been recently reviewed (Tuček, 1978) and is discussed more fully in Section IV.B.4. It has often been suggested (see discussion of Fonnum, 1975) that CAT itself may not control the rate of ACh synthesis since inhibitors of CAT do not alter the *in vivo* rate of ACh synthesis (this rate being apparently below the *in vitro* capacity of the enzyme to produce ACh). Despite reservations such as these on the functional significance of changes in CAT levels in the brain, alterations in the number of enzyme molecules will obviously occur with the loss or regeneration of cholinergic cell processes and as a result of loss of cholinergic neurons. Since the interpretation of variations in CAT levels is not simple, it may be useful to consider changes which occur in pathological conditions in conjunction with the activities of various other cholinergic components.

2. Cholinesterases

There are several types of acylcholinesterases in brain tissue, including the 'specific' or acetylcholinesterase (ACE) which principally hydrolyses ACh (Fig. 1) and 'pseudo' cholinesterases which hydrolyse such esters as butyryl-, propionyl-, or benzoyl-choline (Silver, 1974). For convenience the latter will be referred to here as butyrylcholinesterase (BCE) since it is the enzyme which hydrolyses butyrylcholine which has been investigated in Alzheimer's disease. Regarding the function of these cholinesterases, ACE is probably mainly concerned with the breakdown of ACh released from the nerve terminal (although other functions of the enzyme are suspected) whereas it is not yet known if BCE, which hydrolyses ACh more slowly, plays any part in cholinergic neurotransmission (reviewed by Silver, 1974).

The localization of these enzymes has been inferred from histochemical and subcellular fractionation studies. All cholinergic neurons contain ACE and, although in some brain-regions it is also associated with non-cholinergic neurons, in areas such as the hippocampus (Section II.B.2) the enzyme may be a reliable marker of cholinergic neurons and their processes (Fonnum, 1973). In the brain the greater portion of ACE appears to be associated with the rough endoplasmic reticulum of the nerve cell body and membranous components of the cell processes (Shute and Lewis, 1966a). Neuronal ACE is thought to be synthesized in the cell body, conveyed along the axon by both slow and fast axonal transport systems and probably returned to the cell body by rapid retrograde transport (reviewed by Tuček, 1978). In human brain the enzyme is also distributed in non-neuronal components, such as cerebral blood vessels and some oligodendroglial cells (Perry and coworkers, 1980).

The properties of the pseudocholinesterase (BCE), are not so well characterized in the brain. Most histochemical studies have indicated that it may be associated variously with blood vessels, glial cells of white and grey matter, and neuronal cells of the cortex (reviewed by Silver, 1974), and subcellular fractionation studies have identified the majority of the enzyme with 'myelin membrane' and not 'nerve terminal' fractions (Miller, 1970). Both cholinesterases are clearly associated with several cellular components and the significance of alterations in the enzyme levels may be best assessed in conjunction with the behaviour of other cholinergic activities. In situations where, for example, ACE alters in conjunction with CAT (as in the hippocampus following septal lesions, Section II.B) these changes are likely to reflect specifically the activity of cholinergic neurons.

3. Muscarinic Cholinergic Receptor

There is now substantial evidence to indicate that the *in vitro* binding of muscarinic cholinergic antagonists (measured using radioisotopically labelled ligands) occurs at sites in the brain which are, physiologically and pharmacologically, identical to the muscarinic cholinergic receptor (Birdsall, Burgen, and Hulme, 1978). In areas such as the hippocampus, the *in vitro* binding of the muscarinic antagonist quinuclidinyl benzylate is not significantly affected by destruction of the cholinergic afferent pathway (Yamamura and Snyder, 1974). This observation indicates a post-synaptic localization of receptor binding in at least this brain region, although a pre-synaptic localization of some muscarinic receptor sites is suggested by the experimentally induced release of ACh from cerebral cortex and hippocampus, which is either stimulated by atropine or inhibited by anticholinesterases or oxotremorine (Molenaar and Polak, 1970; Hadhazy and Szerb, 1977). The interpretation of data on muscarinic antagonist binding in brain may, therefore, be complicated by the possible existence of receptor sites which have not been estimated biochemically. A further unknown factor is the precise role in cholinergic transmission of the relatively slow muscarinic response compared with the more rapid action of the nicotinic receptor (Section II.B.4).

B. Some Topographical Aspects

The major histopathological abnormalities of Alzheimer's disease are most prevalent in the cerebral neocortex and archicortical structures such as the hippocampus, cingulum, and entorhinal cortex (Corsellis, 1970; Tomlinson, Blessed, and Roth, 1970; Hooper and Vogel, 1976). In comparable brain areas a combination of biochemical, histochemical, and lesioning procedures, measurements of ACh release and iontophoretic application of ACh have established the existence of an extensive cholinergic network. Some topographical aspects of this cortical cholinergic system are discussed below.

1. Cortical Activities

Biochemical components (Fig. 1) of the cholinergic system have all been demonstrated in the cerebral cortex: acetylcholine (McIntosh, 1941); choline acetyltransferase (Hebb and Silver, 1956); acetylcholinesterase (Koelle, 1954); high-affinity choline uptake (Kuhar and coworkers, 1973); muscarinic cholinergic receptor (MRB) (Hiley and Burgen, 1974; Yamamura and coworkers, 1974); and α-bungarotoxin binding, the latter possibly related to the nicotinic receptor (Polz-Tejera, Schmidt, and Karten, 1975).

These cholinergic components appear, on the basis of present reports on animal (mammalian) brain, to be fairly evenly distributed throughout the different lobes of the neocortex. The transmitter, enzyme and choline uptake systems are, however, generally higher in certain archicortical areas, such as amygdala, hippocampus, cingulum, and entorhinal cortex, compared with neocortical areas (Yamamura and coworkers, 1974; Cheney, Racagni, and Costa, 1976; Fahn, 1976; Vizi and Palkovitz, 1978). In most neocortical regions these cholinergic components are also less concentrated than those in certain underlying structures, such as the caudate nucleus. Activities of ACE, CAT and high-affinity choline uptake are (on a unit weight basis) approximately one tenth of those in caudate nucleus; MRB and the actual levels of ACh itself are between one-half to a third of the caudate levels (Yamamura and coworkers, 1974). In contrast, the putative nicotinic receptor binding is considerably (up to five times) higher in the cortex compared with the caudate, although total α-bungarotoxin binding is much lower than MRB.

The distribution of these various cholinergic activities in the human brain is apparently similar to that in non-human mammalian brain. Thus, CAT is widely distributed in the neocortex and limbic region (Hebb and Silver, 1956), being most active in, for example, the amygdaloid nucleus and superior temporal cortex, and least active in parts of the parietal and occipital lobes (McGeer and McGeer, 1976a). Histochemical (Ishii and Friede, 1967) and biochemical (Domino, Krause, and Bowers, 1973; McGeer and McGeer, 1976a) studies of ACE in human brain tissue also indicate generally higher activities in amygdaloid nucleus and hippocampus compared with neocortex. Compared with ACE, BCE is less active and is distributed more evenly in different regions of the human brain (Foldes and coworkers, 1962; Robinson, 1966; Friede, 1967; Domino, Krause, and Bowers 1973).

2. *Hippocampal Activities*

In contrast to the neocortex, topographical studies of cholinergic 'markers' within the mammalian hippocampus are fairly numerous, presumably reflecting the advantage of being able experimentally to manipulate discrete pathways (in this case the afferent pathway from the septal nucleus to the hippocampus). Examination of cholinergic activities in normal mammalian hippocampus suggests that they are concentrated in particular anatomical layers (Fig. 2); ACE (Shute and Lewis, 1963; Storm-Mathisen, 1970), CAT (Fonnum, 1970), and MRB (Kuhar and Yamamura, 1975) being concentrated in the inner zone of the stratum oriens and the supragranular zone in the fascia dentata, while the putative nicotinic receptor binding is located towards the outer portion of the stratum oriens and dentate hilus (Hunt and Schmidt, 1978). Recent histochemical observations in the human hippocampus have indicated a similar but broader distribution of ACE compared with animal hippocampus (Mellgren, Harkmark, and Srebro, 1977; Perry and coworkers, 1980), and a different distribution for BCE, this enzyme activity being most pronounced in the stratum lacunosum-moleculare and alveus (unpublished observations).

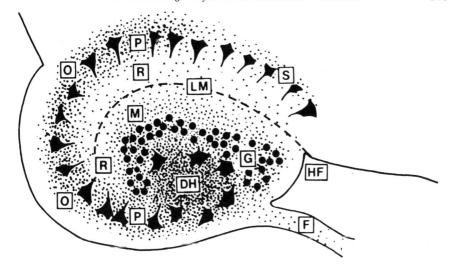

O = Stratum oriens
P = Stratum pyramidale
R = Stratum radiatum
LM = Stratum lacunosum - moleculare

HF = Hippocampal fissure
M = Molecular layer of DH
S = Subiculum
DH = Dentate hilus
F = Fimbria
G = Granular cell layer

Figure 2. Diagram of the mammalian hippocampus showing the major anatomical divisions and different layers. Shaded regions are rich in acetylcholinesterase (considered to contain cholinergic afferent processes)

3. Lesioning Studies

Experimental interruption of the septal input to the hippocampus of animals is followed by accumulation of cholinergic enzymes on the septal side and extensive reductions in hippocampal activities of CAT and ACE, (Lewis, Shute, and Silver, 1967), high-affinity choline uptake (Kuhar and coworkers, 1973), and ACh (Sethy and coworkers, 1973). There are, in contrast, no significant alterations in either MRB (Yamamura and Snyder, 1974) or the putative nicotinic receptor binding (Dudai and Segal, 1978) in the hippocampus following these lesions. Furthermore, kainic acid lesions (which selectively destroy certain cell bodies) do not significantly alter the levels of CAT (Fonnum and Walaas, 1978). These reports suggest that cholinergic enzyme and high-affinity choline uptake activities in the hippocampus are mainly associated with cholinergic afferent processes, whereas cholinergic receptor binding is localized predominantly on the post-synaptic (cholinoceptive) membrane. In contrast to septal lesions, destruction of the entorhinal cortex, which contributes hippocampal afferents via the temporoammonic pathways, results in increased activities of ACE in the molecular layer of the dentate gyrus, a finding which may indicate additional sprouting of the septal afferents (Lynch and coworkers, 1973; Nadler and Cotman, 1978).

Although fewer experiments have been conducted, similar conclusions regarding the nature of the neocortical cholinergic system have been drawn from neocortical undercutting procedures. In these experiments, undercutting of the pericruciate and suprasylvian cortex (Hebb, Krnjević, and Silver, 1963), and of the frontal cortex (Kelly and Moore, 1978) was followed by extensive reductions of ACE and CAT. Such findings suggest that many cholinergic processes innervating the neocortex are afferent fibres arising either from deeper brain nuclei or as projection fibres from other cortical regions.

More specific information concerning the origin of the cortical cholinergic afferents has been obtained by lesioning studies of putative cortical afferent tracts and nuclei. Thus, lesions of the septum result in a loss of cortical ACh (Pepeu, Mulas, and Mulas, 1973) and related cholinergic activities (Kuhar and coworkers, 1973); discrete lesions within the basal ganglia and the septal nuclei deplete cortical CAT (reviewed by Emson and Lindvall, 1978), and trans-section of the pre-optic area results in decreased CAT in the piriform cortex (Wenk, Meyer, and Bigle, 1977). Following such lesioning of afferent fibres, both hippocampal and cortical areas retain a residual cholinergic activity of between 10 and 20 %. A similar percentage is, in fact, lost in the hippocampus treated with kainic acid and presumably represents a smaller population of cholinergic neurons which are either intrinsic to the cortex or which innervate other brain areas.

4. Pharmacological Evidence

Neurophysiological and pharmacological investigations also support the existence of a widespread cholinergic system in the cerebral cortex. Thus, electrical and chemical stimulation influence the release of ACh from the cerebral cortex (McIntosh and Osborin, 1953; Celesia and Jasper, 1966; Hemsworth and Neal, 1968) and hippocampus (Smith, 1972; Rommelspacher and Kuhar, 1974). Iontophoretically applied ACh can excite or inhibit cortical neurons, depending on cellular localization. In the motor cortex for example, Betz cells are excited (Krnjević and Phillis, 1963) whereas other, more superficial neurons are inhibited (Phillis and York, 1967). The post-synaptic response of these cortical neurons may be of the muscarinic type, with a slow onset (5–30 s) or the nicotinic type with a minimum latency of 30 ms. It is believed that inhibitory responses may be primarily of muscarinic type. In the hippocampus electrophysiological recordings indicate that more than 60 % of the neurons (primarily situated in regions rich in biochemical cholinergic activities) are excited by ACh, and the short and long latencies reported (Biscoe and Straughan, 1966; Steiner, 1968) indicate the presence of both muscarinic and nicotinic receptors.

5. *Prospective Pathways*

The evidence that ACh functions as a neurotransmitter in the cerebral cortex of mammalian brain is, if not conclusive, certainly compelling. Neuroanatomical investigations of the precise anatomical pathways of the cholinergic system (to, from, or within the cerebral cortex) have been hampered by the absence of a specific histochemical cholinergic marker. Although Shute and Lewis, in an extensive series of elegant studies (Shute and Lewis, 1963, 1966b; Lewis, Shute, and Silver, 1967), identified ACE containing pathways in the mesencephalic, diencephalic, and cortical regions, uncertainties attached to the use of ACE as a cholinergic neuronal marker have raised questions concerning the specific cholinergic nature of these tracts. Shute and Lewis (1963) described the major ACE-containing ascending systems in the brain, comprising the dorsal and ventral tegmental pathways. The latter pathway has been considered to be responsible (directly and indirectly) for cholinergic innervation of the cerebral cortex, including a probable septal–neocortical connection (Section II.B.3).

The more recent demonstration of monoamine neurotransmitter 'markers' in the ascending mesencephalic (reticular formation) pathways (Fonnum, Walaas, and Iversen, 1977; reviewed by Livett, 1979, Emson and Lindvall, 1978) suggest that, despite their content of ACE, this portion of ascending reticular formation fibres are not primarily cholinergic in nature. In at least the hippocampal region, however, additional biochemical evidence on the distribution and behaviour of other cholinergic components (Sections II.B.2 and II.B.3) strongly supports the validity of the original histochemical observations relating to ACE in animal brains.

In the cerebral cortex itself there is good evidence that at least some of the cholinergic afferent fibres originate in nuclei situated in the septal region and adjacent basal ganglia structures. Emson and Lindvall (1979) have summarized this evidence (based on lesioning, peroxidase tracer studies, and di-isopropylfluorophosphate manipulation of ACE) which suggests that the origin of dorsal and lateral cortical cholinergic afferents may be the pallidum (or substantia innominata), whereas medial frontal cholinergic fibres may arise in the septum (nucleus of the diagonal band). Entorhinal cholinergic afferents have been traced to the lateral pre-optic area and entopeduncular nuclei. These cholinergic cortical pathways are likely to be present in the human brain, although the greater development of the human neocortex may be associated with novel cortical cholinergic pathways, which have not yet been identified.

III. BIOCHEMICAL VARIATIONS IN POST-MORTEM HUMAN BRAIN TISSUE

Routine analysis of the cerebral cholinergic system in Alzheimer's disease is currently confined to post-mortem tissue and requires an assessment of those factors, other than the dementia itself, which contribute to variations in necropsy brain activities. Brain biochemical activities relating to cholinergic and other transmitter systems apparently vary extensively in normal individuals (Bird and Iversen, 1974; McGeer and McGeer, 1976a; Perry and coworkers, 1977b). Although these variations have not been entirely explained, some contributing factors are discussed below.

1. Age

Whereas CAT may be relatively unaffected by ageing, in certain underlying brain regions such as the caudate nucleus it declines significantly in the cerebral cortex from youth to old age (first to ninth decades, McGeer and McGeer, 1976b) and in old age itself (from the seventh decade onwards, Perry and coworkers, 1977b). The enzyme decline in old age is particularly pronounced in the hippocampus (Perry and coworkers, 1977c; Davies, 1978). ACE in the human brain is apparently less affected by the ageing process and fewer significant correlations in the cortex, compared with CAT, have been reported between youth and old age (McGeer and McGeer, 1976b), and no significant correlations between the seventh to tenth decades in the neocortex or hippocampus (Perry and coworkers, 1978a). The effect of age on muscarinic cholinergic receptor binding in human brain is unclear, and both unchanged (Davies and Verth, 1978) and decreased levels (White and coworkers, 1977; Perry, 1980) have been reported. The relatively greater susceptibility of CAT compared with ACE or MRB in normal ageing, has been previously reported (Perry, 1980) and is discussed in Section IV. D.

2. Circadian Variation

Significant variations according to the time of day at which death occurred have been reported for several cholinergic activities of the human cortex, with individual patterns of fluctuation for the different components (Perry and coworkers, 1977d). Recent (unpublished) data suggest that the rhythm of CAT activity may depend on the area of brain investigated, with optimal levels in the hippocampus apparently occurring later in the day compared with those in the frontal cortex (circadian variations in normal cases are illustrated in Fig. 3). Such rhythms, which may differ both in phase and amplitude, could provide information on the functional inter-relationships between different brain regions and, in addition, disrupted or disconnected rhythms may indicate specific abnormalities in pathological conditions such as manic-depressive psychosis and Alzheimer's disease.

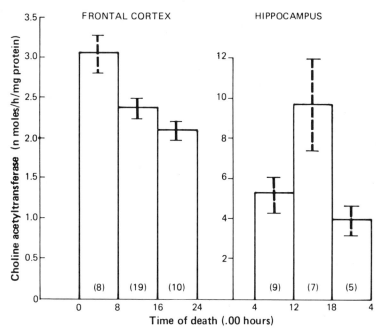

Figure 3. Circadian variation in (normal) human neocortical and hippocampal choline acetyltransferase (CAT, nmol per hour per mg protein). Individuals have been grouped according to the times of day at which death occurred, as indicated. Column heights represent mean values, bars the standard errors, with the numbers of cases in parentheses. The maximum activities are significantly (Student's t-test) different from the two lower activities ($p < 0.02$ and $p < 0.05$ in frontal cortex and hippocampus, respectively)

3. Post-mortem Stability

Although it might be imagined that biochemical investigations in post-mortem tissue would be severely restricted by autolytic change, many enzymes and receptors are apparently quite stable following death. Previous analyses of CAT activity in human brain have not revealed significant alterations according to the post-mortem delay (Bird and Iversen, 1974; McGeer and McGeer, 1976a; Mackay and coworkers, 1978). In the frontal cortex of a recent series of normal and depressed individuals, however (Fig. 4), there was a significant, but not substantial, decline in CAT activity after death. The enzyme loss apparently follows changes in brain temperature after death (Perry and coworkers, 1977e; Spokes and Koch, 1978), being more rapid in the first 20 hours post-mortem during which time the temperature approaches refrigeration temperature. In the same series no significant changes were observed with increasing delays in tissue sampling in ACE, BCE, or MRB (Perry, 1980).

Difficulties attached to the assessment of changes after death include the

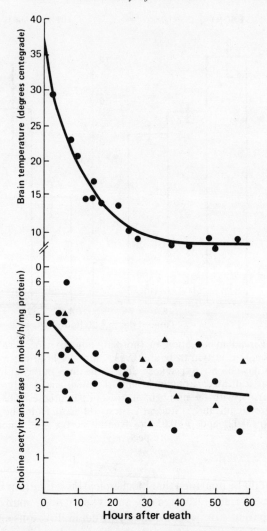

Figure 4. Post-mortem fall in human brain temperature and variation in choline acetyltransferase (CAT). Brain temperature (above) was
recorded in 15 cases in which the interval between
death and autopsy ranged from 4 to 58 hours
(mortuary temperature 6–8°C). CAT activities
(lower graph) in frontal cortex of a separate series
of normal (•) and depressed (▲) cases, in which
the interval between death and tissue storage in
liquid nitrogen ranged from 2 to 59 hours. The
correlation between post-mortem delay and CAT
($r = -0.55$) is significant ($p < 0.01$)

absence of measurements in the immediate post-mortem period and possible differences in stability between activities from normal and pathological brain tissue. Despite these reservations, however, post-mortem stability is unlikely to be a major complication in the investigation of these particular cholinergic activities.

4. Drug Treatments

Brain biochemical observations in mental disease may be complicated by the effects of drug therapy, and a major difference between cases of Alzheimer's disease and normal old people is the long-term administration in the demented group of a neuroleptic drug, usually of the phenothiazine or butyrophenone type. No systematic investigations of the effects of such drugs on cholinergic activities in different regions of animal or human brain have been conducted. Bird and Iversen (1974), in their study of Huntington's disease, found a significant increase in putamen CAT in a group of cases treated with thioridazine compared with groups not treated with this drug. In the rat chronic administration of haloperidol increased striatal but not cortical ACh turnover (Cheney and coworkers, 1978) and putamen CAT was increased after acute and reduced after chronic treatment with thioridazine (Lloyd and coworkers, 1977). Thioridazine does not, apparently, affect animal brain ACE (Sethy and Van Woert, 1974), nor does haloperidol significantly alter MRB (Muller and Seeman, 1977).

Preliminary studies (Fig. 5) have indicated that chronically administered thioridazine (a drug frequently used in senile dementia) but not amitriptyline (an antidepressant) significantly alters CAT activity in rat brain, and that the effect of the drug may depend on the area of brain investigated and the duration of treatment. Throughout the first four weeks, CAT was significantly raised in the caudate and diminished in the cortex, although differences from the placebo group never exceeded 20 %. Neither ACE nor BCE were affected by this drug treatment. There is thus no evidence, as yet, that neuroleptic medication in Alzheimer's disease substantially influences cortical cholinergic enzyme activities, but further investigation of this problem is required. In the interim, a useful approach to assessing drug effects in Alzheimer's disease may be to compare results in Alzheimer's disease with those in other mental disorders, such as schizophrenia and multi-infarct dementia in which a similar drug treatment is often used (Section IV.E.1).

5. Miscellaneous

No significant differences in cholinergic activities between males and females have been reported for human brain tissue, and neither prolonged hospitalization nor coma through illness affect cerebral cholinergic enzymes to any appreciable or significant extent (McGeer and McGeer, 1976a; Perry and coworkers, 1977b).

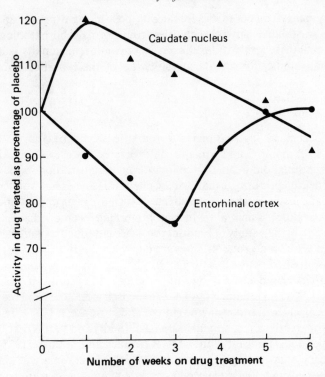

Figure 5. Effects of thioridizine on rat brain choline acetyltransferase (CAT). Pairs of adult rats (one male and one female, Lewis strain), were injected daily (6 out of 7 days) with either thioridazine (4 mg intraperitoneally per kg body weight) or placebo (carrier only) up to the time of death. Two pairs, one drug- and one placebo-treated, were sacrificed after 1–6 weeks on chronic treatment. CAT activities are expressed here as the percentage of mean activity in the drug-treated pair, compared with that in the placebo-treated pair. Between 1 and 4 weeks of treatment, activities in the 8 drug- compared with 8 placebo-treated, animals were significantly (student's t-test) higher in the caudate nucleus ($p < 0.05$) and lower in the entorhinal cortex ($p < 0.05$). (Keith, Perry, and Perry, unpublished data)

IV. CEREBRAL CHOLINERGIC ACTIVITIES IN ALZHEIMER'S DISEASE

A. A Review of the Evidence

In 1964 and 1965 two reports appeared (Pope, Hess, and Lewin, 1964; Friede, 1965) which are consistent with a possible abnormality of ACE in Alzheimer's disease. Over ten years elapsed before these observations were confirmed (biochemically and histochemically—see Table 1) and extended to include a reduction, in necropsy and biopsy brain tissue, of the enzyme which synthesizes ACh: CAT (Davies and Maloney, 1976; Perry and coworkers, 1977a; Spillane and coworkers, 1977; White and coworkers, 1977; Reisine and coworkers, 1978). In addition to these observations of decreased cholinergic enzyme activities, there have now been several reports (Table 1) indicating that the receptor (MRB) is quantitatively unchanged in most brain regions investigated, and that it has normal binding characteristics (Davies and Verth, 1978). In Alzheimer's disease, the pseudocholinesterase (BCE) activity is apparently increased (Table 1).

Table 1. Reports of cholinergic activities in Alzheimer's disease

Acetylcholinesterase	Decreased	Brain biochemistry[a, c, d, e]
		Brain histochemistry[b]
	Increased	
	(in senile plaques)	Brain histochemistry[f, b]
Butyrylcholinesterase	Increased	Brain histochemistry[f]
		Brain biochemistry[c, e]
Choline acetyltransferase	Decreased	Brain biochemistry[d, g, h, i]
Muscarinic receptor	Normal	Brain biochemistry[g, h, j]
	Decreased	Hippocampus only[i]
Choline	Increased	Blood level[k]
	Normal	CSF level[l]

References: [a]Pope, Hess, and Lewin (1964); [b]Perry and coworkers (1980); [c]Op den Velde and Stam (1976); [d]Davies and Maloney (1976); [e]Perry and coworkers (1978b); [f]Friede (1965); [g]Perry and coworkers (1977a); [h]White and coworkers (1977); [i]Reisine and coworkers (1978); [j]Davies and Verth (1978); [k]Aquilonius and coworkers (1975); [l]Christie and coworkers (in press).

Most of the neocortical cholinergic abnormalities in Alzheimer's disease have not so far been observed in other mental disorders (Section IV.E). Furthermore, these abnormalities may be related to the extent of Alzheimer-type pathological changes (see below) occurring in different brain areas (Perry and coworkers, 1977b; Davies, 1978) and different individual cases (Perry and coworkers, 1978b).

Compared with brain tissue, investigations of the cholinergic system in blood and CSF in Alzheimer's disease are sparse (Table 1). There are reports of elevated choline in blood (Aquilonius and coworkers, 1975) and normal CSF choline (including apparently normal exchange between blood and CSF; Christie and coworkers, in press). Resting choline levels in blood or CSF are difficult to interpret in terms of the cholinergic function of the brain, since the concentration in the brain of phosphatidyl choline, which contributes to the choline 'pool', may exceed that of ACh by as much as three orders of magnitude (Ansell and Spanner, 1978), although the turnover rate of the ACh may be relatively much higher.

Preliminary observations (unpublished) on the activities of various different enzymes capable of producing one of the precursors of ACh, acetyl-coenzyme A, in the brain have indicated significant reductions in two particular enzymes, pyruvate dehydrogenase and ATP-citrate lyase in Alzheimer's disease, compared with the normal (Table 2). In this analysis, certain other enzymes, including acetyl-coenzyme A synthetase, carnitine acetyltransferase, and citrate synthase were apparently unchanged (Table 2). In parietal cortex the losses relating to pyruvate dehydrogenase and ATP-citrate lyase were not apparently as extensive (30–40 %) as the reductions in CAT (70 %, see Table 3), an observation which is compatible with selective reductions in cholinergic neuronal processes, activities in other cell types being relatively unaffected.

Table 2. Enzymes* producing acetyl-coenzyme A in necropsy brain tissue in Alzheimer's disease†

	Parietal cortex	Amygdaloid nucleus
Pyruvate dehydrogenase	0.61 ($p < 0.05$)	N.E.
ATP-citrate lyase	0.66 ($p < 0.02$)	0.49 ($p < 0.05$)
Citrate synthase	0.97 (N.S.)	0.81 (N.S.)
Carnitine acetyltransferase	N.E.	0.98 (N.S.)
Acetyl coenzyme A synthetase	N.E.	0.87 (N.S.)

* Estimated by standard spectrophotometric procedures or radiometric methods (pyruvate dehydrogenase, Lefresne, Beaujauan, and Glowinski, 1978; acetylcoenzyme A synthetase, Banns, Hebb, and Mann, 1978).
† Results expressed as the ratio between mean values for the normal group (10 and 7 cases for cortex and amygdala, respectively) and cases of Alzheimer's disease (13 and 7 cases for the two areas). Significance of the difference between the normal and Alzheimer's disease (Student's *t*-test) in parentheses.
N.S., Not significant; N.E., Not estimated.

B. Neuropathological Relationships

1. Differences between Clinical Groups and Brain Regions

If abnormalities of the cholinergic system in Alzheimer's disease are associated with the disease process itself, correlations between biochemical and Alzheimer-type neuropathological changes might be anticipated. When comparisons are made between the activities of CAT and MRB in different brain regions of normal cases, cases of Alzheimer's disease and various other disorders (matched for mean ages and post-mortem sampling delays), CAT (Table 3) is significantly decreased in nearly all regions examined in Alzheimer's disease. These enzyme reductions are generally less extensive in brain areas which are not so obviously affected by Alzheimer-type pathological changes.

Diminished CAT in the neocortex has not been found in the other mental disorders so far investigated, although there is a significant decrease in hippocampal CAT in depression and multi-infarct dementia (Table 3). In the same series (Table 4) there were no significant alterations of MRB in any area examined, although there was a (non-significant) trend towards decreased MRB in the hippocampus and amygdala. Further comparisons of these cholinergic activities in Alzheimer's disease and various other mental disorders are discussed more fully in Section IV.E. From these and results for other brain areas in Alzheimer's disease (Davies, 1978; Davies and Verth, 1978), the pattern of the cholinergic enzyme (CAT) loss appears to resemble that of histopathological changes throughout the brain. Preliminary results do not, however, indicate a similar morphological correlation for the extent of ACE reduction, measured biochemically, although the increase in BCE in different brain regions is more suggestive of a direct relationship between this enzyme abnormality and Alzheimer-type neuropathological changes (Perry and coworkers, 1978a, and unpublished observations).

A possible difficulty associated with comparisons between biochemical activities, measured on a unit weight or protein basis, of different brain areas in Alzheimer's disease is the influence of tissue atrophy. Thus, if certain brain areas are selectively affected by atrophy, comparisons between biochemical activities in the different areas measured in this way may not be valid. It is not, however, possible to make allowances for the degree of atrophy since quantitative estimates of atrophy in white and grey matter have not yet been reported for different brain areas in Alzhemier's disease. A further complication is the presence, in brain tissue, of blood which has intrinsic cholinergic activities such as ACE and BCE. On account of these and other limitations, gross biochemical activities of the brain in Alzheimer's disease are perhaps best regarded as a guide to future microanatomical and subcellular investigations.

2. Quantitative Correlations

A second approach in evaluating the specificity of biochemical changes in Alzheimer's disease is to determine whether or not these changes correlate with the degree of neuropathological abnormalities in different individuals. A number of different histopathological features in Alzheimer's disease can be quantified including, for example, neocortical senile plaques, neurofibrillary tangles, hippocampal granulovacuolar degeneration, and Hirano bodies. Since the neocortical plaque count has been shown to correlate significantly with measures of cognitive function and dementing behaviour (Blessed, Tomlinson, and Roth, 1968), biochemical results were originally examined in relation to plaque numbers. This analysis clearly demonstrated a correlation between decline in CAT activity and increasing plaque numbers in the neocortex of non-demented and demented old people (Fig. 6). Significant correlations were also obtained between the plaque count and both decreased ACE and increased BCE, but not between plaque count and glutamate decarboxylase activity (Perry and co-

Table 3. Choline acetyltransferase activities in necropsy brain tissue (nmol per hour per mg protein)†

Brain region	Normal	Depression	Schizophrenia	Multi-infarct dementia	Alzheimer's disease
Frontal cortex	3.67 ± 0.54 (16)	3.09 ± 0.26 (12)	4.93 ± 0.92 (9)	4.76 ± 1.31 (5)	2.42 ± 0.29 (16)*
Occipital cortex	3.11 ± 0.44 (16)	2.78 ± 0.26 (12)	2.78 ± 0.48 (9)	3.93 ± 0.42 (4)	1.43 ± 0.17 (16)**
Temporal cortex	3.80 ± 0.44 (16)	2.85 ± 0.29 (12)	3.82 ± 0.41 (9)	3.74 ± 0.75 (5)	1.24 ± 0.15 (16)***
Parietal cortex	3.44 ± 0.48 (16)	2.55 ± 0.29 (12)	2.93 ± 0.35 (9)	3.60 ± 0.22 (5)	1.05 ± 0.18 (16)***
Entorhinal cortex	4.75 ± 1.28 (5)	N.E.	N.E.	N.E.	1.47 ± 0.39 (8)*
Hippocampus	7.33 ± 1.12 (16)	4.14 ± 0.94 (12)*	8.24 ± 1.17 (9)	3.44 ± 0.77 (5)**	2.57 ± 0.32 (16)***
Amygdaloid nucleus	14.05 ± 1.57 (5)	12.85 ± 1.59 (3)	12.10 ± 2.84 (8)	N.E.	4.41 ± 1.10 (8)***
Mammillary body	3.84 ± 0.68 (9)	2.75 ± 0.59 (3)	N.E.	3.55 ± 1.10 (5)	1.33 ± 0.12 (6)**
Caudate nucleus	80.50 ± 7.08 (16)	84.08 ± 12.41 (12)	92.05 ± 13.96 (9)	85.8 ± 22.75 (5)	61.80 ± 5.78 (16)*
Substantia nigra	4.67 ± 1.06 (11)	4.29 ± 0.86 (8)	4.78 ± 0.58 (8)	4.97 ± 1.18 (4)	2.50 ± 0.81 (4)
Cerebellum	4.28 ± 1.11 (5)	2.88 ± 1.21 (3)	N.E.	2.85 ± 0.36 (4)	2.56 ± 0.72 (3)

† Clinical categories and biochemical methods as previously described (Perry and coworkers, 1978b)
* ** *** Significantly different (Student's t-test from the normal, $p < 0.05$, 0.02, and 0.001, respectively.
N.E., Not estimated.

Table 4. Muscarinic receptor binding* in necropsy brain tissue[†] (pmol per mg protein)

Brain region	Normal	Depression	Schizophrenia	Alzheimer's disease
Frontal cortex	0.490 ± 0.196 (5)	0.536 ± 0.068 (3)	0.315 ± 0.043 (9)[‡]	0.424 ± 0.071 (5)
Occipital cortex	0.558 ± 0.059 (8)	0.530 ± 0.079 (4)	0.348 ± 0.089 (5)	0.648 ± 0.164 (4)
Temporal cortex	0.648 ± 0.064 (12)	0.675 ± 0.056 (5)	0.381 ± 0.041 (9)[‡]	0.686 ± 0.036 (8)
Parietal cortex	0.553 ± 0.048 (14)	0.572 ± 0.041 (11)	0.376 ± 0.031 (7)[‡]	0.498 ± 0.082 (13)
Hippocampus	0.378 ± 0.055 (12)	0.408 ± 0.185 (5)	0.191 ± 0.036 (9)[‡]	0.302 ± 0.063 (13)
Amygdaloid nucleus	0.340 ± 0.045 (5)	0.430 ± 0.113 (3)	0.255 ± 0.050 (8)	0.241 ± 0.062 (7)
Caudate nucleus	0.886 ± 0.097 (13)	1.053 ± 0.136 (11)	0.678 ± 0.060 (5)	1.282 ± 0.173 (11)
Substantia nigra	0.205 ± 0.085 (3)	0.210 ± 0.056 (3)	0.188 ± 0.023 (4)	N.E.

* Measured from the difference in binding of [3-^{3}H]quinuclidinyl benzilate (10^{-8} mol l^{-1}) in the presence or absence of atropine (10^{-5} mol l^{-1}).

[†] Clinical categories and biochemical method as previously described (Perry and coworkers, 1978b).

[‡] Significantly different from the normal (Student's *t-test*), $p < 0.01$

N.E., Not estimated.

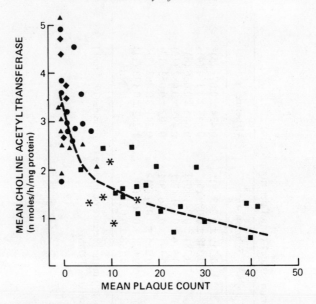

Figure 6. Relation between choline acetyltransferase (CAT)
activity and senile plaque formation in neocortex. Individual
mean plaque counts plotted against mean cortical enzyme
activities in 51 cases. (● , Normal; ▲ , depression; ◆ , multi-
infarct dementia; ■ , Alzheimer's disease; ∗ , dementia of
'mixed' pathology). The correlation between CAT and
plaque count is significant when calculated for the entire
series ($r = 0.82$, $p < 0.001$) and for those 23 cases with
Alzheimer-type pathology ($r = 0.45$, $p < 0.05$). Adapted with
permission, from Perry *et al.*, 1978b.

workers, 1978b), the latter suggesting that the γ-aminobutyric acid system is not
specifically involved in Alzheimer-type pathology. The cholinergic correlations
remained statistically significant if the analysis was restricted to those cases with
Alzheimer-type pathology. Furthermore, the CAT loss was also found to be
significantly correlated with the degree of intellectual impairment in a series of
cases of depression and Alzheimer's disease (Perry and coworkers, 1978b).

Correlations between psychiatric, neuropathological, and biochemical findings, such as these, do not provide any evidence of a direct or close relationship
between the different variables, nor can any conclusions be drawn regarding
cause and effect; but they do suggest that decreased CAT activity may be
particularly associated with the progress of Alzheimer's disease (assessed from
the extent of senile plaque formation and of intellectual impairment). It is not yet
established from these studies whether reduced CAT may be an earlier or later
change in the disease process although, in this respect, comparisons between
alterations in CAT and other cholinergic activities, as a function of increasing

plaque numbers, illustrated that loss of CAT may occur at an earlier stage of Alzheimer-type pathology (Perry and coworkers, 1978b). In contrast, no changes in MRB occur as a function of increasing cortical plaque counts (Perry and coworkers, 1978b).

The extent of Alzheimer-type pathological changes can also be assessed from the degree of neuronal neurofibrillary change. In the neocortex, quantitative estimates of neurofibrillary tangles are less applicable to (biochemical) correlative studies, since severe neocortical tangle formation is restricted to demented individuals (Tomlinson, Blessed, and Roth, 1970) and it is not practical to quantify the small numbers which may be seen in normal (non-demented) cases. In the hippocampus, by comparison, substantial numbers of tangles can occur in the absence of dementia and a semi-quantitative estimate of this histopathological feature can be made (Tomlinson, Blessed, and Roth, 1970). From current biochemical studies (unpublished data) there appears to be a

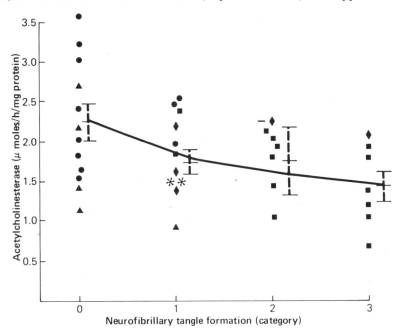

Figure 7. Relation between acetylcholinesterase (ACE) and neurofibrillary tangle formation in hippocampus. ACE is shown for four categories (graded 0, 1, 2, and 3, according to increasing numbers of tangles in the hippocampus). (● , Normal; ▲ , depression; ◆ , multi-infarct dementia; ■ , Alzheimer's disease; * , dementia of 'mixed' pathology). The mean enzyme activities, and standard errors are indicated (bars) in each category, with statistically significant differences between categories 0 and 1 ($p<0.05$) and 0 and 3 ($p<0.01$) and between cases of Alzheimer's disease in categories 1 plus 2 compared with 3 ($p<0.05$)

significant correlation between hippocampal tangle formation and changes in cholinergic enzyme activities (CAT, ACE) and BCE. If the comparison is restricted to cases of Alzheimer's disease (the non-demented group being excluded) this correlation is only statistically significant for the enzyme ACE (Fig. 7).

Granulovacuolar degeneration in the hippocampal pyramidal neurons can also be quantified in both normal cases and in Alzheimer's disease (Tomlinson, Blessed, and Roth, 1970). In Alzheimer's disease the only hippocampal biochemical activity so far investigated, which correlates significantly with granulovacuolar degeneration, is BCE (Fig. 8).

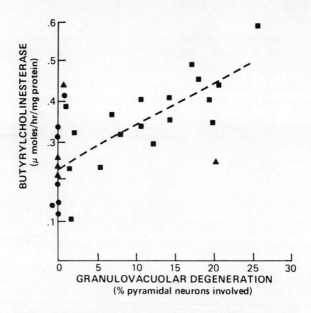

Figure 8. Relation between butyrylcholinesterase (BCE) and granulovacuolar degeneration in hippocampus. Individual enzyme activities are plotted against the percentage of hippocampal pyramidal neurons involved by granulovacuolar degeneration in 30 cases. (●, Normal; ▲, depression; and ■, Alzheimer's disease). The correlation is significant when calculated for the entire series ($r = 0.65$, $p < 0.001$) and for cases of Alzheimer's disease only ($r = 0.68$, $p < 0.01$)

3. Histochemical Observations

Despite its limitations as a 'marker' of cholinergic neurons in certain brain areas the association between ACE and cholinergic neuronal activities in the hippocampus is fairly well established (Section II.B.3). Histochemical observations of ACE in human hippocampus may, therefore, provide useful information concerning the integrity of the cholinergic system in this region of the brain in various mental disorders, and has recently indicated marked abnormalities in Alzheimer's disease (Perry and coworkers, 1980). ACE stains remarkably well in post-mortem hippocampal sections and obvious alterations according to post-mortem delay (6–49 hours) have not so far been observed (Perry and coworkers, 1980). Cross-sections from the hippocampus of a normal case and a well-advanced case of Alzheimer's disease are illustrated in Fig. 9. Normal ACE staining associated with the pyramidal cell layer and adjacent strata (see section II.B.2) is almost absent in this (as other) cases of Alzheimer's disease. Residual ACE staining may be present in the dentate hilus and Rose's areas h_3 to h_5, areas where the cholinergic afferents are believed to enter the hippocampal formation. This residual activity is present in fibre processes, occasional polymorph neurons in the dentate hilus and Golgi type II cells in the stratum oriens, and its cellular localization is similar to that seen in animals following septal lesions (Mellgren and Srebro, 1973). The decreased staining of ACE-containing fine fibres in established cases of Alzheimer's disease is not, apparently, due to the presence of an endogenous enzyme inhibitor or dissociation of ACE from the membrane (unpublished observations), and is compatible with a functional derangement or decline in the numbers of cholinergic afferent processes. A similar, extensive reduction in ACE staining has also been observed in the subiculum, entorhinal, and neocortex (Fig. 9) in Alzheimer's disease, but neither caudate nucleus nor spinal cord are so obviously affected.

As observed by Friede (1965) some, but probably not all, senile plaques are associated with increased ACE activity and this is especially well demonstrated in normal elderly cases (such as in Fig. 9g) in whom small numbers of senile plaques occur. In the particular region of the hippocampus where most ACE fibre-staining is believed to represent a 'cholinergic neuropil' (terminations of afferent processes derived via the septum), the ACE positive processes seen in some senile plaques are probably derived from (axonal) cholinergic afferents. In cases with small numbers of hippocampal neurofibrillary tangles these also stain with ACE (Fig. 9). As neurofibrillary tangle formation increases, in Alzheimer's disease, this ACE histochemical staining apparently decreases (Fig. 9). Whereas not all of the senile plaques appear to stain positively for ACE, it is probable, on the basis of present evidence, that in the early stages of Alzheimer-type pathology (when background fibre-staining is normal) most, if not all tangles, are positively stained (unpublished observations).

Certain deductions can be made from the histochemical observation that neurofibrillary tangles react positively for ACE. In the hippocampus, tangles are predominantly associated with pyramidal neurons, the majority of which are likely to be cholinoceptive (receiving cholinergic afferents via axodendritic synapses; reviewed by Kuhar, 1975). Shute and Lewis (1966a) have suggested that, in general, cholinoceptive neurons may be identified by the presence of ACE on their nuclear membranes and in the human hippocampus pyramidal cell nuclear membranes are, histochemically, ACE-positive (Perry and coworkers, 1979b). On the basis of these various observations, it might be postulated that neurofibrillary tangles in hippocampal pyramidal neurons arise in association with dendritic (cholinoceptive) abnormalities. Before further deductions can be made, further knowledge of cellular mechanisms controlling pre- and post-synaptic ACE is required, as is further knowledge of the precise role of the cholinergic system in Alzheimer-type pathology.

4. Some Interpretations

a. Functional enzyme alterations The interpretation of the biochemical abnormalities in Alzheimer's disease is beset with problems (Section II.B). It is not, for example, possible to say whether changes in enzyme activities represent an alteration in enzyme activities per cell or an actual change in cell numbers or processes. A further complicating factor is the probable existence in the brain of multiple molecular forms of CAT (Fonnum and Malthe-Sørenssen, 1973) and of ACE (Karlson and Fonnum, 1977), which have not yet been investigated in Alzheimer's disease. Nevertheless, certain conclusions may be drawn regarding the functional significance of the cholinergic enzyme abnormalities.

The simplest interpretation of decreased CAT and ACE activity in Alzheimer's disease is that these enzyme abnormalities reflect diminished cholinergic neurotransmission in the brain. This interpretation can, however, be questioned on the grounds that neither enzyme may be rate-limiting, although several animal experiments have suggested that long-term alterations in these enzyme activities may be related to the function of the cholinergic neuron. Thus, exposure to imprinting stimuli is accompanied, in chick brain, by increased CAT and ACE (Rose, Hambley, and Haywood, 1976), and in the rat brain electrical stimulation of the hippocampus (which improves memory function) is accompanied by an increase in CAT activity, especially in those strains with originally higher CAT levels (Jaffard and coworkers, 1977). In the peripheral nervous system CAT activity in the salivary gland is apparently increased by the 'traffic of nerve impulses' (Ekström, 1978). The enzyme changes are, however, relatively

Figure 9. Acetylcholinesterase (ACE) staining in post-mortem human brain. Only minimal counterstain (methyl green) has been used in these sections; details of the methods used are given in Perry and coworkers (1979). Abbreviations used in (a)–(g): A, alveus; O, stratum oriens; P, stratum pyramidale; R, stratum radiatum; LM, stratum lacunosum—moleculare, MG = molecular layer of dentate granular cells, G = dentate granular cells; BV, blood vessel; M, meninges; SP, senile plaques; NT, neurofibrillary tangle.

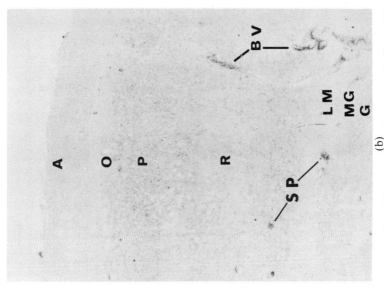

(a)   (b)

(a) and (b) Sections through the hippocampal formation of a normal case (a) (84 years, female; × 38) and a case of Alzheimer's disease (b) (78 years, male; × 28). ACE staining, believed largely to represent an afferent cholinergic neuropil, is concentrated in the stratum oriens, stratum pyramidale, stratum radiatum and granular zone of the dentate fascia. The cytoplasm of pyramidal cells is generally devoid of staining although most pyramidal nuclear membranes show some activity. Occasional cells show intensely stained cytoplasm, probably in Golgi type II cells (indicated with an arrow). In Alzheimer's disease (b) ACE staining is considerably reduced in all areas. Activity is still present in blood vessels

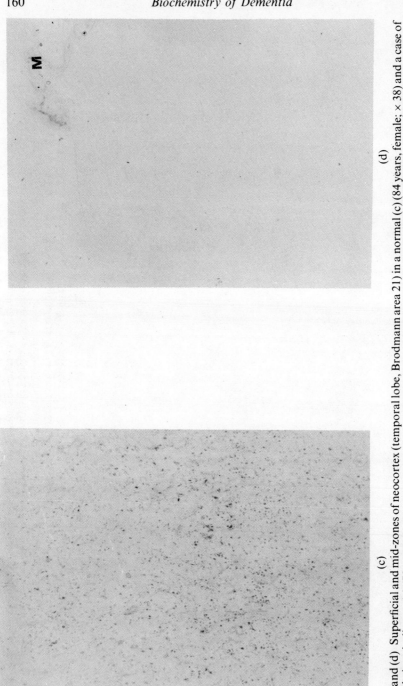

(d)

(c)

(c) and (d) Superficial and mid-zones of neocortex (temporal lobe, Brodmann area 21) in a normal (c) (84 years, female; × 38) and a case of Alzheimer's disease (a) (78 years, male; × 51). In the normal ACE is associated with small nerve processes (from which it may diffuse) and the nuclear membranes of neurons. In Alzheimer's disease ACE activity is greatly diminished and can only be positively identified in the meninges

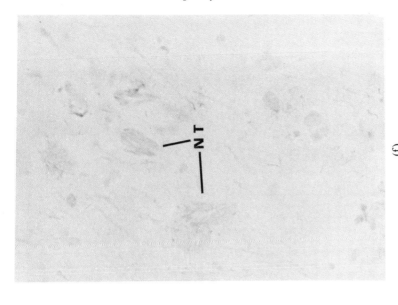

(f)

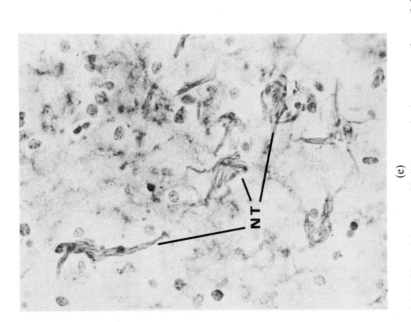

(e)

(e) ACE positive neurofibrillary tangles in a group of superficial neurons in the entorhinal cortex (× 38). Adjacent cortical tissue shows a normal amount of ACE staining (f) Neurofibrillary tangles in the hippocampal pyramidal layer neurons (Roses's area h_3) of a case of Alzheimer's disease (79 years, male) ACE staining of neurofibrillary tangles is considerably reduced or absent in well-established cases of Alzheimer's disease and appears to be reduced to the same extent as the surrounding neuropil (× 375)

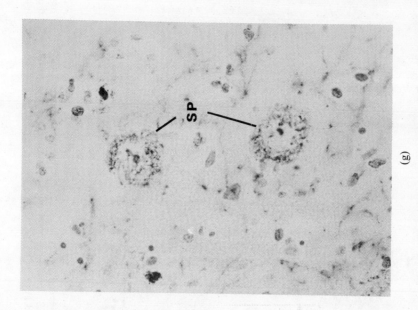

(g)

(g) Senile plaques in the stratum radiatum of a normal case (84 years, female; × 375). In these plaques ACE staining is predominantly located at the periphery of the plaque. In addition to slight, diffuse staining throughout most of the tissue, staining in fine nerve processes can be identified and ACE activity is also present on some nuclear membranes small (20–30 %), which may reflect a 'high safety margin' in the synthesis of ACh (Ekström, 1978).

Experimentally induced enzyme alterations, such as those in the peripheral and central nervous system, presumably reflect changes in enzyme activity or enzyme synthesis in the cell as opposed to major structural changes of the cholinergic neuron. Furthermore, the lack of a substantial variation in CAT according to nervous activity may, perhaps, explain why CAT activity is not significantly affected in conditions which might be expected to reduce mental activity, such as terminal illness or metabolic coma (Section III.E). In contrast to metabolic coma, coma resulting from head injury is apparently associated with substantial CAT losses in the brain (McGeer and McGeer, 1976a) and it may be worth noting that mesencephalic and diencephalic axonal processes are frequently severed as a result of brain trauma.

b. Deafferentation analogies It seems likely, on the basis of the present evidence of extensive CAT reductions in parts of the cortex (Table 3), and depletion of ACE histochemically in the hippocampus (Fig. 9), that these enzyme alterations in Alzheimer's disease reflect a decline in some structural component of the cholinergic neuron. There is a similarity between the behaviour of CAT, ACE, and MRB in Alzheimer's disease and in experimental situations such as septal–hippocampal lesioning and undercutting procedures in the cerebral cortex (Section II.B.3). This similarity suggests that the cholinergic input to areas such as cortex and hippocampus is deranged in Alzheimer's disease, possibly reflecting a degeneration of cholinergic afferent processes to these brain regions. Alternative explanations of the enzyme losses include the possibility that axonal transport along the afferent processes is defective, despite normal enzyme production in the cell body. This explanation would seem unlikely since no increase, or 'pile-up' of the enzyme has been recorded for any single brain area so far investigated in Alzheimer's disease. A possible decline of afferent fibres of the cortex in Alzheimer's disease may partially explain the apparent shrinkage of the cortical lobes in the absence of any alteration in the density of neuronal cell bodies (Tomlinson and Henderson, 1976). If there is, in Alzheimer's disease, a degeneration of cholinergic afferent processes in, for example, the neocortex, it would be important to establish the status of the related nerve cell bodies. The origins of all the cortical cholinergic processes are not yet clearly defined (Section II.B), although they are likely to include underlying nuclei in the septum and adjacent basal ganglia (Section II B.5).

c. Pseudocholinesterase There are several possible explanations for the rise in BCE activity in Alzheimer's disease. Increased BCE, for example, is compatible with axonal degeneration since in rat sciatic nerve enzyme activity increases following axotomy (Ranish, Kiauta, and Dettbarn, 1979). Although butyrylcholinesterase has been associated with glial cells (Section II. A), the increase in BCE activity in Alzheimer's disease is unlikely to be related to an actual increase in glial cell numbers, since the density of glial cells is reported to be unchanged in Alzheimer's disease (Tomlinson and Henderson, 1976) and increased BCE is not seen, histochemically, in glial cells in Alzheimer's disease (Friede, 1965; Perry and Tomlinson, unpublished). An apparent association of BCE activity with components of the blood brain barrier (Silver, 1974) suggests that elevated BCE might reflect changes, possibly secondary to tissue damage, in this barrier. However, major vessel abnormalities at the light microscopic level are not a particular feature of Alzheimer's disease (Corsellis, 1970), although functional changes in the blood-brain barrier might result from neuronal damage. It is of interest that acute experimental infarction is associated with increased BCE in cortical grey matter of animal brains, apparently due to uptake of the enzyme from the blood (Ott and coworkers, 1975).

An alternative explanation for the increase in BCE in Alzheimer's disease derives from the hypothesis (Koelle and coworkers, 1978) that BCE may be a precursor of ACE, with an accumulation of BCE in Alzheimer's disease possibly reflecting decreased production of ACE. However, in the hippocampus (see Fig. 2) BCE and ACE are differentially distributed, the former being apparently associated with the stratum lacunosum-moleculare (Perry and Tomlinson, unpublished) which is unlikely to contain many cholinergic process.

d. Acetyl-coenzyme A The observations (in a limited series) that two of the enzymes which produce acetyl-coenzyme A (pyruvate dehydrogenase and ATP-citrate lyase) are reduced in Alzheimer's disease whereas other enzymes, which could also provide acetyl-coenzyme A for ACh synthesis, are unaffected, require further investigation. In the first place, it would be of interest to establish what relationship, if any, exists between this abnormality and the loss of CAT, particularly whether a possible defect in acetyl-coenzyme A production precedes or follows the defects in the cholinergic system. Secondly, in considering basic cholinergic mechanisms, a 'selective' defect in a particular enzyme or enzymes which synthesize acetyl-coenzyme A, in a disease which apparently involves a cholinergic defect, may provide useful evidence regarding the normal source of acetyl-coenzyme A used in ACh synthesis. In this respect correlations, in different brain regions, between pyruvate dehydrogenase and CAT (Jope, 1978), together with the apparent loss of both enzymes in Alzheimer's disease, are suggestive of a particular role for at least pyruvate dehydrogenase in ACh synthesis.

e. Receptor sensitivities? The apparent normality of MRB, assessed biochemically, is consistent with the ultrastructural observations of preserved post-synaptic membrane 'thickenings' in Alzheimer's disease in the presence of gross morphological abnormalities of the nerve terminal (Gonatas, Anderson, and Evangelista, 1967). Apparently, the muscarinic receptor in the brain (as judged by *in vitro* binding of specific ligands) does not respond to denervation with a large increase in receptor numbers (Section II.B. 3). In this respect it differs from nicotinic receptors in muscle which increase following denervation. A difficulty in interpreting MRB activities is the pharmacological evidence in favour of a population of pre-synaptic muscarinic receptors (Section II.A.3) which indicates that present biochemical analysis may not be estimating pre-synaptic receptor sites. These pre-synaptic receptor sites, if they exist, might be expected to decline in Alzheimer's disease in conjunction with axonal terminal abnormalities. A further unknown factor relating to cholinergic activities in Alzheimer's disease is the status of the nicotinic receptor. Preliminary investigations of α-bungarotoxin binding in rat and human brain tissue have indicated post-mortem instability of the binding (Barnard and Perry, unpublished observations). It might be predicted, by analogy with cholinergic deafferentation (Section II.B.3) that nicotinic receptor binding in Alzheimer's disease may be normal in, for example, the hippocampus.

C. Comparisons with other Transmitter Systems

Of the different neurotransmitter systems in the brain, investigations in Alzheimer's disease have so far included only the noradrenaline (NE), dopamine (DA), 5-hydroxytryptamine (5-HT), γ-aminobutyric acid (GABA), and ACh systems. In contrast to the biochemical observations on cerebral cholinergic activities (Table 1), reports relating to these other (non-cholinergic) transmitter systems have not generally been consistent.

a. Noradrenaline Original reports of noradrenergic abnormalities in Alzheimer's disease have, to a certain extent, been supported recently (Adolfsson and coworkers, 1978), although significant reductions were observed in only 2 out of 10 areas investigated (putamen and frontal cortex) and the diagnosis of the disease was apparently based on clinical data. Biochemical findings indicating normality of the noradrenergic system include those discussed in a preliminary report (Davies and Maloney, 1976) in which dopamine β-hydroxylase and monoamine oxidase (two enzymes involved in noradrenergic metabolism) were apparently unchanged in Alzheimer's disease and in those of Yates (personal communication), indicating no significant reduction of noradrenaline in the amygdaloid or caudate nuclei. In histochemical studies, no relationship between senile plaques and monoamine oxidase activity was observed by Friede (1965), although Berger, Escourolle, and Moyne (1976) reported an apparent loss of noradrenergic-like fibre fluorescence in the cerebral cortex and fluorescent varicosities associated with plaques (Berger, Escourolle, and Moyne 1976).

b. Dopamine There have also been a number of inconsistent findings relating to this transmitter system in Alzheimer's disease, with reports of no significant alterations in DA or homovanillic acid (Davies, 1979; Yates, personal communication), but of significant losses of DA in 2 out of 10 areas (thalamus and pons) investigated (Adolfsson and coworkers, 1978). Spiroperidol binding (a measure of dopamine receptor activity in the brain) was apparently reduced in one of four areas recently investigated (caudate nucleus, Reisine and coworkers, 1978).

c. 5-Hydroxytryptamine No significant alterations in 5-HT, were originally observed in any of the 10 brain areas investigated by Adolfsson and coworkers (1978), although more recent observations (Gottfries, Chapter 10) indicate losses of 5-HT and 5-hydroxyindoleacetic acid in Alzheimer's disease. Bowen (Chapter 5) has observed a reduction in 5-HT receptor binding, using the ligand lysergic acid diethylamide whereas, using as a ligand 5-HT itself, preliminary observations (Marshall and Perry, unpublished observations) suggest the receptor binding is not significantly different from the normal.

d. γ-Aminobutyric Acid Decreased glutamate decarboxylase in necropsy tissue in Alzheimer's disease (Bowen and coworkers, 1974) was found to occur in various other mental diseases (Perry and coworkers, 1977b), and to bear no apparent relation to the extent of Alzheimer-type neuropathological abnormalties (Perry and coworkers, 1978b). Furthermore, a significant reduction in this enzyme (which synthesizes GABA) was not observed in biopsy tissue (Spillane and coworkers, 1977). Reisine and coworkers (1978) have recently reported significant decreases in GABA receptor binding, in two of four regions of the brain investigated, a decrease which did not, apparently, correlate with decreased CAT.

5. Controversial Evidence

On the basis of the present evidence, a particular abnormality of the dopamine, 5-hydroxytryptamine, or γ-aminobutyric acid systems in Alzheimer's disease is not, so far, clearly indicated. Possible abnormalities of the noradrenergic system and the reported alteration in GABA receptor binding in Alzheimer's disease merits further investigation. It will be of interest to establish whether the receptor alteration reflects abnormalities in some non-cholinergic neurons in Alzheimer's disease or is, alternatively, related to the apparent 'susceptibility' of the GABA system (as assessed by GAD activity) to a variety of pre-mortem changes connected with illness and coma (Perry and coworkers, 1977b).

Reported losses in non-cholinergic transmitter activities, so far investigated, are apparently neither consistent nor, where recorded, as extensive as the loss of CAT, and do not obviously follow the distribution of neuropathological changes in Alzheimer's disease. Thus, Adolfsson and coworkers (1978) did not observe significant losses of DA or NA in two areas of the brain which are usually severely affected by Alzheimer-type neuropathological abnormalities (hippocampus and adjacent gyrus). Regarding the specificity of possible catecholamine abnormalities, it is not yet clear to what extent catecholamine activities in Alzheimer's disease may be influenced by factors unrelated to dementia, such as physical illness or coma. Dopamine, for example, has been reported to be significantly, though not extensively, reduced in all types of coma (Jellinger and coworkers, 1978), and noradrenaline in cortical biopsy tissue was not demonstrated histochemically in one case of subarachnoid haemorrhage who was in a deep coma (Nyström, Olson, and Ungerstedt, 1972).

D. Comparisons with 'normal' Old Age

A detailed comparison between the behaviour of the cholinergic system in normal old age and in Alzheimer's disease has been made elsewhere (Perry, 1980). Whereas significant losses of both CAT and ACE occur in Alzheimer's disease, only the former (in some brain areas) declines significantly in old age itself (Section II.A). Consistent reductions in ACE, measured biochemically and histochemically (unpublished), are not seen in old age. These observations are compatible with a relative susceptibility in old age of the nerve terminal itself (in which most CAT may be localized) and with a more extensive involvement in Alzheimer's disease of the cholinergic neuron (ACE being more widely distributed in the cell than CAT).

The extent to which Alzheimer's disease may consist of an accentuation of the 'normal' ageing process, in certain brain regions, is not known. If the disease is simply an extension of age-related changes in brain biochemistry, these should all be apparent to a greater extent in Alzheimer's disease. With respect to transmitter systems this does not appear to be the case since most transmitter-related activities (in, for example, the DA, NA, GABA, and ACh systems) apparently decline with increasing age in the human brain (McGeer and McGeer, 1976b; McGeer, 1978); but a specific abnormality in all of these systems in Alzheimer's disease has not been established (Section IV.D).

There may be an association between age-related reductions in MRB (almost certainly localized on non-cholinergic cell processes) and the reported effects of age on non-cholinergic transmitter systems. Conversely, the normality of MRB in Alzheimer's disease may reflect a relative sparing of these other cell-types in the disease. These various observations are compatible with a 'particular' abnormality of the cholinergic system in Alzheimer's disease, as opposed to a generalized exacerbation of ageing changes.

E. Comparisons with other Cerebral Disorders

1. A Specific Question

Comparisons of cholinergic brain biochemistry in Alzheimer's disease, and in various neurological and psychiatric disorders, is a useful means of assessing the cholinergic changes in Alzheimer's disease. Observations relating to neocortical CAT, ACE, and MRB activities in dementia, depression, schizophrenia, Huntington's and Parkinson's diseases, are summarized in Table 5. In the latter two disorders investigations have obviously concentrated on measurements in brain regions other than the neocortex. Despite this reservation, sufficient data exist (Table 5) to indicate that reductions in neocortical CAT and ACE measured in Alzheimer's disease do not occur to any significant extent in these other diseases. If various 'non-specific' factors, such as drug treatment, hospitalization, physical inactivity, or generalized deranged mental function contributed to the cortical enzyme changes in Alzheimer's disease, similar changes might be expected in some of the other disorders. The absence of such changes (Table 5), together with a correlation between CAT loss and intellectual impairment (Perry and coworkers, 1978b), suggests that the widespread loss of neocortical cholinergic enzymes in Alzheimer's disease may be related to a selective global impairment of cognitive function. This is a predominant feature of Alzheimer's disease but not of the other neurological and psychiatric diseases (Table 5).

In brain regions other than the neocortex, such as the hippocampus, cholinergic abnormalities (at least with respect to CAT) are not confined to Alzheimer's disease and occur, to a lesser extent (Section IV.B.1), in depression

Table 5. Neocortical cholinergic activities in cerebral disorders

Condition	Choline acetyl- transferase	Acetyl cholin- esterase	Muscarinic receptor binding
Alzheimer's disease	Reduced[a, b, c, d]	Reduced[a, e]	Normal[b, c, f, d]
Multi-infarct dementia	Normal[b]	Normal[e]	Normal[g]
Depression	Normal[b]	Normal[e]	Normal[g]
Renal encephalopathy	Normal[b]	–	–
Parkinson's disease	Normal[h]	Normal[i]	Normal[h]
Huntington's disease	Normal[j]	Increased[i]	Normal[k]
Schizophrenia	Normal[l, g]	Normal[l] Increased[m, g]	Decreased[g]

References: [a] Davies and Maloney (1976); [b] Perry and coworkers (1977); [c] White and coworkers (1977); [d] Reisine and coworkers (1978); [e] Perry and coworkers (1978a); [f] Davies and Verth (1978); [g] Perry and coworkers (1980); [h] Reisine and coworkers (1977); [i] McGeer and McGeer (1976); [j] Bird and Iversen (1974); [k] Wastek and coworkers (1976); [l] Domino, Kranse, and Bowers (1979); [m] McGeer and McGeer (1977).

and multi-infarct dementia, conditions in which memory impairment (one of the clinical features of Alzheimer's disease) also occurs. Since some of the histopathological features of Alzheimer's disease are also present in such diseases as Down's syndrome (in cases reaching middle age), dementia pugilistica, progressive supranuclear palsy, and the Guam–Parkinson dementia complex (Tomlinson, Chapter 2), neurochemical investigations in these disorders will be of great interest.

2. Depression

The behavioural effects of certain cholinergic drugs indicate an involvement of the cholinergic system in some of the features of manic depressive illness (reviewed by Davis, Hollister, and Berger, 1977). Thus, physostigmine may counter manic symptoms (Janowsky and coworkers, 1973) and choline may induce depression (Tamminga and coworkers, 1976). Post-mortem investigations of brain tissue in depression have previously indicated no significant reductions in CAT or ACE in the neocortex (Table 5), although a non-significant trend towards decreased cerebral CAT was observed (Perry and coworkers, 1977b). In a further series (Section IV.B.1) this trend reached statistical significance in the hippocampus, and there may be a relationship between decreased neocortical CAT and impaired cognitive function in some cases of depression (Perry and coworkers, 1978b). These biochemical observations are consistent with a disturbance of cognitive function (including memory) in depression (Folstein and McHugh, 1978). This cognitive impairment is apparently reversible since physostigmine increases I.Q. score in manic depressive patients (Telford and Worrall, 1978) and cognitive function is restored on recovery from the illness itself. The absence of a permanent intellectual impairment in depression may, in contrast to Alzheimer's disease, reflect a relative integrity of cholinergic neuronal processes since the enzyme ACE (contained in cholinergic fibres, Section II.A.2) is unchanged in depression (Perry and coworkers, 1978a).

3. Schizophrenia

In schizophrenia, early pharmacological observations suggested that cholinergic agonists may counter certain clinical symptoms (Pfeiffer and Jenney, 1957), and a major disturbance of cholinergic function has been postulated in this disorder (Neubauer, 1975). Biochemical observations (Table 5) relating to cholinergic activities in the brains of chronic schizophrenic cases, include increased ACE and decreased MRB. If these observations are substantiated and shown to be unrelated to drug effects, they would warrant further investigation of the cholinergic system in schizophrenia.

V. PSYCHOPHARMACOLOGICAL OBSERVATIONS

Since one of the earliest and most prominent features of Alzheimer's disease consists of a short-term memory defect, physiological mechanisms and pharmacological aspects of short-term memory are obviously relevant to an understanding of the disease, especially with respect to possible therapeutic measures.

A. Memory and the Cholinergic System

There are likely to be many stages involved in the processing of (memory) information, involving diverse brain areas and chemical processes. In Alzheimer's disease, the particular neuropathological involvement of the hippocampus (Corsellis, 1970) and apparent abnormality of the cholinergic system (Section IV.A), raise the question of the anatomical role of the hippocampus and the biochemical role of the cholinergic system in memory functions. Numerous experiments on animals have now demonstrated a central role for the cholinergic system in memory and learning (reviewed by Deutsch, 1973; Brimblecombe, 1974; De Feudis, 1974; Karczmar, 1975). The effects of drugs, surgical lesioning, and electrical stimulation have indicated that the hippocampus may be a critical structure in the short-term storage of information, although the evidence relating to this function of the hippocampus is not always straightforward in these animal experiments (Black, 1978). Nevertheless, during learning the 'trial response' may be impaired through lesioning or application of muscarinic antagonists and improved by electrical stimulation of the septal pathway (Warburton and Russel, 1969; Singh, Ott, and Matties, 1974; Gralewicz and coworkers, 1978; Jaffard and coworkers, 1977).

In man, an involvement of the hippocampus in short-term memory has frequently been inferred from various clinical and neuropathological observations (reviewed by Dejong, 1973), although there are obviously hazards attached to the assignment of specific functions to brain regions, such as the hippocampus, as a result of behavioural disorders following their destruction (Horel, 1978). Similarly, from a neurochemical point of view, it may be naive to draw conclusions on the chemical processes involved in memory from the behavioural effects of apparently specific drugs. Nevertheless, experiments in man on the effects of various cholinergic drugs have demonstrated significant alterations in memory and other cognitive functions (reviewed by Davis and Yamamura, 1978). Thus, learning is apparently impaired following the administration of the muscarinic cholinergic antagonist, scopolamine (Crow and Grove-White, 1973; Drachman and Leavitt, 1974; Peterson, 1977). This impairment may primarily involve the capacity to store new information, leaving long-term memory function intact (Peterson, 1977), and is reported to mimic some of the cognitive defects common to senile dementia (Drachman, 1977). Furthermore, these drug-induced changes which may, according to Drachman (1978), provide an experimental model for Alzheimer's disease, are apparently reversed by physostigmine but not by amphetamine (Drachman, 1977, 1978). In contrast to the effects of antagonists, cholinergic agonists, such as choline or arecoline and physostygmine may enhance certain aspects of learning in normal subjects (Sitaram, Weingartner, and Gillin, 1978; Mohs and Davis, in press), and in one pathological situation (herpes encephalopathy) physostygmine has been reported to improve short-term memory function (Peters and Levin, 1977).

B. Cholinergic Agonists in Alzheimer's Disease

These psychopharmacological data (above), implicating the cholinergic system in memory function, together with the biochemical observations of a cerebral cholinergic abnormality in Alzheimer's disease, have led to the formulation of a cholinergic hypothesis of the memory disorder in the disease (Smith and Swash, 1978) and have recently prompted several trials of cholinergic agonists in suspected cases of Alzheimer's disease. Oral choline, reported by some investigators (Wurtman and Growdon, 1978) but not others (Flentge and Van den Berg, 1979) to increase the levels of ACh in animal brain tissue including the hippocampus (Hirsch, Growdon, and Wurtman, 1977) has not, in trials so far conducted, resulted in significant clinical improvement in cases of Alzheimer's disease (Boyd and coworkers, 1977; Etienne and coworkers, 1978a; Signoret, Whitely, and Lhermitta, 1978; Smith and coworkers, 1978). Some effects of lecithin, the natural dietary source of choline, are somewhat more positive, with reports of significant cognitive improvements in certain cases (Etienne and coworkers, 1978b) and of a reduction in further deterioration in the long term (Christie and coworkers, in press).

Interpretation of the clinical effects of choline compounds in Alzheimer's disease is complicated by the number of unknown factors. Biochemically, ACh turnover (as opposed to levels of the transmitter) may not be increased in the brain by oral choline (Eckernäs, 1977), and theoretical comparisons of the kinetics of low- and high-affinity choline uptake suggest that elevations in brain choline may actually stimulate the former rather than the latter (Jenden, 1977). Consequently, choline may need to be provided in higher doses or for longer periods in order to influence ACh levels in the nerve terminal. In this connection, the possible development of tolerance may have to be considered (Davis and coworkers, 1978). On the pathological side, it is not yet known whether ACh release is impaired in Alzheimer's disease, nor whether production of the other ACh precursor, acetyl-coenzyme A, is normal. This last question may be answered by further investigation of the various enzymes which may provide acetyl-coenzyme A for ACh synthesis (Section IV. A).

An alternative approach to cholinergic 'potentiation' in the brain is the use of ACE inhibitors, such as physostygmine, which raise the content of cerebral ACh (Bartholini, Bartholini, and Domino, 1973). In a case of familial Alzheimer's disease, physostygmine significantly reduced the false-positive (intrusion) errors during recall (Smith and Swash, 1979). This observation raises the interesting possibility that the memory defect in Alzheimer's disease may include the inability to suppress inappropriate information and that this particular component of memory function might be under cholinergic control. Obviously, the effects of cholinergic drugs in Alzheimer's disease are worth investigating further, and there are many other cholinergic agonists which might be employed in future trials. These include other inhibitors of ACE (Comfort, 1978), muscarinic agonists such as arecoline, the various analogues of oxotremorine (Davis, Hollister, and Berger, 1977; Jenden, 1977), and guanidine which promotes ACh release in the Eaton–Lambert syndrome (Van Woert, 1976).

VI. OVERVIEW

A. A Cholinergic Involvement

The concept of a cholinergic involvement in the pathology of Alzheimer's disease is now supported by a variety of consistent biochemical and psychopharmacological evidence. It is, however, unlikely that Alzheimer's disease is primarily due to widespread cholinergic dysfunction, since some of the most active cholinergic brain regions (such as caudate-putamen) are not obviously involved at the histopathological level. Cerebral cholinergic abnormalities may, therefore, be the result of some other, as yet unidentified, pathological process in Alzheimer's disease. In this respect, it is worth considering various possible modulators of cholinergic function and possible reasons for a particular susceptibility of the cholinergic system in the brain.

B. Some Cholinergic Modulators

Numerous interactions exist between the different transmitter systems in the brain and include, in the cortex, modulation of ACh levels or ACh release by 5-hydroxytryptamine (Samanin and coworkers, 1978), dopamine (Mantovani and Pepeu, 1978), and noradrenaline (Vizi and coworkers, 1978). The extent to which these, and other non-cholinergic transmitter systems, may be involved in Alzheimer's disease is not yet clear, although present evidence (Section II. C) suggests that abnormalities of, at least, dopamine and γ-aminobutyric acid systems are not specifically related to the disease itself. There are obviously many other transmitter and related systems which require to be investigated in Alzheimer's disease, including the polypeptide hormone and 'neuromodulator' groups. These neuropeptides are unevenly distributed in the brain, and increasing evidence suggests that some may be released from nerve terminals to act directly as neuromodulators (Gainer, 1977). Certain of these peptides, including thyrotropin-releasing hormone, somatostatin, neurotensin, angiotensin, substance p and β-endorphin, influence the turnover of ACh in discrete brain areas including, in some instances, cortex and hippocampus (Cheney and coworkers, 1978; Malthe-Sørenssen and coworkers, 1978). There may also be a functional link between growth hormone and the cholinergic system, since cholinergic drugs apparently control the release of this hormone (Bruni and Merties, 1978). This latter observation is of particular interest in view of the emaciated state of many patients with Alzhemier's disease.

C. Cholinergic Susceptibilities

One possible mechanism of selective cholinergic vulnerability consists of the interference by an autoimmune or toxic element in normal cholinergic transmitter function. Examples of this mechanism include the putative immunological abnormality in myasthenia gravis (affecting the nicotinic receptor) and the postulated toxin production (inhibiting ACh release) in the Eaton–Lambert syndrome associated with undifferentiated small cell lung carcinoma (Van Woert, 1976). In experimental situations the effects on cholinergic transmission of a broad range of neurotoxins (Howard, 1978) suggest that the cholinergic synapses may be particularly vulnerable in this respect.

The cholinergic system may also be particularly sensitive to metabolic disturbances on account of its absolute dependence on *de novo* transmitter synthesis. Unlike many other neurotransmitter systems, in which reuptake into the nerve terminal may contribute to the provision of transmitter for further release, recycling of this kind in the cholinergic system is probably confined to choline and a constant supply of newly-synthesized acetyl-coenzyme A is required to maintain transmitter release. These characteristics of the cholinergic system may partly account for the apparently greater rate of ACh turnover (Hanin and Costa, 1976) compared with that of, for example, the catecholamines (Cooper, Bloom, and Roth, 1974) in brain tissue.

Recent observations (Blass, Chapter 7) indicate an apparent susceptibility of cholinergic neurons to minor metabolic restrictions. Thus, impairment of carbohydrate utilization in even mild hypoxia substantially reduced the incorporation of radioisotopically labelled glucose into ACh, an effect which was more pronounced in hippocampus and neocortex, compared with striatum (Blass and coworkers, Chapter 7). In this respect it will be interesting to determine the relation, if any, between the reductions in particular enzymes which may provide acetyl-coenzyme A for ACh synthesis (Section IV.A) and in CAT activity in Alzheimer's disease. It is, on the whole, unlikely that 'hypoxia' primarily accounts for the cholinergic abnormalities of Alzheimer's disease, since the cholinergic enzyme activities are not decreased in multi-infarct dementia (Sections IV.B and IV.E) nor in experimental infarction (Ott and coworkers, 1975; Bowen and coworkers, 1976). Nevertheless, the possibility of a relatively stricter dependence of the cholinergic system on transmitter synthesis could account for a comparative sensitivity to other types of metabolic derangement in certain brain areas.

D. Conclusion

Although present biochemical evidence is compatible with a 'cholinergic hypothesis' in Alzheimer's disease, current research continues to raise more questions than it answers. Our knowledge not only relating to brain biochemistry in Alzheimer's disease but also to many fundamental aspects of the cerebral cholinergic system will, no doubt, expand rapidly in the future. The advent of a reliable histochemical 'marker' and of a 'probe' of cerebral cholinergic function, which can be used in human subjects, will open new avenues in the investigations of cholinergic mechanisms in mental disorders such as Alzheimer's disease.

VII. SUMMARY

Recent biochemical and psychopharmacological observations have indicated an involvement of the cholinergic system in senile dementia of Alzheimer-type (Alzheimer's disease). In biochemical analysis of post-mortem brain tissue from established cases of Alzheimer's disease, cholinergic enzyme activities are consistently abnormal and, psychopharmacologically, cholinergic antagonists (such as scopolamine) induce in normal individuals cognitive impairments, including short-term memory defects reminiscent of those in Alzheimer's disease. From comparisons between the biochemistry of the cholinergic system in Alzheimer's disease, various other mental disorders, and normal old age, the evidence suggests a specific involvement of the cholinergic system in Alzheimer's disease. Biochemically, the enzyme (choline acetylase and cholinesterase) abnormalities correlate with the extent of certain Alzheimer-type neuro-pathological changes and histochemically acetylcholinesterase activity is decreased in Alzheimer's disease, although neurofibrillary tangles and a proportion of senile (neuritic) plaques stain positively. The behaviour of the cortical cholinergic system (loss of choline acetylase and acetylcholinesterase with apparently no alteration in muscarinic receptor binding) is similar in both Alzheimer's disease and in experimental animals following surgical lesioning of cholinergic afferent processess. The cholinergic defect of Alzheimer's disease is, therefore, compatible with a decline in normal cholinergic afferent function, a decline which may in turn reflect an abnormality of a cholinergic 'modulator' in the brain. Among the numerous potential 'modulators' of cholinergic neuronal function only various other neurotransmitter systems have, to date, been examined in Alzheimer's disease, and consistent reports of extensive abnormalities (related to neuropathological changes) of the γ-aminobutyric acid, dopamine, 5-hydroxytryptamine, and noradrenaline systems have not yet appeared. There are, however, many other transmitter and neuropeptide systems which remain to be investigated in Alzheimer's disease.

ACKNOWLEDGEMENTS

The work reported here was carried out in collaboration with Professor B. E. Tomlinson, Drs G. Blessed, K. Bergmann, and P. Gibson, and their permission to use some unpublished data is much appreciated. The assistance of Mrs P. Taylor, Mr J. McClennan and Mr A. B. Keith is gratefully acknowledged, as are biochemical facilities provided by Dr R. N. J. Pennington and the financial support of the Newcastle Area Health Authority (Teaching) Research Committee and the Wellcome Foundation (Grant 7596/1.24). We are indebted to all of these.

REFERENCES

Adolfsson, R., C. G. Gottfries, L. Oreland, B. E. Roos and B. Winblad (1978). Reduced levels of catecholamines in the brain and increased activity of monoamine oxidase in platelets in Alzheimer's disease: therapeutic implications. In R. Katzman, R. D. Terry, and K. L. Bick (Eds) *Alzheimer's Disease: Senile Dementia and Related Disorders*, Raven Press, New York. pp. 441–451.

Ansell, G. B. and S. Spanner (1978). The source of choline for acetylcholine synthesis. In D. J. Jenden (Ed.) *Cholinergic Mechanisms and Psychopharmacology*, Plenum Press, New York. pp. 431–445.

Aquilonius, S. M., G. Ceder, U. Lying-Tunell, H. O. Malmlund, and J. Schuberth (1975). The arteriovenous difference of choline across the brain of man. *Brain Res.*, **99**, 430–433.

Banns, H., C. Hebb, and S. P. Mann (1978). Synthesis of acetyl-CoA and acetyl-dephospho-CoA by acetyl-CoA synthetase in the rat. *J. Neurochem.*, **30**, 915–916.

Bartholini, A., R. Bartholini, and E. F. Domino (1973). Effects of physostigmine on brain acetylcholine content and release. *Neuropharmacology*, **12**, 12–25.

Berger, B., R. Escourolle, and M. A. Moyne (1976). Axones, caticholaminerques du cortex cerebral humain. *Rev. Neurol. (Paris)*, **136**, 183–194.

Bird, E. D. and L. L. Iversen (1974). Huntington's chorea—postmortem measurement of glutamic acid decarboxylase, choline acetyltransferase and dopamine in basal ganglia. *Brain*, **97**, 457–472.

Birdsall, N. J. M., A. S. V. Burgen, and E. C. Hulme (1978). Correlation between the binding properties and pharmacological responses of muscarinic receptors. In D. J. Jenden (Ed.) *Cholinergic Mechanisms and Psychopharmacology*, Plenum Press, New York. pp. 25–33.

Biscoe, T. J. and D. W. Straughan (1966). Microelectrophoretic studies of neurones in the cat hippocampus. *J. Physiol. (London)*, **183**, 341–59.

Black, A. H. (1978). Functions of the septal-hippocampal system. *Nature (London)*, **271**, 208–9.

Blessed, G., B. E. Tomlinson, and M. Roth (1968). The association between quantitative measures of dementia and of senile change in the cerebral grey matter of elderly subjects. *Brit. J. Psychiat.*, **114**, 797–811.

Bowen, D. M., M. J. Goodhardt, A. J. Strong, C. B. Smith, P. White, N. M. Branston, L.

Symon, and A. N. Davison (1976). Biochemical indices of brain structure, function and 'hypoxia' in cortex from baboons with middle cerebral artery occlusions. *Brain Res.*, **117**, 503–7.

Bowen, D. M., P. White, R. H. A. Flack, C. B. Smith, and A. N. Davison (1974). Brain decarboxylase activities as indices of pathological changes in senile dementia. *Lancet*, **1**, 1247–9.

Boyd, W. D., J. Graham-White, G. Blackwood, I. Glen, and J. McQueen (1977). Clinical effects of choline in Alzheimer senile dementia. *Lancet*, **2**, 711.

Brimblecombe, R. W. (1974). *Drug Action on Cholinergic Systems*. Macmillan, London.

Browning, E. T. (1976). Acetylcholine synthesis: substrate availability and the synthetic reaction. In A. M. Goldberg and I. Hanin (Eds) *Biology of Cholinergic Function*, Raven Press, New York. pp. 187–201.

Bruni, J. F. and J. Merties (1978). Effects of cholinergic drugs on growth hormone release. *Life Sci.*, **23**, 1351–8.

Celesia, C. and G. H. H. Jasper (1966). Acetylcholine released from cerebral cortex in relation to the state of activation. *Neurology*, **16**, 1053–63.

Cheney, D. L., F. Moroni, D. Malthe-Sørenssen, and E. Costa (1978). Endogenous modulators of acetylcholine turnover rate. In D. J. Jenden (Ed.) *Cholinergic Mechanisms and Psychopharmacology*, Plenum Press, New York. pp. 551–63.

Cheney, D. L., G. Racagni, and E. Costa (1976). Distribution of acetylcholine and choline acetyltransferase in specific nuclei and tracts of rat brain. In A. M. Goldberg and I. Hanin (Eds) *Biology of Cholinergic Function*, Raven Press, New York. pp. 655–81.

Christie, J. E., E. I. M. Blackburn, A. I. M. Glen, A. Shering, C. M. Yates, E. H. Jellinek, and S. Zeisel (In press). In L. J. Whalley, and A. I. M. Glen (Eds) *Alzheimer's Disease, Early Recognition of Potentially Reversible Deficits*, Churchill Livingstone, Edinburgh.

Comfort, A. (1978). Cholinesterase inhibition in treatment of Alzheimer's disease. *Lancet*, **1**, 659–60.

Cooper, J. R., F. E. Bloom, and R. H. Roth (1974). The biochemical basis of neuropharmacology. Oxford University Press, Oxford.

Corsellis, J. A. N. (1970). The limbic areas in Alzheimer's disease and in other conditions associated with dementia. In G. E. W. Wolstenholme and M. O'Connor (Eds) *Alzheimer's Disease and Related Conditions*, J. & A. Churchill, London. pp. 37–50.

Crow, T. J. and I. G. Grove-White (1973). An analysis of the learning deficit following hyoscine administration to man. *Brit. J. Pharmacol.*, **49**, 322–7.

Davis, K. L., P. A. Berger, L. E. Hollister, and J. D. Barchas (1978). Cholinergic involvement in mental disorders. *Life Sci.*, **22**, 1865–72.

Davis, K. L. and H. I. Yamamura (1978). Cholinergic underactivity in human memory disorders. *Life Sci.*, **23**, 1729–34.

Davis, K. L., L. E. Hollister, and P. A. Berger (1977). Cholinergic mechanisms in neurological and psychiatric disorders. In E. Usdin, D. A. Hamburg, and J. D. Barchas (Eds) *Neuroregulators and Psychiatric Disease*, Oxford University Press, Oxford. pp. 442–50.

Davies, P. (1978). Studies on the neurochemistry of central cholinergic systems in Alzheimer's disease. In R. Katzman, R. D. Terry, and K. L. Bick (Eds) *Alzheimer's Disease: Senile Dementia and Related Disorders*, Raven Press, New York. pp. 453–459.

Davies, P. (1979). Biochemical changes in Alzheimer's disease—senile dementia: neurotransmitters in senile dementia of Alzheimer's type. In R. Katzman (Ed.) *Congenital and Acquired Cognitive Disorders*, Raven Press, New York. pp. 153–60.

Davies, P. and A. J. F. Maloney (1976). Selective loss of cholinergic neurons in Alzheimer's disease. *Lancet*, **2**, 1403.

Davies, P. and A. H. Verth (1978). Regional distribution of muscarinic acetylcholine receptor in normal and Alzheimer-type dementia brains. *Brain Res.*, **138**, 385–92.

De Feudis, F. V. (1974). *Central Cholinergic Systems and Behaviour*, Academic Press, New York.

Dejong, R. N. (1973). The hippocampus and its role in memory. *J. Neurol. Sci.*, **19**, 73–83.

Deutsch, J. A. (1973). The cholinergic synapse and the site of memory. In J. A. Deutsch (Ed.) *The Physiological Basis of Memory*, Academic Press, New York. pp. 59–74.

Domino, E. F., R. R. Krause, and J. Bowers (1973). Various enzymes involved with putative neurotransmitters. *Arch. Gen. Psychiat.*, **29**, 195–201.

Drachman, D. A. (1977). Cognitive function in man. Does the cholinergic system have a special role? *Neurology*, **27**, 783–90.

Drachman, D. A. (1978). Memory, dementia and the cholinergic system. In R. Katzman, R. D. Terry, and K. L. Bick (Eds) *Alzheimer's Disease: Senile Dementia and Related Disorders*, Raven Press, New York. pp. 141–8.

Drachman, D. A. and J. Leavitt (1974). Human memory and the cholinergic system, a relationship to ageing? *Arch. Neurol.*, **30**, 113–21.

Dudai, Y. and M. Segal (1978). α-Bungarotoxin binding sites in rat hippocampus; localisation in post-synaptic cells. *Brain Res.* **154**, 167–71.

Eckernäs, S.-A. (1977). Plasma choline and cholinergic mechanisms in the brain. *Acta Physiol. Scand.*, **449**, (Suppl.), 1–62.

Ekström, J. (1978). Acetylcholine synthesis and its dependence on nervous activity. *Experientia*, **34**, 1247–51.

Emson, P. C. and O. Lindvall (1979). Distribution of putative neurotransmitters in the neocortex. *Neuroscience*, **4**, 1–30.

Etienne, P., S. Gauthier, G. Johnson, B. Collier, T. Mendis, D. Dastoor, M. Cole, and H. F. Muller (1978a). Clinical effects of choline in Alzheimer's disease. *Lancet*, **1**, 508–9.

Etienne, P., S. Gauthier, D. Dastoor, B. Collier, and J. Ratner (1978b). Lecithin in Alzheimer's disease. *Lancet*, **2**, 1206.

Fahn, S. (1976). Regional distribution of GABA and other putative neurotransmitters and their enzymes. In E. Roberts, T. N. Chase, and D. B. Towers (Eds) *GABA in Nervous System Function*, Raven Press, New York. pp. 169–86.

Flentge, F. and C. J. Van Den Berg (1979). Choline administration and acetylcholine in brain. *J. Neurochem.*, **32**, 1331–3.

Foldes, F. F., E. K. Zsigmond, V. P. Foldes, and E. G. Erdös (1962). The distribution of acetylcholinesterase and butyrylcholinesterase in the human brain. *J. Neurochem.*, **9**, 559–72.

Folstein, M. F. and P. R. McHugh (1978). Dementia syndrome of depression. In R. Katzman, R. D. Terry, and K. L. Bick (Eds) *Alzheimer's Disease: Senile Dementia and Related Disorders*, Raven Press, New York. pp. 87–96.

Fonnum, F. (1970). Topographical and subcellular localisation of choline acetyltransferase in rat hippocampal region. *J. Neurochem.*, **17**, 1029–37.

Fonnum, F. (1973). Recent developments in biochemical investigations of cholinergic transmission. *Brain Res.*, **62**, 497–507.

Fonnum, F. (1975). Review of recent progress in synthesis, storage and release of acetylcholine. In P. Waser (Ed.) *Cholinergic Transmission*, Raven Press, New York. pp. 145–59.

Fonnum, F. and D. Malthe-Sørenssen (1973). Membrane affinities and subcellular distribution of the different molecular forms of choline acetyltransferase in rat. *J. Neurochem.*, **20**, 1351–9.

Fonnum, F. and I. Walaas (1978). The effect of intrahippocampal kainic acid injections and surgical lesions on neurotransmitters in hippocampus and septum. *J. Neurochem.*, **31**, 1173–81.

Fonnum, F., I. Walaas, and E. Iversen (1977). Localization of GABAergic, cholinergic and aminergic structures in the mesolimbic system.*J. Neurochem.*,**29**, 221–30.

Friede, R. L. (1965). Enzyme histochemical studies of senile plaques. *J. Neuropath. Exp. Neurol.*, **24**, 477–91.

Friede, R. L. (1967). A comparative mapping of the distribution of butyryl cholinesterase in the brains of four species of mammals including man. *Acta Anatomica*, **66**, 161–177.

Gainer, H. (Ed.) (1977). *Peptides in Neurobiology*, Plenum Press, New York.

Gonatas, N. K., A. Anderson, and I. Evangelista (1967). The contribution of altered synapses in the senile plaque—an electron microscope study in Alzheimer's dementia. *J. Neuropath. Exp. Neurol.*, **26**, 25–39.

Gralewicz, S., K. Gralewicz, H. Ciborska-Jabukowska, and H. Ziemska (1978). Proactive and retroactive effects of hippocampal stimulation on active avoidance learning, hippocampal EEG and brain acetylcholinesterase activity in cats. *Acta Neurobiol. Exp.*, **38**, 45–61.

Hadhazy, P., and J. C. Szerb (1977). The effect of cholinergic drugs on (^{3}H)-acetylcholine release from slices of rat hippocampus, striatum and cortex. *Brain Res.*, **123**, 311–22.

Hanin, I. and E. Costa (1976). Approaches used to estimate acetylcholine turnover *in vivo*: effects of drugs on brain acetylcholine turnover. In A. M. Goldberg and I. Hanin (Eds) *Biology of Cholinergic Function*, Goldberg, Raven Press, New York. pp. 355–94.

Hebb, C. (1963). Formation, storage and liberation of acetylcholine. In G. B. Koelle (Ed.) *Cholinesterases and Anticholinesterase Agents*, Springer-Verlag, Berlin. pp. 55–88.

Hebb, C. O., K. Krnjević, and A. Silver (1963). Effect of undercutting on the acetylcholinesterase and choline acetyltransferase activity in the cat's cerebral cortex. *Nature (London)*, **198**, 692.

Hebb, C. O. and A. Silver (1956). Choline acetylase in the central nervous system of man and some other mammals. *J. Physiol.*, **134**, 718–28.

Hemsworth, B. A. and M. J. Neal (1968). The effect of central stimulation drugs on acetylcholine release from rat cerebral cortex. *Brit. J. Pharmacol.*, **34**, 543–50.

Hesse, H. (1943). *The Glass Bead Game*, translated from German by R. & C. Winston (Penguin Books, England, 1972).

Hiley, C. R. and A. S. V. Burgen (1974). The distribution of muscarinic receptor sites in the nervous system of the dog. *J. Neurochem.*, **22**, 159–62.

Hirsch, M. J., J. H. Growdon, J. Wurtman (1977). Increase in hippocampal acetylcholine after choline administration. *Brain Res.*, **125**, 383–5.

Hooper, M. W. and F. S. Vogel (1976). The limbic system in Alzheimer's disease. *Amer. J. Path.*, **85**, 1–20.

Horel, J. A. (1978). The neuroanatomy of amnesia. A critique of the hippocampal memory hypothesis. *Brain*, **101**, 403–46.

Howard, B. (1978). Effects of polypeptide neurotoxins on acetylcholine storage and release. In D. J. Jenden (Ed.) *Cholinergic Mechanisms and Psychopharmacology*, Plenum Press, New York. pp. 565–85.

Hunt, S. P. and J. Schmidt (1978). The electron microscopic autoradiographic localisation of α-bungarotoxin binding sites within the central nervous system of the rat. *Brain Res.*, **142**, 152–9.

Ishii, T. and R. L. Friede (1967). Comparative histochemical mapping of the distribution of acetyl-cholinesterase and nicotinamide adenine-diaphorase activities in the human brain. *Int. Rev. Neurobiol.*, **10**, 231–75.

Jaffard, R., A. Ebel, C. Destrade, T. Durkin, P. Mandel, and B. Cardo (1977). Effects of hippocampal electrical stimulation on long-term memory and on cholinergic mechanisms in three inbred strains of mice. *Brain Res.*, **133**, 277–89.

Janowsky, D. S., M. K. El-yousef, J. M. Davis, and H. J. Sekerke (1973). Parasympathetic suppression of manic symptoms by physostigmine. *Arch. Gen. Psychiat.*, **28**, 542–7.

Jellinger, K., P. Riederer, G. Kleinberger, S. Wuketich, and P. Kothbauer (1978). Brain monoamines in human hepatic encephalopathy. *Acta Neuropath.*, **43**, 63–8.

Jenden, D. J. (1977). Some recent developments in the biochemical pharmacology of cholinergic systems. In E. Usdin, D. A. Hamburg, and J. D. Barchas (Eds) *Neuroregulators and Psychiatric Disorders*, Oxford University Press, Oxford. pp. 425–33.

Jenden, D. J. (Ed.) (1978). *Cholinergic Mechanisms and Psychopharmacology*, Plenum Press, New York.

Jope, R. S. (1978). Pyruvate utilisation, choline uptake and acetylcholine synthesis. In D. J. Jenden (Ed.) *Cholinergic Mechanisms and Psychopharmacology*, Plenum Press, New York. pp. 497–509.

Karczmar, A. G. (1975). Cholinergic influences on behaviour. In P. G. Waser (Ed.) *Cholinergic Mechanisms*, Raven Press, New York. pp. 501–29

Karlson, R. L. and F. Fonnum (1977). Properties of the external acetylcholinesterase in guinea-pig iris. *J. Neurochem.*, **29**, 151–6.

Kelly, P. H. and K. E. Moore (1978). Decrease of neocortical choline acetyltransferase after lesion of the globus pallidus in the rat. *Exp. Neurol.*, **61**, 479–84.

Koelle, G. B. (1954). The histochemical localisation of cholinesterases in the CNS of the rat. *J. Comp. Neurol.*, **100**, 211–35.

Koelle, G. B., W. A. Koelle, E. G. Smyrl, R. Davis, and A. F. Nagle (1978). Histochemical and pharmacological evidence of the function of butyrylcholinesterase. In D. J. Jenden (Ed.) *Cholinergic Mechanisms and Psychopharmacology*, Plenum Press, New York. pp. 125–37.

Krnjević, K. and J. W. Phillis (1963). Acetylcholine-sensitive cells in the cerebral cortex. *J. Physiol. (London)*, **166**, 296–327.

Kuhar, M. J. (1975). Cholinergic neurons: septal-hippocampal relationships. In R. L. Isaacson and K. H. Pribram (Eds) *The Hippocampus*, Vol. I, Plenum Press, New York. pp. 269–83.

Kuhar, M. J. and S. F. Atweh (1978). Distribution of some suspected neurotransmitters in the central nervous system. *Rev. Neurosci.* **3**, 35–76.

Kuhar, M. J., V. H. Sethy, R. H. Roth, and G. K. Aghajanian (1973). Choline: selective accumulation by central cholinergic neurons. *J. Neurochem.*, **20**, 581–93.

Kuhar, M. J. and H. Yamamura (1975). Cholinergic muscarinic receptors in rat brain, light autoradiographic localisation by the specific binding of a potent antagonist. *Nature (London)*, **253**, 560–1.

Lefresne, P., J. C. Beaujouan, and J. Glowinski (1978). Origin of the acetyl moiety of acetylcholine in rat striatal synaptosomes: a specific pyruvate dehydrogenase involved in ACh synthesis. *Biochimie*, **60**, 479–87.

Lewis, P. R., C. C. D. Shute, and A. Silver (1967). Confirmation from choline acetylase analyses of a massive cholinergic innervation to the rat hippocampus. *J. Physiol.*, **191**, 215–24.

Livett, B. G. (1978). Immunohistochemical localization of nervous system—specific proteins and peptides. *Int. Rev. Cytol.*, **7**, 33–218.

Lloyd, K. G., A. Shibuya, L. Davidson, and O. Hornykiewicz (1977). Chronic neuroleptic therapy: Tolerance and GABA systems. *Adv. Biochem. Psychopharmacol.*, **16**, 409–13.

Loewi, O. (1921). Überhumorale Übertragbarkeit der Herznervenwirkung, *Pflügers Archiv für die gesamte Physiologie des Menschen und der Tiere*, **189**, 239–42.

Lynch, G. S., S. Masko, T. Parks, and C. W. Cotman (1973). Relocation and hyperdevelopment of the dentate gyrus following entorhinal lesions in immature rats. *Brain Res.*, **50**, 174–8.

Mackay, A. V. P., P. Davies, A. J. Dewar, and C. M. Yates (1978). Regional distribution of enzymes associated with neurotransmission by monoamines, acetylcholine and GABA in the human brain. *J. Neurochem.*, **30**, 827–39.

Malthe-Sørenssen, D., P. L. Wood, D. L. Cheney, and E. Costa (1978). Modulation of the turnover rate of acetylcholine in rat brain by intraventricular injections of thyrotropin releasing hormone, somatostatin, neurotensin and angiotensin II. *J. Neurochem.*, **31**, 685–91.

Mantovani, P. G. Pepeu (1978). Influence of dopamine agonists on cholinergic mechanisms in the cerebral cortex. In S. Gatattini, J. F. Pujol, and R. Samanin (Eds) *Interactions between Putative Transmitters in the Brain*, Raven Press, New York. pp. 53–9.

Mautner, H. G. (1977). Choline acetyltransferase. *C.R.C. Critical Review of Biochemistry*, **4**, 341–70.

McGeer, E. G. (1978). Ageing and neurotransmitter metabolism in the human brain. In R. Katzman, R. D. Terry, and K. L. Bick (Eds) *Alzheimer's Disease: Senile Dementia and Related Disorders*, Raven Press, New York. pp. 427–40.

McGeer, P. L. and E. G. McGeer (1976a). Enzymes associated with the metabolism of catecholamines, acetylcholine and GABA in human controls and patients with Parkinson's disease and Huntington's chorea. *J. Neurochem.*, **26**, 65–76.

McGeer, E. G. and P. L. McGeer (1976b). Neurotransmitter metabolism in the ageing brain. In R. D. Terry and S. Gershon (Eds) *Neurobiology of Ageing*. Raven Press, New York. pp. 389–403.

McGeer, P. L. and E. G. McGeer (1977). Possible changes in striatal and limbic cholinergic systems in schizophrenia. *Arch. Gen. Psychiat.*, **34**, 1319–23.

McIntosh, F. C. (1941). The distribution of acetylcholine in the peripheral and the central nervous system. *J. Physiol.*, **99**, 436–42.

McIntosh, F. C. and P. E. Osborn (1953). Release of acetylcholine from intact cerebral cortex. *Prose. XIX International Physiology Congress*, pp. 580–1.

Mellgren, S. I., W. Harkmark, and B. Srebro (1977). Some enzyme histochemical characteristics of the human hippocampus. *Cell and Tissue·Research*, **181**, 450–71.

Mellgren, S. I. and B. Srebro (1973). Changes in acetylcholinesterase and distribution of degenerating fibres in the hippocampal region after septal lesions in the rat. *Brain Res.*, **52**, 19–36.

Miller, E. K. (1970). *Phospholipid Assembly and Exchange in Cerebral Membranes*. Ph.D. Thesis, University of Cambridge.

Mohs, R. C. and K. L. Davis (In press). Psychometric aspects of studies on drugs used to improve memory function in Alzheimer's disease. In *Alzheimer's Disease, Early Recognition of Potentially Reversible Deficits.* Churchill Livingstone, Edinburgh.

Molenaar, P. C. and R. L. Polak (1970). Stimulation by atropine of acetylcholine release and synthesis in cortical slices from rat brain. *Brit. J. Pharmacol.*, **40**, 406–17.

Morley, B. J., J. F. Lorden, G. B. Brown, G. E. Kemp, and R. J. Bradley (1977). Regional distribution of nicotinic acetylcholine receptor in rat brain. *Brain Res.*, **134**, 161–6.

Muller, P. and P. Seeman (1977). Brain neurotransmitter receptors after long-term haloperidol. *Life Sci.*, **21**, 1751–8.

Nachmanson, D. and A. L. Michado (1943). The formation of acetylcholine. A new enzyme: 'choline acetylase'. *J. Neurophysiol.*, **6**, 397–403.

Nadler, J. V. and C. W. Cotman (1978). Interaction between afferents to the dentate gyrus after entorhinal lesion during development: long-term regulation of choline acetyltransferase. *Brain Res.*, **142**, 174–81.

Neubauer, H. (1975). The role of central cholinergic mechanisms of schizophrenia. *Medical Hypothesis*, **1**, 32–4.

Nyström, B., L. Olson, and U. Ungerstedt (1972). Noradrenaline nerve terminals in human cerebral cortex. *Science*, **176**, 924–6.

Op Den Velde, W. and F. C. Stam (1976). Some cerebral proteins and enzyme systems in Alzheimer's presenile and senile dementia. *J. Amer. Geriat. Soc.*, **24**, 12–6.

Ott, E. O., J. Abraham, J. S. Meyer, A. N. Achari, A. N. C. Chee, and N. T. Mathew (1975). Disordered cholinergic neurotransmission and dysautoregulation after acute cerebral infarction. *Stroke*, **6**, 172–80.

Pepeu, G., A. Mulas, and M. L. Mulas (1973). Changes in the acetylcholine content in the rat brain after lesions of the septum, fimbria and hippocampus. *Brain Res.*, **57**, 153–64.

Perry, E. K. (1980). The cholinergic system in normal old age and dementia. *Age and Aging*. **9**, 1–8.

Perry, R. H., G. Blessed, E. K. Perry, and B. E. Tomlinson (1980). Histochemical observations on cholinesterase activities in the brains of elderly normal and demented (Alzheimer-type) patients. *Age and Aging*. **9**, 9–16.

Perry, E. K., R. H. Perry, G. Blessed, and B. E. Tomlinson (1977a). Necropsy evidence of central cholinergic deficits in senile dementia. *Lancet*, **1**, 189.

Perry, E. K., P. H. Gibson, G. Blessed, R. H. Perry, and B. E. Tomlinson (1977b). Neurotransmitter enzyme abnormalities in senile dementia. *J. Neurol. Sci.*, **34**, 247–65.

Perry, E. K., R. H. Perry, P. H. Gibson, G. Blessed, and B. E. Tomlinson (1977c). A cholinergic connection between normal ageing and senile dementia in the human hippocampus. *Neurosci. Lett.*, **6**, 85–9.

Perry, E. K., R. H. Perry, and B. E. Tomlinson (1977d). Circadian variations in cholinergic enzymes and muscarinic receptor binding in human cerebral cortex. *Neurosci. Lett.*, **4**, 185–9.

Perry, R. H., B. E. Tomlinson, M. J. Taylor, and E. K. Perry (1977e). Human brain temperature at necropsy, a guide in post-mortem biochemistry. *Lancet*, **1**, 38.

Perry, E. K., R. H. Perry, G. Blessed, and B. E. Tomlinson (1978a). Changes in brain cholinesterases in senile dementia of Alzheimer type. *Neuropath. Appl. Neurobiol.*, **4**, 273–7.

Perry, E. K., B. E. Tomlinson, G. Blessed, K. Bergmann, P. H. Gibson, and R. H. Perry (1978b). Correlation of cholinergic abnormalities with senile plaques and mental test scores in senile dementia. *Brit. Med. J.*, **2**, 1457–9.

Peters, B. H. and H. S. Levin (1977). Memory enhancement after physostigmine treatment in the amnesic syndrome. *Arch. Neurol.*, **34**, 215–9.

Peterson, R. C. (1977). Scopolamine-induced learning failures in man. *Psychopharmacology*, **52**, 283–9.

Pfeiffer, C. F. and E. H. Jenney (1957). The inhibition of the conditioned response and the counteraction of schizophrenia by muscarinic stimulation of the brain. *Ann. N. Y Acad. Sci.*, **66**, 753–64.

Phillis, J. W. and D. H. York (1967). Cholinergic inhibition in the cerebral cortex. *Brain Res.*, **5**, 517–20.

Polz-Tejera, G., J. Schmidt, and H. J. Karten (1975). Autoradiographic localisation of α-bungarotoxin-binding sites in the central nervous system. *Nature (London)*, **258**, 349–51.

Pope, A., H. H. Hess, and E. Lewin (1964). Studies on the microchemical pathology of human cerebral cortex. In M. M. Cohen and R. S. Snider (Eds) *Morphological and Biochemical Correlates of Neural Activity*, Harper and Row, New York. pp. 98–111.

Ranish, N. A., T. Kiauta, and W.-D. Dettbarn (1979). Axotomy-induced changes in cholinergic enzymes in rat nerve and muscle. *J. Neurochem.*, **32**, 1157–64.

Reisine, T. D., J. Z. Fields, H. I. Yamamura, E. D. Bird, E. Spokes, P. S. Schreiner, and S. J. Enna (1977). Neurotransmitter receptor alterations in Parkinson's disease. *Life Sci.*, **21**, 335–44.

Reisine, T. D., H. I. Yamamura, E. D. Bird, E. Spokes, and S. J. Enna (1978). Pre- and post-synaptic neurochemical alterations in Alzheimer's disease. *Brain Res.*, **159**, 477–80.

Robinson, N. (1966). Friedreich's ataxia: a histo-chemical and biochemical study. II. Hydrolytic enzymes. *Acta Neuropath.*, **6**, 34–45.

Rommelspacher, H. and M. J. Kuhar (1974). Effects of electrical stimulation on acetylcholine levels in central cholinergic nerve terminals. *Brain Res.*, **81**, 243–51.

Rose, S. P. R., J. Hambley, and J. Haywood (1976). Neurochemical approaches to developmental plasticity and learning. In M. R. Rosenzweig and E. L. Bennet (Eds) *Neural Mechanisms of Learning and memory*, M.I.T. Press, Cambridge, Massachusetts.

Rossier, J. (1977). Choline acetyltransferase; a review with special reference to its cellular and subcellular localization. *Int. Rev. Neurobiol.*, **20**, 284–337.

Samanin, R., A. Quattrone, G. Peri, H. Ladinsky, and S. Consolo (1978). Evidence of an interaction between serotonergic and cholinergic neurons in the corpus striatum and hippocampus of the rat. *Brain Res.*, **151**, 73–82.

Sethy, V. H., R. H. Roth, M. J. Kuhar, and M. H. Van Woert (1973). Choline and acetylcholine: regional distribution and effect of degeneration of cholinergic nerve terminals in the rat hippocampus. *Neuropharmacology*, **12**, 819–23.

Sethy, V. H. and M. H. Van Woert (1974). Brain acetylcholine and cholinesterase: effect of phenothiazines and physostigmine interaction in rats. *J. Neurochem.*, **23**, 105–9.

Shute, C. C. D. and P. R. Lewis (1963). Cholinesterase-containing systems of the brain of the rat. *Nature (London)*, **199**, 1160–4.

Shute, C. C. D. and P. R. Lewis (1966a). Electron microscopy of cholinergic terminals and acetylcholinesterase-containing neurones in the hippocampal formation of the rat. *Zeitschrift für Zellforschung*, **69**, 334–43.

Shute, C. C. D. and P. R. Lewis (1966b). Cholinergic and monoaminergic pathways in the hypothalamus. *Brit. Med. Bull.*, **22**, 221–6.

Signoret, J. L., A. Whitely, F. Lhermitta (1978). Influence of choline on amnesia in early Alzheimer's disease. *Lancet*, **2**, 837.

Silver, A. (1974). *Biology of Cholinesterases*, North-Holland, Amsterdam.

Singh, H. K., T. Ott, and H. Matties (1974). Effect of intrahippocampal injection of atropine on different phases of a learning experiment. *Psychopharmacologia*, **38**, 247–56.

Sitaram, N., H. Weingartner, and J. C. Gillin (1978). Human serial learning: Enhancement with arecholine and choline and impairment with scopolamine. *Science*, **201**, 274–6.

Smith, C. M. (1972). The release of acetylcholine from rabbit hippocampus. *Brit. J. Pharmacol.*, **45**, 172.

Smith, C. M. and M. Swash (1978). Possible biochemical basis of memory disorder in Alzheimer's disease. *Ann. Neurol.*, **3**, 471–3.

Smith, C. M. and M. Swash (1979). Physostigmine in Alzheimer's disease. *Lancet*, **1**, 42.

Smith, C. M., M. Swash, A. N. Exton-Smith, M. J. Phillips, P. W. Overstall, M. E. Piper, and M. R. Bailey (1978). Choline in Alzheimer's disease. *Lancet*, **2**, 318.

Spillane, J. A., P. White, M. J. Goodhardt, R. H. A. Flack, D. M. Bowen, and A. N. Davison (1977). Selective vulnerability of neurons in organic dementia. *Nature (London)*, **266**, 558–9.

Spokes, E. G. and D. J. Koch (1978). Post-mortem stability of dopamine, glutamate decarboxylase and choline acetyltransferase in the mouse brain under conditions simulating the handling of human autopsy material. *J. Neurochem.*, **31**, 381–3.

Steiner, F. A. (1968). Influence of microelectrophoretically applied acetylcholine on responsiveness of hippocampal and lateral geniculate neurons. *Pfleugers Archiv: Eur. J. Physiol.*, **303**, 173–80.

Storm-Mathisen, J. (1970). Quantitative histochemistry of acetylcholinesterase in rat hippocampal region correlated to histochemical staining. *J. Neurochem.*, **17**, 739–50.

Tamminga, C., R. C. Smith, S. Chang, J. S. Haraszti, and J. M. Davis (1976). Depression associated with oral choline. *Lancet*, **2**, 905.

Telford, R. and E. P. Worrall (1978). Cognitive functions in manic depressives—effects of lithium and physostigmine. *Brit. J. Psychiat.*, **133**, 424–8.

Tomlinson, B. E., G. Blessed, and M. Roth (1970). Observations on the brains of demented old people. *J. Neurol. Sci.*, **11**, 205–42.

Tomlinson, B. E. and G. Henderson (1976). Some quantitative cerebral findings in normal and demented old people. In R. D. Terry and S. Gerschon (Eds) *Neurobiology of Ageing*, Raven Press, New York. pp. 183–227.

Tuček, S. (1978). *Acetylcholine Synthesis in Neurons*, Chapman and Hall, London.

Van Woert, M. H. (1976). Myasthenia gravis, Eaton–Lambert syndrome and familial dysautonomia. In A. M. Goldberg and I. Hanin (Eds) *Biology of Cholinergic Function*, Raven Press, New York. pp. 567–81.

Vizi, S. E. and M. Palkovits (1978). Acetylcholine content in different regions of the rat brain. *Brain Res. Bull.*, **3**, 93–6.

Vizi, E. S., A. Ronai, L. G. Harsing, and J. Knoll (1978). Presynaptic modulation by norepinephrine and dopamine of acetylcholine release in the peripheral and central nervous system. In D. J. Jenden (Ed.) *Cholinergic Mechanisms and Psychopharmacology*, Plenum Press, New York. pp. 587–603.

Warburton, D. M. and R. W. Russel, (1969). Some behavioural effects of cholinergic stimulation in the hippocampus *Life Sci.*, **8**, 617–27.

Wastek, G. J., L. Z. Stern, P. C. Johnson, and H. I. Yamamura (1976). Regional alteration in muscarinic cholinergic receptor binding in human brain. *Life Sci.*, **19**, 1033–40.

Wenk, H., U. Meyer, and V. Bigle (1977). Centrifugal cholinergic connections in the olfactory system of the rat. *Neuroscience*, **2**, 797–800.

White, P., C. R. Hiley, M. J. Goodhardt, L. H. Carrasco, J. P. Keet, I. E. I. Williams, and D. M. Bowen (1977). Neocortical cholinergic neurons in elderly people. *Lancet*, **1**, 668–70.

Wurtman, R. J. and J. H. Growdon (1978). Dietary enhancement of CNS neurotransmitters. *Hospital Practice*, **March**, 71–7.

Yamamura, H. I., M. J. Kuhar, D. Greenberg, and S. H. Snyder (1974). Muscarinic cholinergic receptor binding—regional distribution in monkey brain. *Brain Res.*, **66**, 541–6.

Yamamura, H. I. and S. H. Snyder (1974). Post-synaptic localisation of muscarinic cholinergic receptor binding in rat hippocampus. *Brain Res.*, **78**, 320–6.

Biochemistry of Dementia
Edited by P. J. Roberts
© 1980, John Wiley & Sons Ltd.

Chapter 9

Clinical and Biochemical Studies in Alzheimer's Disease

C. M. YATES, I. A. BLACKBURN, J. E. CHRISTIE,
A. I. M. GLEN, A. SHERING, J. SIMPSON,
I. J. WHALLEY, and S. ZEISEL*

*M. R. C. Brain Metabolism Unit, Department of Pharmacology, University of
Edinburgh, 1 George Square, Edinburgh, EH8 9JZ, U.K.*

Massachusetts Institute of Technology, Cambridge, Massachusetts, U.S.A.

I. INTRODUCTION

Alzheimer's disease, or Alzheimer-type dementia, describes a dementing condition which is characterized by a large increase in the number of senile plaques and neurofibrillary tangles demonstrated at post-mortem. The pre-senile form of this disease refers to an onset before age 65 years and the senile form to onset after 65 years.

Drugs used in the treatment of Alzheimer's disease may be divided into two categories: (a) alleviation of distress, and (b) attempts to treat an underlying cause. Included in (a) are antidepressants to treat a frequently coexisting depression, and tranquillizers. The latter, particularly certain of the pheno-thiazines, are used to sedate patients who are restless and difficult to manage. Category (b) includes agents designed to increase cerebral oxygenation or to effect central cholinergic stimulation.

A. Attempts to Increase Cerebral Oxygenation

Intermittent exposure to hyperbaric oxygen was reported by Jacobs and coworkers (1969) to improve cognitive function in patients with chronic brain syndrome, which included patients with Alzheimer's disease. Thompson and coworkers (1976), however, in a more controlled study, could not reproduce these observations and were unable to demonstrate any improvement in cerebral blood flow. They also noted that patients with cerebrovascular disease, who might be expected to have reduced cerebral oxygenation, did not respond to hyperbaric oxygen. Two drugs claimed by the manufacturers to improve cognition and memory in the elderly, by stimulating the cerebral circulation, are piracetam (1-acetamido-2-pyrrolidone) and Hydergine (a mixture of halogenated ergot alkaloids). However, in two double-blind studies, piracetam was found to have no effect on dementia (Dencker and Lindberg, 1977) nor on mental function and cerebral blood flow (Gustafson and coworkers, 1978). In a review article, Hughes, Williams, and Currier (1976) concluded that the small magnitude of expected improvement combined with the absence of indications of long-term benefits suggested that Hydergine was of minor clinical value in the treatment of dementia. Thus, no agent has as yet been shown to counteract the reduction in cerebral blood flow which Ingvar and his colleagues have demonstrated in Alzheimer's disease (Editorial, *Brit. Med. J.*, 1976).

B. Attempts to Stimulate Cholinergic Transmission in the Central Nervous System

Pfeiffer and Jenney, in 1957, described 'lucid intervals' in schizophrenics given arecoline and atropine methylnitrate. In a search for longer-acting cholinergic agonists or precursors of acetylcholine, they discovered that 2-dimethylaminoethanol (deanol) increased motor and verbal activity and insomnia in schizophrenia (Pfeiffer and coworkers, 1957). Dimethylaminoethanol is incorporated into liver and brain phospholipids (Groth, Bain, and Pfeiffer, 1958; Ansell and Spanner, 1962) and has been reported to increase the concentrations of choline and acetylcholine in rat brain (Haubrich and coworkers, 1975). The *p*-chlorophenoxyacetic acid ester of dimethyl aminoethanol (centrophenoxine or meclofenate; Thuillier, Rumpf, and Thuillier, 1959) was reported to relieve confusional states, memory, and intellectual disturbance in senescence (Nandy and Bourne, 1966). These early reports have not been confirmed in a large double-blind trial, although a significant improvement in learning was observed in a small double-blind trial (Gedye, Exton-Smith, and Wedgwood, 1972). Nandy and Bourne (1966) suggested that the clinically beneficial effects of centrophenoxine might be related to its ability to reduce lipofuscin accumulation in senescent guinea-pigs and rats (Riga and Riga, 1974). An age-related increase in intracellular oxidation, indicated by the age-related increase in deposition of lipofuscin (Brody, 1960; Mann and Yates, 1974), might result in oxidation of the thiol groups of the microtubules and the formation of the abnormal twisted tubules of Alzheimer's disease (Terry and Wisniewski, 1969). Deaner[R], the ester of dimethylaminoethanol and *p*-acetamidobenzoic acid, has been used with varied success to treat tardive and L-dopa-induced dyskinesias (Miller, 1974; Casey and Denney, 1975; Fann and coworkers, 1975; Klawans, Topel, and Bergen, 1975). In view of the subsequent discovery of a loss of choline acetyltransferase activity in Alzheimer brain tissue (Davies and Maloney, 1976; Perry and coworkers, 1977), the action and use of deanol as a central cholinergic stimulant requires reappraisal.

C. Clinical Implications of Post-mortem Studies of Alzheimer's Disease

Until the advent of biochemical examination of post-mortem brain tissue, no marked biochemical abnormalities which could be related to the illness had been found in patients with Alzheimer's disease (Embree, Bass, and Pope, 1972). Early studies on post-mortem brain showed increased lysosomal enzyme activity which could be related to gliosis (Bowen, Smith, and Davison, 1973) and reduction in acidic, neuronin-type proteins (Smith and Bowen, 1976). However, these changes, unlike more recent studies of the cholinergic system, did not suggest a mode of treatment. The presence in Alzheimer brain tissue of muscarinic receptors in normal numbers and showing normal affinity (Perry and coworkers, 1977; Davies and Verth, 1978) suggests that the presumed deficit in cholinergic transmission, caused by a reduction in choline acetyltransferase activity (Davies and Maloney, 1976; Perry and coworkers, 1977; White and coworkers, 1977), might be remedied by increasing the amount of acetylcholine at the receptor. Oral administration of choline (Cohen and Wurtman, 1976) and lecithin (Hirsch and Wurtman, 1978) to rats increases the concentration of choline and acetylcholine in brain. We have, therefore, attempted to treat patients with Alzheimer's disease by administration of choline and lecithin. Our first study was of seven severely demented in-patients, five over 80 years old and two aged over 70. Choline chloride (5 g per day or 10 g per day), given for two weeks, produced no improvement, as measured by psychometric tests or nurses' behavioural ratings (Boyd and coworkers, 1977). Some patients did, however, appear to be more manageable and more aware of their surroundings. We considered that treatment should be attempted in younger patients in whom the dementing process was not so far advanced. Psychometric tests, which were almost impossible in the older patients, should be more satisfactory in younger, less demented patients. We also investigated the possibility that Alzheimer's disease might be related to a deficit of choline uptake. Cholinergic neurons have a sodium-dependent, high-affinity choline uptake system which is believed to be the rate-limiting step in the synthesis of acetylcholine (Haga and Noda, 1973; Yamamura and Snyder, 1973; Simon, Atweh, and Kuhar, 1976) and appears to be coupled to choline acetyltransferase (Barker and Mittag, 1975). Choline is transported from blood plasma to brain by a system which resembles an amino acid transport mechanism (Cornford, Braun, and Oldendorf, 1978). Thus, a deficit of choline uptake at the nerve cell or the blood-brain barrier might produce the well-documented loss of brain choline acetyltransferase activity in Alzheimer's disease.

The aims of the present study were:

(i) To observe the clinical effects of choline and lecithin in a carefully selected group of patients with pre-senile Alzheimer dementia.

(ii) To measure serum and CSF choline levels to determine if there was any abnormality in the basal levels, and to observe the effect of choline and lecithin treatment.

(iii) To compare choline uptake by Alzheimer erythrocytes (RBCs) with the uptake by age and sex-matched controls.

II. CLINICAL EFFECTS OF CHOLINE AND LECITHIN IN PRE-SENILE ALZHEIMER'S DEMENTIA

Patients with a progressive history of dysmnesia, commencing before 65 years of age, were admitted to the research ward of the Medical Research Council Brain Metabolism Unit in the Royal Edinburgh Hospital. They were assessed over a three-week period during which they received no medication. During this period, which also allowed the patients to adapt to the ward environment, basal scores for behavioural and psychometric performance and samples of blood for determination of basal levels of serum choline and RBC choline uptake were obtained. A diagnosis of Alzheimer's disease was based largely on the dysmnesia and the exclusion of other conditions such as alcoholism (Table 1). Fulfilment of criteria A to E in Table 1 was considered essential for a firm diagnosis and admission to the trial. Neurological examination was performed by a neurologist independent of the ward psychiatrists. Informed consent was obtained from the patient or the nearest relative if the patient was unable to understand what was involved. The study protocol was approved by the Ethics Committee of the Royal Edinburgh Hospital.

Following admission to the trial, choline chloride was administered in a syrup, as 0.6 g given four times a day. The dose was increased over a four-day period to 1.5 g given four times a day. This daily dose of 6 g was maintained for five days. Choline chloride was then withdrawn and the patients remained drug-free for seven days. Lecithin granules (G. R. Lane Health Products Ltd) were then given, at a starting dose usually of 10 g given four times a day. The dose was increased over four days to a maintenance dose of 25 g given four times a day. This maintenance dose, of 100 g daily, was continued for 7–10 days until the patient was discharged. The preparation of lecithin granules contained between 20 and 30 % phosphatidyl choline and an estimated 3.5 % free choline. Thus, the full daily doses of choline chloride and lecithin granules contained approximately 4.5 g and 3.5 g free choline, respectively, calculated as base. The first two patients were started on 7 g lecithin four times daily and maintained on this dose. Five patients were discharged on 100 g lecithin daily and one patient was discharged on 28 g lecithin daily.

Table 1. Diagnosis of Alzheimer pre-senile dementia

A. Onset under the age of 65 years with dysmnesia as the initial feature. Progressing dementia

B. History. Absence of:

Alcoholism	Cardiovascular disease (acquired)
Head injury	Peripheral vascular disease
Pre-existing epilepsy	Cerebrovascular accident
Mental handicap	Family history suggestive of other causes of dementia

C. Physical and neurological examination. Absence of:

Hypertension	Fundal hypertensive change
Peripheral vascular disease	Cerebellar signs
Pyramidal tract signs	Cranial nerve signs

D. CAT scan evidence of cerebral atrophy and absence of additional pathology

E. The following investigations within normal limits:

Haemoglobin	Chest X-ray
ESR	Skull X-ray
B_{12}	ECG
Folate	CSF: VDRL
Urea and electrolytes	Pressure
Liver function tests	Protein
Fasting blood glucose	Gamma globulin
T4	
VDRL	

F. Additional features which provide support to the diagnosis of Alzheimer's disease:

Dyspraxia	Expressive dysphasia
Paraphasia	Pallilalia
Logoclonia	Echolalia
Stiff gait, generalized tone increase	

A. Patient Assessment

Global assessment of the degree of dementia, based on history, clinical features, and behaviour, was made by a psychiatrist using a 1–10 scale. A rating of 1 corresponded to slight dysmnesia which was apparent on testing and a rating of 10 to a completely incapacitated, bed-ridden, mute patient.

Patients were assessed daily throughout their stay in the ward by specially trained nursing staff, using the modified Stockton Rating Scale (Meer and Baker, 1966; Gilleard and Pattie, 1977). This scale itemizes 12 aspects of self-care and behaviour, such as dressing, helpfulness, irritability, and sociability, which are rated on a three-point scale. The higher the score, the greater the disability. During the study the nursing staff felt that the scale was not sufficiently sensitive and it was therefore expanded to five points. Individual patients were scored using one scale only.

A psychologist administered a battery of tests (Eisenson, 1954; Weschsler, 1955; Kimura and Archibald, 1974) to assess the following: (i) orientation and memory, which included forward and backward digit span and logical memory; (ii) agnosia for (a) common objects, (b) pictures, (c) colours, (d) auditory agnosia, (e) tactile agnosia, (f) naming of body parts; (iii) dyspraxia for (a) draw and copy, (b) hand position, (c) finger flexion, (d) use of objects, (e) intransitive gestures. The test, which took 30–45 min to complete, was given on two occasions while the patients were in the ward. Base-line scores were obtained 2–3 weeks after admission (i.e. after the patients had had time to become accustomed to the ward) but before starting choline therapy. Patients were retested about four weeks later, just before discharge, when they had been on 100 g lecithin daily for 7–10 days. In six patients the test was repeated three months after discharge.

B. Effects of Treatment

Twelve patients, seven women and five men, satisfied the diagnostic criteria for Alzheimer pre-senile dementia (Table 2). One patient (AR) was too demented and unco-operative to participate in the trial. His behaviour was, however, assessed while in the ward and receiving no treatment. The mean age of the 11 patients admitted to the trial, was 60 with a range of 53–67 years and a mean time since onset of 3.8 years. A further patient (MS), diagnosed as suffering from Pick's disease (Sim, Turner and Smith, 1966), is included separately in some of our results. Choline chloride and lecithin were well-tolerated and caused few side-effects. Transient diarrhoea was common and in two patients this resulted in occasional faecal incontinence. There was, however, no increase in urinary incontinence or other signs of stimulation of peripheral cholinergic synapses, and

Table 2. Patients with pre-senile Alzheimer dementia

Patient	Sex	Age	Age of onset of dysmnesia	Global rating of dementia (1–10)
GY	M	61	60	1
JH	F	58	54	3
AH	F	53	50	4
CR	F	57	54	4
JS	F	64	61	4
JP	M	57	53	4
MH	F	54	51	5
SH	F	67	58	5
TH	M	62	59	6
JK	M	66	61	7
MF	F	61	57	7
Mean	7F, 4M	60	56	

no noticeable fishy odour. The patients tended to become mildly irritated on both choline and lecithin and some appeared to have improved mood. In one patient (JK) lecithin had to be discontinued because of aggressive behaviour. Of the six patients interviewed after three months on lecithin, one showed a marked gain in weight.

The overall global assessment and the nurses' ratings on the Stockton scale are shown in Table 3. The mean daily rating over three consecutive days was calculated for six periods as follows:

- (i) Admission—first three drug-free days in the ward.
- (ii) Pre-choline—three drug-free days immediately before starting choline.
- (iii) Choline—three days while on 6 g choline chloride daily.
- (iv) Pre-lecithin—three drug-free days immediately before starting lecithin.
- (v) Lecithin—three days immediately following establishment of maintenance dose of 100 g lecithin daily.
- (vi) Discharge lecithin—three days on 100 g or 28 g (JH and MH only) lecithin daily just before discharge. The higher the score, the greater the disability.

The admission (i) and pre-choline (ii) scores, representing baseline behaviour, did not differ by more than two points in 6 out of the 11 patients. Of the remaining five patients, four showed a reduced score at the pre-choline test compared with

Table 3. Nurses' ratings of Alzheimer patients using the modified Stockton scale

Patient	Sex	Age	Global Rating	Mean daily rating over 3 days					
				Ad-mission	Pre-choline	Chol-ine	Pre-lecithin	Leci-thin	Discharge lecithin
GY	M	61	1	1	1	1	1	0	1
JH	F	58	3	2	3	7	5	3†	3†
CR*	F	57	4	16	12	13	7	4	4
AH	F	53	4	14	13	11	7	6	6
JP*	M	57	4	15	17	11	16	13	9
JS	F	64	4	13	16	15	12	13	13
MH	F	54	5	13	8	18	12	12†	12†
SH	F	67	5	18	19	19	19	19	19
TH	M	62	6	16	13	14	17	13	15
JK	M	66	7	19	21	22	20	19	19
MF*	F	61	7	29	23	22	25	28	27
AR	M	64	8	22	No treatment				24
MS*	M	63	Pick's disease	16	12	14	16	18	19

* Stockton ratings measured on a 5-point scale.
† Only 28 g lecithin granules per day.

the admission test, presumably representing adaptation to the ward environment, and one patient (JS) had a higher score at the pre-choline test. Scores at periods (iii), (iv), (v), and (vi) were compared with the base-line scores at periods (i) and (ii). Three patients (CR, AH, and JP) improved on lecithin and two of these (AH and JP) showed some improvement on choline. CR and AH improved in the pre-lecithin drug-free week. Patients showing improvement all rated 4 on the global scale. Patient AR, who was severely demented and was not treated, and patient MS who had Pick's disease, worsened during their six weeks in the ward.

The results of psychological testing are given in Table 4. A high score indicates a good response. The patients are arranged in the table in order of increasing disability, as assessed by the global rating score. Two of the patients who showed improvement on the behavioural scale (JS and CR, Table 3) and one patient (MF) who showed no change in behavioural score, had increased psychometric scores when on lecithin. In all three patients, this improvement was due to a diminution of apraxia. One patient's apraxia (JP) worsened during lecithin treatment. Of the six patients tested three months after discharge, two (JS and CR) had stopped taking lecithin. One of these patients (CR) had a score indicating increased dyspraxia. The four patients who continued to take lecithin showed no improvement but, on the other hand, had not deteriorated since their last testing.

It would thus appear that neither choline nor lecithin had a dramatic effect on the function of the group as a whole. There was, however, a suggestion of improvement in three patients (CR, AH, and JP) with a mild to moderate dementia when treated with lecithin. Particular aspects which were improved were speech, orientation, and lessening of dyspraxia. Two mildly affected patients (global ratings 1 and 3) and severely affected patients with ratings of more than 6 showed no detectable improvement, although one of the mildly affected (GY) reported a reduced reliance on note-taking. The nurses' ratings gave a better indication of the patient's overall behaviour and function than did the psychological tests. We have found in many studies that daily behavioural ratings by trained nursing staff are an extremely sensitive assessment technique. The psychological tests we used covered a wide area of possible defects. In order to keep the duration of testing to a reasonable time of 30–45 min, the individual components of the test battery had to be kept short and were thus not sufficiently sensitive for patients with mild dysmnesia, or proved too difficult for severely affected patients. An alternative technique would be to tailor the tests to each patient and measure his response over a period of time. An estimate of rate of deterioration and effect of treatment on this rate could then be established. This approach is particularly suitable for the assessment of Alzheimer-type dementia because of the extreme variability in the level of functioning. Table 5 summarizes studies in which choline (four reports) and lecithin (one report) have been given to patients with Alzheimer's disease. In only one study were the effects of active

Table 4. Scores of psychological testing of Alzheimer patients

Patient	Global score	Pre-treatment				Lecithin prior to discharge				3 Months on lecithin				
		A	B	C	Total	A	B	C	Total	A	B	C	Total	
GY	1	36	70	62	168	33	70	66	169	32	70	66	168	
JH	3	27	70	60	157					26	70	66	162	28 g only
AH	4	11	65	66	142	9	65	66	140	9	68	64	141	
JS	4	16	63	58	137	13	68	66	147	11	68	62	141 ⎱ lecithin
CR	4	4	68	50	122	6	70	62	138	9	61	45	115 ⎰ stopped
JP	4	11	62	53	126	6	53	37	96	12	53	39	104	
SH	5	9	40	30	79	12	43	20	75					
MF	7	0	11	3	14	3	8	19	30					

A: Orientation, digit score, logical memory; maximum score 45.
B: Agnosia; maximum score 70.
C: Dyspraxia, maximum score 66.

Table 5. Choline and lecithin in Alzheimer's disease

Authors	Patients	Treatment	Response
Choline:			
Boyd and coworkers (1977)	7 Advanced cases, aged over 70 yr	Choline chloride 5 g per day for 2 wk 10 g per day for 2 wk	No change in psychological tests; some patients more manageable
Etienne and coworkers (1978)	3 Advanced cases, aged 76–88 yr	Choline bitartrate 8 g per day for 8 wk	One patient slightly better on nurses' rating
Smith and coworkers (1978)	10 Cases, mean age 77 yr	Choline bitartrate 9 g per day for 2 wk, double-blind placebo	No improvement in psychological tests; 3 patients less confused
Signoret, Whiteley, and Lhermitte (1978)	8 Mixed cases, aged 59–78 yr	Choline citrate 9 g per day for 3 wk	3 Younger patients had improved short-term recall
Lecithin:			
Etienne and coworkers (1979)	7 Cases onset within 3 yr, aged 42–81 yr	Lecithin granules 25–100 g per day for 4 wk	3 Patients had improved new learning

treatment compared with the effects of a placebo, in a double-blind trial by Smith and coworkers (1978). No measurable improvement, using behavioural and psychological tests, was found in ten patients given 9 g choline bitartrate daily for two weeks, but three patients seemed less confused. The duration of illness was not stated. Signoret, Whiteley, and Lhermitte (1978) found that choline produced some improvement in learning in three younger patients who had a short duration of illness. Etienne and coworkers (1978) found choline had no effect in three patients with moderately advanced dementia. In the present study we found very little improvement on choline, but the patients received choline for only one week and there was a suggestion of improved behaviour in the drug-free week following choline. Etienne and coworkers (1979) gave lecithin, 25–100 g daily, to seven out-patients with pre-senile and senile dementia of less than three years' duration; three patients showed an improvement in learning. Lecithin, 25 g daily, was well-tolerated but reduction in appetite and diarrhoea, not a marked problem in our younger patients, was more pronounced in the older patients. Thus, the evidence to date suggests that administration of choline or lecithin for 2–4 weeks may effect improvement in Alzheimer dementia of less than three years' duration. However, long-term double-blind trials are required to determine if the rate of deterioration of these patients is reduced by choline and lecithin. The sensitivity of nurses' behavioural ratings, found by ourselves and

Etienne and coworkers (1978), suggests that behavioural measures, e.g. by relatives in the home, could be of great value in the assessment of Alzheimer patients on chronic therapy.

III. EFFECT OF CHOLINE AND LECITHIN ON CHOLINE LEVELS IN CSF AND SERUM IN ALZHEIMER PATIENTS

On the morning before starting choline treatment, the patients were fasted and kept in bed. Diagnostic lumbar puncture was performed using a standardized technique. The first 5 ml cerebrospinal fluid (CSF) was collected in a glass testtube and immediately frozen, and a further 5 ml CSF taken for routine investigations. Venous blood, 5–10 ml, was also taken and stored at 4°C for up to 6 h prior to separation of the serum by centrifugation at 7–10°C. Serum and CSF were stored at −20°C until assayed for free choline. After four days on choline chloride, 6 g daily, samples of CSF and serum were obtained under exactly the same conditions, except that the first daily dose of 1.5 g choline chloride was given one hour before lumbar puncture and venepuncture. The following day, the patient was allowed to get up and have breakfast, and a blood sample was taken 3 h after the first daily dose of choline. The same procedures were repeated after four and five days on the maintenance dose of lecithin, 100 g daily.

A. Assay of Free Choline

Serum ultrafiltrates were prepared using a membrane cone with a cut-off at mol. wt 25 000 (Amicon, High Wycombe, Berks) and stored at −20 °C (Eckernäs and Aquilonius, 1977). Free choline was measured in CSF and serum ultrafiltrates, using a preparation of choline acetyltransferase (CAT), specific activity 2.39 μmol per mg protein per hour, derived from sheep caudate nucleus (Mannervik and Sorbo, 1970; Shea and Aprison, 1973) and stored in liquid nitrogen at pH 6.0 in 500-μl portions. Assays were carried out in 1.5 ml stoppered polypropylene tubes using a modification of the method of Fonnum (1975). To 10 μl CSF or serum ultrafiltrate and 5 μl CAT, was added 5 μl buffered substrate to give final concentrations, in the reaction medium, of sodium phosphate buffer pH 7.4, 50 mmol l^{-1}; albumin, 550 μg l^{-1}; eserine, 100 μmol l^{-1} and ^{14}C-acetyl-coenzyme A, 100 μmol l^{-1} (equivalent to 0.02 μCi per tube). After incubation at 37 °C for 60 min, the reaction was stopped by removing the lid of the polypropylene tube and dropping the tube into a scintillation vial containing 10 ml 0.425 % 2,5-diphenyloxazole (PPO) in toluene; 5 ml sodium phosphate buffer pH 7.4, 10 mmol l^{-1}, containing acetylcholine, 200 μmol l^{-1} and 2 ml acetonitrile containing sodium tetraphenylboron (Sigma), 27.3 mmol l^{-1}. The vial was shaken briefly, centrifuged to separate the phases and ^{14}C counted for 10 min in a Nuclear Chicago Mark II scintillation counter. The enzymatic reaction was linear to 600 pmol choline. The reagent blank gave a reading equivalent to about 10 pmol choline. The CSF estimations were repeated blind using choline kinase and ^{32}P by Dr S. Zeisel, Massachusetts Institute of Technology, Cambridge, U.S.A. Samples of CSF from nine patients under investigation in a neurological ward, who showed no signs of organic brain disease, served as controls.

B. Choline Levels in CSF

The mean concentration ($\pm$ S.D.) of choline in CSF from 11 fasting Alzheimer patients was 2.9 ± 0.3 nmol ml^{-1}. One hour after administration of 1.5 g choline chloride or 25 g lecithin, the CSF levels were increased to 5.1 ± 0.8 nmol ml^{-1} ($n = 8$, $p < 0.001$) and 4.0 ± 0.9 nmol ml^{-1} ($n = 7$, $p < 0.01$), respectively. The CSF choline levels after administration of choline chloride and lecithin did not differ significantly at the 5 % level. There was no correlation between choline levels in serum and CSF before or after either treatment. Lower absolute values for CSF choline were found when choline kinase was used to assay choline, but similar increases were detected following administration of choline chloride and lecithin (Figs 1 and 2). The mean concentration of choline in CSF from nine neurological

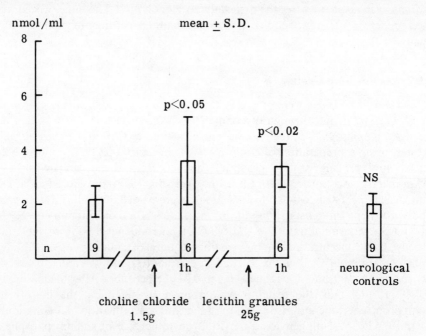

Figure 1. Effect of oral administration of choline and lecithin on CSF levels of choline in patients with pre-senile Alzheimer dementia. CSF taken from fasting patients before, and 1 h after, 1.5 g choline chloride or 25 g lecithin. Neurological controls not fasted. Assay using choline acetyltransferase

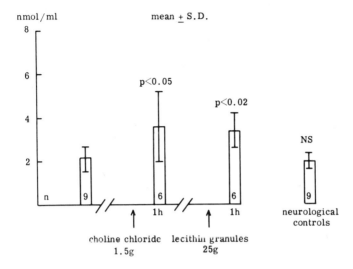

Figure 2. Effect of oral administration of choline and lecithin on CSF levels of choline in patients with pre-senile Alzheimer dementia. CSF taken from fasting patients before, and 1 h after, 1.5 g choline chloride or 25 g lecithin. Neurological controls not fasted.
Assay using choline kinase

controls was 2.3 ± 0.6 nmol ml^{-1} by the choline acetyltransferase method. Aquilonius and coworkers (1972) and Growdon, Cohen, and Wurtman (1977), using this method of assay, reported mean values of CSF choline in controls of 2.5 ± 0.4 nmol ml^{-1} (S.D., $n = 19$) and 2.2 ± 0.7 nmol ml^{-1} (S.D., $n = 5$), respectively. CSF choline levels, measured by choline acetyltransferase, were higher ($p < 0.05$) in the Alzheimer than in the control patients; using the choline kinase method there was no significant difference between the two groups. It may be of significance that the control samples had been stored at $-20\,°$C for 1–2 years, whereas the Alzheimer samples were stored for a maximum of one year before assay. Growdon, Cohen, and Wurtman (1977) found a mean increase of 74% in CSF choline one hour after administration of a mean dose of 3.75 g choline base to eight patients with Huntington's chorea. In the eight Alzheimer patients, a mean increase in CSF choline of 72% was found one hour after administration of 1.5 g choline chloride (equivalent to 1.1 g choline base), indicating that passage of choline from plasma to CSF is no lower in patients with Alzheimer's disease than in patients with Huntington's chorea. The resting concentration of choline in CSF from the patient with Pick's disease was 3.2 nmol ml^{-1}; this was increased to 7.0 and 6.4 nmol ml^{-1}, respectively, after choline chloride and lecithin. The relationship of CSF choline levels to plasma choline and acetylcholine metabolism in the brain is not fully understood, but it appears that CSF choline represents precursor choline, originating from plasma or brain phospholipids

(Schuberth and Jenden, 1975; Growdon, Cohen, and Wurtman, 1977), and not choline derived from the metabolism of acetylcholine in the brain. Thus, after stopping intravenous infusion of labelled choline into rabbits, the rate of fall of labelled choline in cisternal CSF differed from the rate of fall of labelled acetylcholine in brain (Schuberth and Jenden, 1975), and drugs which interfere with brain acetylcholine turnover did not alter choline levels in dog ventricular CSF (Aquilonius, Schuberth, and Sundwall, 1970). Schuberth and Jenden (1975) showed that, at physiological plasma choline levels in the rabbit, 60 % of plasma choline passed into the cisternal CSF, presumably via the carrier-mediated blood-brain barrier transport system demonstrated by Cornford, Braun, and Oldendorf (1978). In cats, ventricular CSF choline levels were, however, increased by less than two-fold despite a ten-fold increase in plasma choline concentration (Gardiner and Domer, 1968). This suggests that choline is rapidly removed from the CSF, possibly by active transport into the choroid plexus (Aquilonius and Winbladh, 1972), and that measurement of CSF choline levels after a choline load can give only an approximate estimate of choline transport into brain. We can, therefore, deduce that there is no gross defect of choline transport into brain in Alzheimer's disease.

C. Choline Levels in Serum

Fasting serum levels of choline in the 11 Alzheimer patients ranged from 5.7 to 16.3 nmol ml^{-1}, with a mean ($\pm$ S.D.) of 11.5 ± 3.2 nmol ml^{-1}. One hour after administration of 1.5 g choline chloride or 25 g lecithin granules, serum choline levels were significantly increased to 30.9 ± 4.3 nmol ml^{-1} ($p < 0.001$) and 33.7 ± 10.3 nmol ml^{-1} ($p < 0.001$), respectively. Three hours after administration of 1.5 g choline chloride or 25 g lecithin, in patients allowed to have breakfast, the mean levels remained significantly elevated at 32.4 ± 5.0 nmol ml^{-1} ($n = 10$, $p < 0.001$) and 35.6 ± 7.0 nmol ml^{-1} ($n = 9$, $p < 0.001$), respectively (Fig. 3). There was no correlation between disability, as measured by the global rating score, and fasting serum choline levels. There was no significant difference between the levels in the four male patients (12 ± 2.5 nmol ml^{-1}) and in the seven female patients (11.3 ± 2.5 nmol ml^{-1}). Eckernäs and Aquilonius (1977), using the same method of assay, found a mean concentration of 10.6 ± 0.4 nmol ml^{-1} in sera from 23 fasting controls aged 24–74 years. These control values were not significantly different from fasting choline levels in the Alzheimer patients. Serum choline levels at 1 h and 3 h after administration of 1.5 g choline chloride (equivalent to 1.1 g choline base) or 25 g lecithin granules (equivalent to approximately 0.9 g choline base) were almost identical, indicating that the serum choline levels after lecithin granules are related to the free choline content of the granules. Wurtman, Hirsch, and Growdon (1977) observed that 100 g lecithin granules produced higher serum choline levels in fasted volunteers than did an equivalent dose of choline base. They attributed this difference to breakdown of

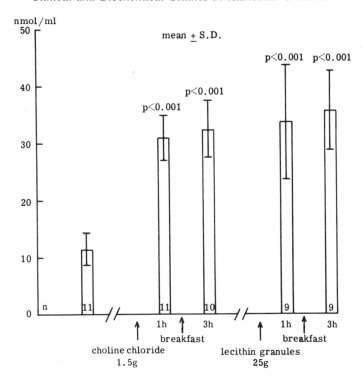

Figure 3. Effect of oral administration of choline and lecithin on serum levels of choline in patients with pre-senile Alzheimer dementia. Blood samples taken from fasted patients before, and 1 h after, 1.5 g choline chloride or 25 g lecithin. Samples also taken 3 h after 1.5 g choline chloride or 25 g lecithin in patients who had had breakfast

choline in the gut to trimethylamine derivatives (Marks, Dudley, and Wan, 1978) which are responsible for the fishy odour of patients given high doses of choline (Etienne and coworkers, 1978). The odour was not noticeable with the doses we used, possibly because the choline was administered in a syrup. Fairly steady levels of serum choline of about 30 nmol ml^{-1} were maintained throughout the day in an Alzheimer patient given four daily doses of 1.5 g choline chloride interspersed with hospital meals. Similar levels were found by Hirsch, Growdon, and Wurtman (1978) in volunteers given a total of 5 g choline as egg yolk and lecithin granules in three separate meals in one day. This suggests that lecithin or choline chloride administered 3–4 times a day are equally effective in maintaining serum choline levels. We did not find, as reported by Etienne and coworkers (1979), that a good clinical response to lecithin was associated with high serum choline levels. We observed no correlation between gastrointestinal side-effects and serum choline levels, possibly because some of these effects were due to a direct action, particularly of lecithin granules, on the gut. The bulky nature of lecithin granules makes them less acceptable than choline, the bitter taste of which can be successfully masked in a syrup. It is also much more difficult to prepare a placebo for the granules than for the choline syrup. Manufacture of granules containing 80–100% phosphatidylcholine instead of, as at present, 20–30% phosphatidylcholine, should considerably reduce the bulk. In rats, serum levels of 20–30 nmol ml^{-1} choline, about the same concentrations as were reached in our patients, are associated with a 100% increase in brain choline and a 20% increase in brain acetylcholine. The latter increase was not augmented by raising the dose of choline (Cohen and Wurtman, 1975). High digh doses of choline, which produce parasympathomimetic side-effects, (Etienne and coworkers, 1978; Signoret, Whiteley, and Lhermitte, 1978) may, therefore, be no more effective in treatment than lower doses.

D. Source of Choline used in Synthesis of Brain Acetylcholine

Adult brain cannot synthesize choline (Bremner and Greenberg, 1961) and therefore relies on a supply from the blood. Several workers have demonstrated that labelled choline injected intravenously is rapidly transported into brain (Schuberth, Sparf, and Sundwall, 1969; Diamond, 1971; Haubrich, Reid, and Gillette, 1972), probably via a carrier-mediated blood-brain barrier transport mechanism (Cornford, Braun, and Oldenfeld, 1978). Using labelled choline, Freeman, Choi, and Jenden (1975) demonstrated that uptake of choline into brain continued in the presence of a net efflux from the brain. They concluded that a source of choline within the brain was responsible for the arteriovenous difference in choline concentration reported by Dross and Kewitz (1972). Since labelled acetylcholine is found in the brain within minutes of the intravenous injection of labelled choline, it would appear that brain acetylcholine can be synthesized directly from free choline (Haubrich, Reid, and Gillette 1972; Choi, Freeman, and Jenden, 1975; Schuberth and Jenden, 1975). Following the suggestion by Ansell and Spanner (1971) that choline containing lipid can pass into brain, Illingworth and Portman (1972) demonstrated transfer of labelled lysophosphatidylcholine from plasma to brain and its subsequent conversion in brain to acetylcholine in the squirrel monkey. Studies by Schuberth and Jenden (1975) and Ceder and Schuberth (1977) indicate that the relative proportions of free and bound plasma choline used by brain to synthesize acetylcholine may be species-dependent. Choline containing lipids in the plasma may, therefore, serve as an additional or alternative source of brain acetylcholine in humans. If this is so, one might expect Alzheimer patients to respond better to administration of lecithin than to free choline. In the present study, lecithin appeared to be more effective than choline, but a true comparison is not possible because the two treatments were not continued for the same length of time. In the one other report of lecithin in the treatment of dementia (Etienne and coworkers, in press), three out of seven cases of onset within three years had improved learning. A direct comparison of choline and lecithin in the treatment of early pre-senile Alzheimer dementia is called for.

IV. CHOLINE UPTAKE BY ERYTHROCYTES (RBCs)

Human RBCs possess a transport system for choline which, at micromolar concentrations, appears to follow Michaelis–Menten kinetics and has a K_m for choline of 20–30 μmol (Askari, 1966; Martin, 1972; Lee and coworkers, 1974). We therefore measured choline influx into RBCs from patients with Alzheimer's disease and also in patients with mongolism (Down's syndrome). Mongols who die over the age of 40 years have the histological features of Alzheimer's disease (Olson and Shaw, 1969; Burger and Vogel, 1973; Ellis, McCulloch, and Corley, 1974) and have been reported to exhibit dementia (Olson and Shaw, 1969; Wisniewski and coworkers, 1978).

A. Measurement of Choline Influx into RBCs

10 ml of blood was collected into sodium heparin tubes from the trial patients during the initial assessment period. Samples were also obtained from five male and three female patients who fulfilled our diagnostic criteria for Alzheimer's disease, who were not on drugs and were in-patients in other wards of the Royal Edinburgh Hospital or in other hospitals. Ten in-patients with Down's syndrome, aged at least 40 years, from Gogarburn Hospital, Edinburgh, were also investigated. Permission to take blood samples was obtained from the patients' nearest relatives. All Down's syndrome patients were drug-free and had Trisomy 21 anomaly. Hospital and laboratory staff and volunteers from old-age pensioner day centres served as controls.

Choline uptake was measured by the method of Lee and coworkers (1974). The blood was stored at 4 °C for not more than 24 h before the red cells were isolated by centrifugation for 10 min at 1400 g and 4 °C. The cells were then washed four times with 3 vol. buffer and incubated overnight at 37 °C in 30 vol. buffer to remove intracellular choline. The buffer was 5 mmol l^{-1} Tris-HCl, pH 7.4 at 37 °C, containing 155 mmol l^{-1} sodium chloride, 1 g l^{-1} D-glucose and 200 mg l^{-1} chloramphenicol. The supernatant was discarded after centrifugation (10 min, 1400 g, 4 °C) and the cells washed once more with 5 vol. buffer and centrifuged. 200 μl packed RBCs were equilibrated for 5 min at 37 °C with 0.8 ml buffer at 37 °C. 40 μl of an aqueous solution of methyl-^{14}C-choline chloride (59 mCi mmol^{-1}, Amersham) was then added to give a final concentration of 1 μmol l^{-1} choline (0.13 μCi per tube). After 5 min, uptake of choline was stopped by the addition of 5 ml ice-cold buffer containing 200 μmol l^{-1} hemicholinium-3 (Aldrich). After centrifugation (5 min, 1400 g, 4 °C) the cells were washed a further three times with 5 ml buffer containing 100 μmol l^{-1} hemicholinium-3.

Blanks were prepared by adding the ^{14}C-choline at the same time as 200 μmol l^{-1} hemicholinium-3 to 200 μl packed cells from two blood samples chosen at random from the samples being analysed. In the Down's series and its age-matched controls, hemicholinium-3 was not present in the stopping buffer and blanks were prepared for each sample because the blank values differed between samples. Intracellular ^{14}C-choline was released by precipitating the cells with 2 ml 5% (w/v) trichloroacetic acid (TCA) containing 1 mmol l^{-1} cold choline. One ml of the TCA supernatant was added to 10 ml NE 260 Micellar Scintillant (Nuclear Enterprises, Edinburgh) and counted for 10 min in a Nuclear Chicago Mark II Scintillation Counter. The results were expressed as nmol choline taken up by one litre cells per min at 37 °C and were not corrected for the intracellular water liberated during TCA precipitation.

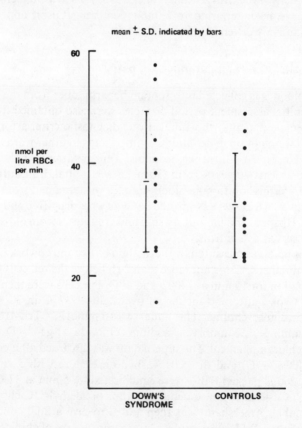

Figure 4. Choline influx into erythrocytes from patients with Down's syndrome and age- and sex-matched controls

B. Choline Influx into RBCs from Patients with Alzheimer's Disease and Down's Syndrome

The mean (±S.D.) age of the five men and five women with Down's syndrome was 52 ± 6 years. The mean ($\pm$ S.D.) age of the age- and sex-matched controls with which the Down's patients were compared was 51 ± 8 years. There was no significant difference between choline influx into RBCs from the Down's patients (36.7 ± 12.6 nmol per litre per min) and from the control patients (32.4 ± 9.2 ± 9.2 nmol per litre per min) (Fig. 4).

The mean ($\pm$ S.D.) choline influx into RBCs from ten male Alzheimer patients aged between 57 and 68 years with a mean age ($\pm$ S.D.) of 63 ± 3 years, was 31.8 ± 8.9 nmol per litre per min. Influx into RBCs from 14 male controls of the same mean age and same age range was 34.0 ± 8.0 nmol per litre per min. There was no significant difference between the male Alzheimer and the control groups (Fig. 5). The mean ($\pm$ S.D.) choline influx into RBCs from ten female Alzheimer

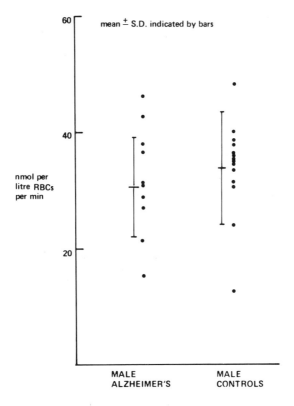

Figure 5. Choline influx into erythrocytes from male patients with pre-senile Alzheimer dementia and age-matched controls

patients was 25.1 ± 10.2 nmol per litre per min. The ages of the female Alzheimer patients ranged from 53 to 77 years, with a mean ($\pm$ S.D.) of 65 ± 7 years. Nineteen female controls of the same age range and with a mean age ($\pm$ S.D.) of 61 ± 6 years had a mean ($\pm$ S.D.) choline uptake of 25.1 ± 14.8 nmol per litre per min. There was no significant difference between the female Alzheimer patients and the female controls (Fig. 6). Choline influx into RBCs from the Alzheimer patients was not related to the global rating score. Uptake by RBCs from the patient with Pick's disease was only 7.9 nmol per litre per min, which was outside

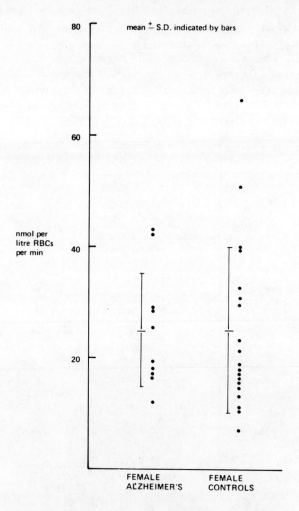

Figure 6. Choline influx into erythrocytes from female patients with pre-senile Alzheimer dementia and age-matched controls

the 95 % confidence limits obtained for the male Alzheimer patients and the male controls. The coefficients of variation of estimates of choline uptake were 6 % and 13 % in two controls sampled four and eight times, respectively, over a period of 4–8 months. This indicates that the wide range in choline uptake values observed in patients and controls is due to differences between individuals and not to differences within individuals. The results from two larger control groups, of 40 men aged between 27 and 83 years, and 43 women aged between 25 and 80 years, are plotted as a frequency histogram in Fig. 7. There was no correlation in either sex, between RBC choline influx and age. Choline uptake was normally distributed in the male controls and in the male Alzheimer patients. However, in both the female controls and female Alzheimer patients, the distribution was skewed towards lower values. This accounts for the wider variance observed in women compared to men. The skewed distribution was also apparent in women aged over 50 years and is therefore unlikely to be due to a direct hormonal effect. Lee and coworkers (1974) commented on the wide variation in choline uptake between individuals but did not describe the different distributions found in men and women. Reasons for the different sex distribution, as for the presence of a choline transport system in the RBC, remain obscure. We found no difference in the apparent K_m of choline influx into RBCs from a lithium-treated patient, a patient with Alzheimer's disease, and a control, the mean K_m being 46 μmol estimated at 1 and 25 μmol choline under steady-state conditions. Lee and coworkers (1974) and Martin (1977) reported a K_m of 20–30 μmol for RBC choline uptake, which is higher than the K_m for high-affinity uptake into synaptosomes (Yamamura and Snyder, 1973, K_m = 1.4–3.1 μmol; Simon, Atweh, and Kuhar, 1976, K_m = 0.8 μmol) and lower than the K_m of the blood-brain barrier transport mechanism (Cornford, Braun, and Oldenfeld, 1978, K_m = 400 μmol). Choline influx into RBCs differs in other respects, including non-dependence on sodium, from neuronal high-affinity choline uptake (Martin, 1977). The K_m of RBC choline uptake more closely resembles the K_m of choline transport into the choroid plexus (K_m = 40 μmol, Aquilonius and Winbladh, 1970), and the K_m of low-affinity, sodium-independent choline transport into synaptosomes (Haga and Noda 1973, K_m = 40 μmol; Yamamura and Snyder, 1973, K_m = 33–93 μmol). Low-affinity choline uptake has not been as rigorously investigated as the high-affinity system, but it is of interest that Diamond and Kennedy (1969) showed that lithium was a potent inhibitor of low-affinity transport of choline into guinea-pig synaptosomes (Martin, 1977). Choline influx into human RBCs is markedly inhibited *in vitro* and almost abolished *in vivo* by lithium (Lee and coworkers, 1974). The latter effect, which we observed in two patients, is irreversible (Lingsch and Martin, 1976).

C. Choline Transport into Neurons

In vitro, choline transported by the sodium-dependent high-affinity carrier is

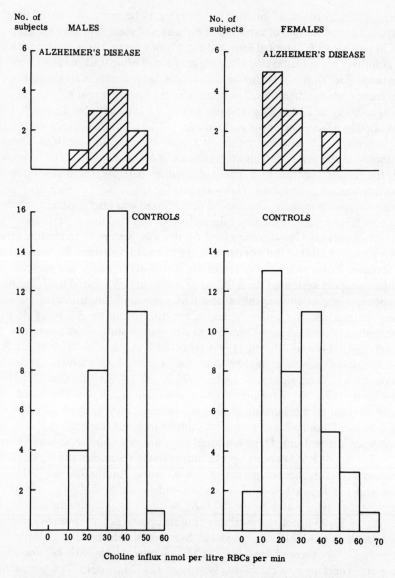

Figure 7. Frequency distribution of choline influx into erythrocytes from male and female patients with pre-senile Alzheimer dementia and from male and female controls

the major source of acetylcholine synthesized within the synaptosomes (Haga and Noda, 1973; Yamamura and Snyder, 1973) and of acetylcholine released by potassium depolarization from hippocampal slices (Mulder and coworkers,

1974) and retina (Massey and Neal, 1979). The levels of choline normally present in brain tissue (17–44 nmol g^{-1}, Haubrich and Chippendale, 1977) and ventricular CSF 5 μM, Aquilonius and Winbladh, 1972) would saturate high-affinity choline uptake. However, the increases in whole brain (Cohen and Wurtman, 1975; Haubrich and coworkers, 1975) and hippocampal (Hirsch, Growdon, and Wurtman, 1977) acetylcholine concentrations following administration of choline suggests that, *in vivo*, high-affinity choline uptake is not saturated by concentrations of choline present at the nerve cell membrane or that low-affinity uptake can supply choline for the synthesis of acetylcholine. There is some *in vitro* evidence to support the latter contention (Diamond and Milfay, 1972; Carroll and Goldberg, 1975). The observation by Ulus and Wurtman (1976) of an increased activity of tyrosine hydroxylase in striata of rats given choline suggests that the choline-induced increase in acetylcholine levels is accompanied by an increase in acetylcholine release. The report by Bowen and coworkers (1977), of a reduced choline uptake into synaptosomes prepared from an Alzheimer brain, has not been repeated. Bowen and coworkers (1977) commented on the marked reduction in uptake with increase in post-mortem interval, possibly related to the post-mortem rise in brain choline (Ceder and Schuberth, 1977). Thus, in the absence of any evidence of a deficit in high- or low-affinity choline uptake, or, as indicated by our CSF results, of a deficiency in the transport of choline from plasma to brain, it would seem reasonable to attempt to increase cholinergic transmission in Alzheimer's disease by administration of the precursors choline or lecithin.

V. OBSERVATIONS OF THE TREATMENT OF ALZHEIMER'S DISEASE

Lesions of the hippocampus caused by physical damage or alcohol poisoning (Korsakoff's syndrome) produce memory impairment which is similar, but not identical, to the memory loss observed in Alzheimer's disease (Smith and Swash, 1978). In normal volunteers serial word learning was reduced by scopolamine and enhanced by choline or arecoline given in combination with a peripheral anticholinesterase (Sitaram, Weingartner, and Gillin, 1978). This evidence of a link between the hippocampus, memory, and cholinergic function indicates a causal relationship between the loss of hippocampal choline acetyltransferase and the memory deficit of Alzheimer's disease (Davis and Yamamura, 1978). The question is whether treatment with precursor is the best way of counteracting the cholinergic deficit. Choline and lecithin appear to be effective only in the early stages of the disease, when there are presumably sufficient functioning cholinergic neurons to convert choline to acetylcholine. This same restriction would apply to treatment with deanol, another possible form of precursor therapy. Deanol, however, has the disadvantage that it competes with choline for transport into the brain (Cornford, Braun, and Oldendorf, 1978; Millington,

McCall, and Wurtman, 1978). An alternative treatment of early Alzheimer's disease would be to protect released acetylcholine from destruction by administration of a centrally acting anticholinesterase. For effective therapy, a long-acting anticholinesterase which penetrates the brain is required. The effect of an anticholinesterase could be potentiated by the concomitant administration of choline. In view of the normal numbers and affinity of muscarinic receptors in Alzheimer brain (Davies and Verth, 1978) cholinergic agonists should, theoretically, be effective in both early and late forms of the disease. The duration of action of currently available centrally acting cholinergic agonists is, however, too short for their use as therapeutic agents. Short-acting agonists or anticholinesterases could, however, be given to Alzheimer patients as a challenge to determine if the cholinergic receptors are still functionally capable of responding to stimulation. Intravenous infusion of low doses of physostigmine, which improves memory in control subjects (Davis and coworkers, 1978), would be a suitable test procedure.

Finally we need to know more about the state of other neurotransmitter systems in Alzheimer's disease. Drug-induced alterations of systems other than the cholinergic system may provide additional or alternative methods of treatment.

ACKNOWLEDGEMENT

We are grateful to Mrs Yvonne Allison for technical assistance.

REFERENCES

Ansell, G. B. and S. Spanner (1962). The effects of 2-dimethylaminoethanol on brain phospholipid metabolism. *J. Neurochem.*, **9**, 253–63.
Ansell, G. B. and S. Spanner (1971). Studies on the origin of choline in the brain of the rat. *Biochem. J.*, **122**, 741–50.
Aquilonius, S-M., B. Nyström, J. Schuberth, and A. Sundwall (1972). CSF choline in extrapyramidal disorders. *J. Neurol., Neurosurg. Psychiat.*, **35**, 720–5.
Aquilonius, S-M., J. Schuberth, and A. Sundwall (1970). Studies on choline in cerebrospinal fluid. *Acta Pharmacol. Toxicol*, **28** (Suppl. 1), 35.
Aquilonius, S-M. and B. Winbladh (1972). CSF clearance of choline and some other amines. *Acta Physiol. Scand.*, **85**, 78–90.
Askari, A. (1966). Uptake of some quaternary ions by human erythrocytes. *J. Gen. Physiol.*, **49**, 1147–60.
Barker, L. A. and T. W. Mittag (1975). Comparative studies of substrates and inhibitors of choline transport and choline acetyltransferase. *J. Pharmacol. Exp. Therap.*, **192**, 87–94.
Bowen, D. M., C. B. Smith, and A. M. Davison (1973). Molecular changes in senile dementia. *Brain*, **96**, 849–56.
Bowen, D. M., C. B. Smith, P. White, M. J. Goodhardt, J. A. Spillane, R. H. A. Flack, and A. N. Davison (1977). Chemical pathology of the dementias. *Brain*, **100**, 397–426.
Boyd, W. D., J. Graham-White, G. Blackwood, I. Glen, and J. McQueen (1977). Clinical

effects of choline in Alzheimer senile dementia. *Lancet*, **ii**, 711.

Bremner, J. and D. M. Greenberg (1961). Methyl transferring enzyme system of microsomes in the biosyntheses of lecithin (phosphatidylcholine). *Biochim. Biophys. Acta*, **46**, 205–16.

Brody, H. (1960). The deposition of aging pigment in the human cerebral cortex. *J. Gerontol.*, **15**, 258–61.

Burger, P. G. and F. S. Vogel (1973). The development of the pathologic changes of Alzheimer's disease and senile dementia in patients with Down's syndrome. *Amer. J. Path.*, **73**, 457–68.

Carroll, P. T. and A. M. Goldberg (1975). Relative importance of choline transport to spontaneous and potassium release of Ach. *J. Neurochem.*, **25**, 523–7.

Casey, D. E. and D. Denney (1975). Deanol in the treatment of tardive dyskinesia. *Amer. J. Psychiat.*, **132**, 864–7.

Ceder, G. and J. Schuberth (1977). *In vivo* formation and post-mortem changes of choline and acetylcholine in the brain of mice. *Brain Res.*, **128**, 580–4.

Choi, R. L., J. J. Freeman, and D. J. Jenden (1975). Kinetics of plasma choline in relation to turnover of brain choline and formation of brain acetylcholine. *J. Neurochem.*, **24**, 735–41.

Cohen, E. L. and R. J. Wurtman (1975). Brain acetylcholine: increase after systemic choline administration. *Life Sci.*, **16**, 1095–102.

Cohen, E. L. and R. J. Wurtman (1976). Brain acetylcholine: Control by dietary choline. *Science*, **191**, 561–2.

Cornford, E. M., L. D. Braun, and W. H. Oldendorf (1978). Carrier-mediated blood-brain barrier transport of choline and certain choline analogues. *J. Neurochem.*, **30**, 299–308.

Davies, P. and A. F. J. Maloney (1976). Selective loss of central cholinergic neurones in Alzheimer's disease. *Lancet*, **ii**, 1403.

Davies, P. and A. H. Verth (1978). Regional distribution of muscarinic acetylcholine receptor in normal and Alzheimer's-type dementia brains. *Brain Res.*, **138**, 385–92.

Davis, K. L., R. C. Mohs, J. R. Tinklenberg, L. E. Hollister, A. Pfefferbaum, and B. S. Kopell (1978). Physostigmine: enhancement of long-term memory functions in normal subjects. *Science*, **201**, 274–6.

Davis, K. L. and H. I. Yamamura (1978). Cholinergic underactivity in human memory disorders. *Life Sci.*, **23**, 1729–34.

Dencker, S. J. and D. Lindberg (1977). A controlled double-blind study of piracetam in the treatment of senile dementia. *Nord. Psykiatr. Tidskaft.*, **31**, 48–52.

Diamond, I. (1971). Choline metabolism in brain. The role of choline transport and the effects of phenobarbital. *Arch. Neurol. (Chicago)*, **24**, 233–9.

Diamond, I. and E. P. Kennedy (1969). Carrier-mediated transport of choline into synaptic nerve endings. *J. Biol. Chem.*, **244**, 3258–63.

Diamond, I. and D. Milfay (1972). Uptake of ^{3}H-methyl choline by microsomal, synaptosomal, mitochondrial and synaptic vesicle fractions of rat brain. *J. Neurochem.*, **19**, 1899–1909.

Dross, K. and H. Kewitz (1972). Concentration and origin of choline in the rat brain. *Naunyn-Schmiedebergs Arch. Pharmac.*, **274**, 91–106.

Eckernäs, S-A. and S-M. Aquilonius (1977). Free choline in human plasma analysed by simple radio-enzymatic procedure: age distribution and effect of a meal. *Scand. J. Clin. Lab. Invest.*, **37**, 183–7.

Editorial (1976). Cerebral blood flow in dementia. *Brit. Med. J.*, **1**, 1487–8.

Eisenson, J. (1954). *Examination for Aphasia*, The Psychological Corporation, New York.

Ellis, W. G., J. R. McCulloch, and C. L. Corley (1974). Presenile dementia in Down's syndrome. *Neurology*, **24**, 101–6.

Embree, L. J., N. H. Bass, and A. Pope (1972). Biochemistry of middle and late life dementias. In A. Lajtha (Ed.) *Handbook of Neurochemistry*, Vol. VII, Plenum Press, New York. pp. 329–69.

Etienne, P., S. Gauthier, D. Dastoor, B. Collier, and J. Ratnor (1979). Alzheimer's disease, clinical effect of lecithin treatment. In A. Barbeau, J. Growdon, and R. J. Wurtman (Eds) *Choline and Lecithin in Brain Diseases*, Raven Press, New York.

Etienne, P., S. Gauthier, G. Johnson, B. Collier, T. Mendis, D. Dastoor, M. Cole, and H. F. Muller (1978). Clinical effects of choline in Alzheimer's disease. *Lancet*, i, 508–9.

Fann, W. E., J. L. Sullivan III, R. D. Miller, and G. M. McKenzie (1975). Deanol in tardive dyskinesia: a preliminary report. *Psychopharmacologia (Berl.)*, 42, 135–137.

Fonnum, F. (1975). A rapid radiochemical method for the determination of choline acetyltransferase. *J. Neurochem.*, 24, 407–9.

Freeman, J. J., R. L. Choi, and D. J. Jenden (1975). Plasma choline: its turnover and exchange with brain choline. *J. Neurochem.*, 24, 729–34.

Gardiner, J. E. and F. R. Domer (1968). Movement of choline between the blood and CSF in the cat. *Arch. Int. Pharmacodyn. Ther.*, 175, 482–96.

Gedye, J. L., A. N. Exton-Smith, and J. Wedgwood (1972). A method for measuring mental performance in the elderly and its use in a pilot clinical trial of meclofenate in organic dementia. *Age and Ageing*, 1, 74–80.

Gilleard, C. J. and A. H. Pattie (1977). The Stockton geriatric rating scale: a shortened version with British normative data. *Brit. J. Psychiat.*, 131, 90–4.

Groth, D. P., J. A. Bain, and C. C. Pfeiffer (1958). The comparative distribution of C^{14}-labelled dimethylamino-ethanol and choline in the mouse. *J. Pharmacol. Exp. Ther.*, 124, 290–5.

Growdon, J. H., E. L. Cohen, and R. J. Wurtman (1977). Effects of oral choline administration on serum and CSF choline levels in patients with Huntington's disease. *J. Neurochem.*, 28, 229–31.

Gustafson, L., J. Risberg, M. Johanson, M. Fransson, and V. A. Maximillan (1978). Effects of piracetam on regional cerebral blood flow and mental functions in patients with organic dementia. *Psychopharmacology*, 56, 115–7.

Haga, T. and H. Noda (1973). Choline uptake systems of rat brain synaptosomes. *Biochim. Biophys. Acta*, 291, 564–75.

Haubrich, D. R. and T. J. Chippendale (1977). Regulation of acetylcholine synthesis in nervous tissue. *Life Sci.*, 20, 1465–78.

Haubrich, D. R., W. D. Reid, and J. R. Gillette (1972). Acetylcholine formation in mouse brain and effect of cholinergic drugs. *Nature (New Biol.)*, 238, 88–9.

Haubrich, D. R., P. F. L. Wang, D. E. Clody, and P. W. Wedeking (1975). Increase in rat brain acetylcholine induced by choline or deanol. *Life Sci.*, 17, 975–80.

Hirsch, M. J., J. H. Growdon, and R. J. Wurtman (1977). Increase in hippocampal acetylcholine after choline administration. *Brain Res.*, 125, 383–5.

Hirsch, M. J., J. H. Growdon, and R. J. Wurtman (1978). Relations between dietary choline or lecithin intake, serum choline levels, and various metabolic indices. *Metabolism*, 27, 953–60.

Hirsch, M. J. and R. J. Wurtman (1978). Lecithin consumption elevates acetylcholine concentrations in rat brain and adrenal gland. *Science*, 202, 223–4.

Hughes, J. R., J. G. Williams, and R. D. Currier (1976). An ergot alkaloid preparation (Hydergine) in the treatment of dementia: Critical review of the clinical literature. *J. Amer. Geriat. Soc.*, 24, 490–7.

Illingworth, D. R. and O. W. Portman (1972). The uptake and metabolism of plasma lysophosphatidylcholine *in vivo* by the brain of squirrel monkeys. *Biochem. J.*, 130, 557–67.

Jacobs, E. A., P. M. Winter, H. J. Alvis, and S. M. Small (1969). Hyperoxygenation effects on cognitive functioning in the aged. *New Engl. J. Med.*, **281**, 753–7.

Kimura, D. and Y. Archibald (1974). Motor functions of the left hemisphere. *Brain*, **97**, 337–50.

Klawans, H. L., J. L. Topel, and D. Bergen (1975). Deanol in the treatment of levodopa-induced dyskinesias. *Neurology*, **25**, 290–3.

Lee, G., C. Lingsch, P. T. Lyle, and K. Martin (1974). Lithium treatment strongly inhibits choline transport in human erythrocytes. *Brit. J. Clin. Pharmacol.*, **1**, 365–70.

Lingsch, C. and K. Martin (1976). An irreversible effect of lithium administration to patients. *Brit. J. Pharmacol.*, **57**, 323–7.

Mann, D. M. A. and P. O. Yates (1974). Lipoprotein pigments—their relationship to ageing in the human nervous system. *Brain*, **97**, 481–8.

Mannervik, B. and B. Sorbo (1970). Inhibition of choline acetyltransferase from bovine caudate nucleus by sulfhydryl reagents and reactivation of the inhibited enzyme. *Biochem. Pharmacol.*, **19**, 2509–16.

Marks, R., F. Dudley, and A. Wan (1978). Trimethylamine metabolism in liver disease. *Lancet*, **i**, 1106–7.

Martin, K. (1972). Extracellular cations and the movement of choline across the erythrocyte membrane. *J. Physiol.*, **224**, 207–30.

Martin, K. (1977). Choline transport in red cells. In J. C. Ellory and V. C. Lew (Eds) *Membrane Transport in Red Cells* Academic Press, London. pp. 101–13.

Massey, S. C. and M. J. Neal (1979). Release of ^{3}H-acetylcholine from the isolated retina of the rat by potassium depolarisation: dependence on high affinity choline uptake. *Brit. J. Pharmacol.*, **65**, 271–6.

Meer, B. and J. A. Baker (1966). The Stockton geriatric rating scale. *J. Gerontol.*, **21**, 393–403.

Miller, Edith (1974). Deanol in the treatment of levodopa-induced dyskinesias. *Neurology*, **24**, 116–9.

Millington, W. R., A. L. McCall, and R. J. Wurtman (1978). Deanol acetamidobenzoate inhibits the blood brain barrier transport of choline. *Ann. Neurol.*, **4**, 293–301.

Mulder, A. H., H. I. Yamamura, M. J. Kuhar, and S. H. Snyder (1974). Release of acetylcholine from hippocampal slices by potassium depolarisation: dependence on high affinity choline uptake. *Brain Res.*, **70**, 372–6.

Nandy, K. and G. H. Bourne (1966). Effect of centrophenoxine on the lipofuchsin pigments in the neurons of senile guinea-pigs. *Nature (London)*, **210**, 313–4.

Olson, M. I. and C-M. Shaw (1969). Presenile dementia and Alzheimer's disease in mongolism. *Brain*, **92**, 147–56.

Perry, E. K., R. H. Perry, G. Blessed, and B. E. Tomlinson (1977). Necropsy evidence of central cholinergic deficits in senile dementia. *Lancet*, **i**, 189.

Pfeiffer, C. C. and E. H. Jenney (1957). The inhibition of conditioned response and the counter action of schizophrenia by muscarinic stimulation of the brain. *Ann. N.Y. Acad. Sci.*, **66**, 753–64.

Pfeiffer, C. C., E. H. Jenney, R. P. Smith, W. Bevan, K. F. Killam, E. U. Killam, and W. Blackmore (1957). Stimulant effect of 2-dimethyl-aminoethanol—possible precursor of brain acetylcholine. *Science*, **126**, 610–2.

Riga, S. and D. Riga (1974). Effects of centrophenoxine on the lipofuscin pigments in the nervous system of old rats. *Brain Res.*, **72**, 265–75.

Schuberth, J. and D. J. Jenden (1975). Transport of choline from plasma to CSF in the rabbit with reference to the origin of choline and to acetylcholine metabolism in brain. *Brain Res.*, **84**, 245–56.

Schuberth, J., B. Sparf, and A. Sundwall (1969). A technique for the study of acetylcholine turnover in mouse brain *in vivo*. *J. Neurochem.*, **16**, 695–700.

Shea, P. A. and M. H. Aprison (1973). An enzymatic method for measuring picomole quantities of acetylcholine and choline in CNS tissue. *Anal. Biochem.*, **56**, 165–77.

Signoret, J. I., A. Whiteley, and F. Lhermitte (1978). Influence of choline on amnesia in early Alzheimer's disease. *Lancet*, **ii**, 837.

Sim, M., E. Turner, and W. T. Smith (1966). Cerebral biopsy in the investigation of presenile dementia. *Brit. J. Psychiat.*, **112**, 119–25.

Simon, J. R., S. Atweh, and M. J. Kuhar (1976). Sodium-dependent high affinity choline uptake: a regulatory step in the synthesis of acetylcholine. *J. Neurochem.*, **26**, 909–22.

Sitaram, N., H. Weingartner, and J. C. Gillin (1978). Human serial learning: enhancement with arecholine and choline and impairment with scopolamine. *Science*, **200**, 274–6.

Smith, C. B. and D. M. Bowen (1976). Soluble proteins in normal and diseased human brain. *J. Neurochem.*, **27**, 1521–8.

Smith, C. M. and M. Swash (1978). Possible biochemical basis of memory disorder in Alzheimer disease. *Ann. Neurol.*, **3**, 471–2.

Smith, C. M., M. Swash, A. N. Exton-Smith, M. J. Phillips, P. W. Overstall, M. E. Piper, and M. R. Bailey (1978). Choline therapy in Alzheimer's disease. *Lancet*, **ii**, 318.

Terry, R. D. and H. Wisniewski (1969). The ultrastructure of the neurofibrillary tangle and the senile plaque. In G. E. W. Wolstenholme and M. O'Connor (Eds) *Alzheimer's disease and related conditions*, J. & A. Churchill, London. pp. 145–65.

Thompson, L. W., C. D. Glenn, W. D. Obrist, and A. Heymann (1976). Effects of hyperbaric oxygen on behavioural and physiological measures in elderly demented patients. *J. Gerontol.*, **31**, 23–8.

Thuillier, G., J. Rumpf, and J. Thuillier (1959). Préparation et étude pharmacologique préliminaire des esters diméthyl amino ethyliques de divers acides agissant comme regulateurs de croissance des végétaux. *Comptes Rendu de L'Acad. des Sci.*, **249**, 2081–3.

Ulus, I. H. and R. J. Wurtman (1976). Choline administration: activation of tyrosine hydroxylase in dopaminergic neurons of rat brain. *Science*, **194**, 1060–1.

Wechsler, D. (1955). *Manual for Wechsler Memory Scale*, The Psychological Corporation, New York.

White, P., C. R. Hiley, M. J. Goodhardt, L. M. Carasco, J. P. Keet, I. E. Williams, and D. M. Bowen (1977). Neocortial cholinergic neurons in elderly people. *Lancet*, **i**, 668–70.

Wisniewski, K., J. Howe, D. G. Williams, and H. M. Wisniewski (1978). Precocious aging and dementia in patients with Down's syndrome. *Biol. Psychiat.*, **13**, 619–27.

Wurtman, R. J., M. J. Hirsch, and J. H. Growdon (1977). Lecithin consumption raises serum-free choline levels. *Lancet*, **ii**, 68–9.

Yamamura, H. I. and S. H. Snyder (1973). High affinity transport of choline into synaptosomes of rat brain. *J. Neurochem.*, **21**, 1355–74.

Biochemistry of Dementia
Edited by P. J. Roberts
© 1980, John Wiley & Sons Ltd.

Chapter 10

Amine Metabolism in Normal Ageing and in Dementia Disorders

C. G. GOTTFRIES

*University of Göteborg, Psychiatric Research Centre,
St. Jörgen's Hospital, Hisings Backa, Sweden*

Impairment of psychic functions in old age can be due to normal ageing (physiological ageing or orthoinvolution) and to dementia disorders (pathological ageing or pathoinvolution). Normal ageing will produce no severe mental impairment. Intellectual functions can be divided into subfunctions; common functions such as logical and spatial capacities and psychic tempo, and more specific functions based on knowledge and experience such as verbal and numerical capacities. From psychological tests it is evident that normal ageing does not mean a general impairment of all psychic functions. It is mainly the common intellectual functions which are reduced in relation to age, while the specific functions are more resistant to normal ageing. This is of interest when discussing ageing from a biochemical viewpoint.

Dementia means a more severe impairment of mental functions. It is a condition which may be irreversible and progressive. Dementia may develop at any age but is most common later in life and therefore the old age dementias are most discussed in the context of dementia disorders.

From a clinical point of view it may be difficult to distinguish normal ageing from pathological ageing. With regard to structural changes as well as biochemical it has been shown that normal ageing and some dementia disorders have features in common. Therefore, the question of whether there is a continuity between orthoinvolution and pathoinvolution has not yet been settled.

There are two main groups of dementia disorders: the cerebrovascular diseases and degenerative disorders with no obvious vascular disease. It is now accepted that the dementia caused by vascular disease is due to infarctions or hemorrhage. As infarctions of the brain tissue seem to be the most common cause the term 'multi-infarction dementia' has been suggested (Hachinski and coworkers, 1974).

The non-vascular diseases are senile dementia and the pre-senile dementias. If the dementia has its onset after 65 years of age the condition is called senile dementia. Whether senile dementia is a homogeneous group is still under discussion.

The pre-senile dementias are Alzheimer's disease, Pick's disease, Huntington's chorea, and the spongiform encephalopathies (Jakob–Creutzfeldt's disease). Alzheimer's disease has many features in common with senile dementia, but genetic investigations (Larsson and coworkers, 1963) do not support the assumption that these are the same type of disorder. The distinction between senile dementia and Alzheimer's disease is difficult and may be impossible. The group senile dementia, therefore, may very well include patients with Alzheimer's disease when the disease has a late onset. Senile dementia and Alzheimer's disease are usually grouped together under the name 'dementia of Alzheimer type'.

I. MONOAMINES

The following monoamines and their associated enzymes of synthesis and degradation have been identified as transmitters in the mammalian brain:

Active amines	*Related enzymes*	*Metabolites*
Dopamine (DA)	Tyrosine hydroxylase (TH)	Homovanillic acid
	Dopa decarboxylase (DOD)	(HVA)
	Monoamine oxidase (MAO)	
	Catechol-*o*-methyl-transferase (COMT)	
	Dopamine- β-hydroxylase	
Noradrenaline (NA)		3-Methoxy-4-hydroxy-phenethyleneglycol (MHPG)
	MAO	
	COMT	
5-Hydroxytrypt-amine (5-HT)	Tryptophane hydroxylase	5-Hydroxyindoleacetic acid (5-HIAA)
	5-Hydroxytryptophane decarboxylase	
	MAO	

By the use of a histochemical method it is possible to visualize the monoamines DA, NA, and 5-HT (Carlsson and coworkers, 1962). This has focussed interest on monoamine functions in the brain. Studies in mental disorders strongly suggest that estimation of the monoamines and their metabolites has given important information about psychiatric and neurologic diseases. It is conceivable that disturbances of monoamine systems may have pathogenetic importance for affective disorders (Schildkraut, 1965; Coppen, 1967; Weil-Malherbe, 1972). There are also results which indicate that an increased activity in the dopaminergic system may have importance for the schizophrenic psychoses (Bird and coworkers, 1977).

A. Monoamines and Normal Ageing

Experience with animals has shown that the synthesis of NA and DA is reduced in senescent rats, as is the activity of TH (Finch, 1973; Algeri and coworkers, 1978). The activities of TH as well as DOD have been examined post-mortem in human subjects in the substantia nigra, the caudate nucleus, the putamen, and the hypothalamus. There were highly significant age declines of TH and DOD in the substantia nigra, the caudate nucleus, and the putamen. The TH activity in the hypothalamus, however, did not change with increasing age (Cote and Kremzner, 1974). In an investigation by McGeer and coworkers (1971) and McGeer and McGeer (1973) the TH activity was investigated in six human subjects (age range 5–57 years) and an age-related decline could be confirmed. As the TH activity is the rate-limiting step in the synthesis of catecholamines, the age-related reduced activity of TH is of special interest. In post-mortem investigations on the human brain, declines in DOD have been reported in relation to age by Lloyd and Hornykiewicz (1970).

Carlsson and Winbladh (1976) found a negative correlation between DA levels in the human basal ganglia and age in subjects over 20 years. Gottfries and coworkers (1979) studied a group of patients with an age range of 23–92 years. A significant decline in the DA concentration in the caudate nucleus, globus pallidus, mesencephalon, hippocampus, and cortex gyrus hippocampus was observed with age. The HVA levels were 0-correlated to age in this investigation, but Carlsson (1978) reported a weak negative correlation in the caudate nucleus. In another investigation a negative correlation between age and brain tissue levels of HVA was reported (Livrea and coworkers, 1978). A negative correlation between age and the levels of NA was also found by us (Gottfries and coworkers, 1979). The end-metabolite of NA is MHPG and this metabolite was negatively correlated to age in the caudate nucleus (Gottfries and coworkers, 1979).

As has been suggested by MacLean and coworkers (1965), there is a significant positive correlation between age and concentration of 5-HT in the brain stem; this finding was confirmed by Pare and coworkers (1969). In our own investigations we also found increased levels of 5-HT with increasing age in the mesencephalon and the medulla oblongata, but in the globus pallidus and in the cortex gyrus hippocampus the correlation between 5-HT and age was negative at a statistically significant level (Gottfries and coworkers, 1979). Carlsson (1978) also reported a negative correlation when DA and NA levels in brain tissue were correlated to age. When 5-HT and age were studied there was a positive correlation in the medulla oblongata, while the correlation was negative in the hippocampus. The correlation between 5-HIAA and age was positive at a significant level in the caudate nucleus, the hippocampus, the cortex gyrus cinguli, and the cerebellum according to our investigations (Gottfries and coworkers, 1979). In Table 1 the correlations between age and monoamines and their metabolites are presented according to our previous findings and findings from an on-going investigation in Sweden (Gottfries and coworkers, 1979; Carlsson, 1978).

In investigations on the cerebrospinal fluid (CSF), a positive correlation has been found between age and the metabolites HVA and 5-HIAA (Fig. 1) (Bowers and Gerbode, 1968; Gottfries and coworkers, 1971).

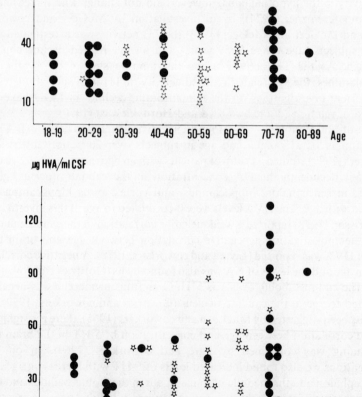

Figure 1. Homovanillic acid (HVA) and 5-hydroxyindoleacetic acid (5-HIAA) in the cerebrospinal fluid (CSF) related to age. ●, Healthy volunteers; ☆, schizophrenic patients

Table 1. Product-moment correlations (*r*) between dopamine (DA), homovanillic acid (HVA), noradrenaline (NA), 3-methoxy-4-hydroxy-phenetylene-glycol (MHPG), 5-hydroxytryptamine (5-HT), and 5-hydroxyindoleacetic acid (5-HIAA) in brain tissue and age

Part of brain	DA/age r	DA/age n	HVA/age r	HVA/age n	NA/age r	NA/age n	MHPG/age r	MHPG/age n	5-HT/age r	5-HT/age n	5-HIAA/age r	5-HIAA/age n
Hypothalamus	-0.18, -0.31†	24, a	-0.16	19	-0.14	28	-0.37	11	0.40†	21	0.29	21
Nucleus caudatus	-0.33*, -0.41**	23, a	-0.01, -0.43†	44, a	-0.19	42	-0.51*	11	0.12	41	0.32*	41
Putamen	-0.19, -0.42**	24, a	0.06	44	-0.22†	42	0.27	11	0.14	41	0.12	41
Globus pallidus	-0.41*	18	0.28	18	-0.36†	18			-0.46*	20	0.10	20
Thalamus	-0.08	18	-0.27	18	0.15	36	0.09	11	-0.02	45	0.22	45
Mesencephalon	-0.41*, -0.51**	18, a	-0.34	17	-0.20	36	-0.38	11	0.48**	25	0.22	45
Pons	0.16	18	0.09	17	0.03	37	0.26	11	0.08	24	0.13	26
Medulla oblongata	0.34	18	0.03	18	-0.22†	37	0.16	11	0.44*, 0.50**	24, a	0.22	40
Hippocampus	-0.37*	18	-0.04	18	-0.10, -0.42*	34, a	-0.40	11	0.32, -0.42*	21, a	0.47**	26
Cortex gyrus hippocampus	-0.38*	18	0.35	18	-0.32†	18	-0.17	11	-0.36*	36	0.18	37
Cortex gyrus cinguli	0.10	18	0.11	18	-0.29	18	-0.45	11	-0.01	42	0.35*	39
Cortex gyrus frontalis	-0.25	18	0.35	18	0.07	32	-0.19	11	0.15	38	0.16	44
Cortex gyrus occipitalis	-0.14	18	-0.01	18	-0.08	36	-0.14	11	-0.08	38	0.01	39
Cortex gyrus temporalis	-0.03	18	-0.01	19	-0.17	20			0.04	18	-0.03	18
Cortex gyrus parietalis	0.04	18	0.23	18	-0.11	17			-0.25	17	-0.13	17
Cerebellum	0.05	18	0.14	18	-0.01	38	0.02	11	-0.02	16	0.43*	18
Medulla spinalis									0.08	16	0.01	19

n, Number of cases; † *p* < 0.10; * *p* < 0.05; ** *p* < 0.01.
(One-sided test for DA/age and NA/age.)
Values from Gottfries and coworkers (1979); and (*a*) from an on-going Swedish investigation, *n* = 17–54 (Carlsson, 1978).

The activity of MAO, which deaminates the monoamines, has been shown to be increased in relation to age (Robinson and coworkers, 1972, 1977; Gottfries and coworkers, 1975). It seems that the correlation between age and MAO estimated with β-phenylethylamine as substrate (MAO-B) is stronger than that with serotonin as substrate (MAO-A) (Table 2) (Gottfries and coworkers, 1979). There is also an age-related increase in the activity of platelet-MAO (Robinson and coworkers, 1972).

Table 2. Product-moment correlations between different forms of MAO activity in human brain and age. One-sided test of significance (from Gottfries and coworkers, 1979)

Part of brain	MAO-A (serotonin)	MAO-AB (tryptamine)	MAO-B (β-phenylethylamine)
Hypothalamus	−0.07	0.10	0.44**
Nucleus caudatus	0.03	−0.20	0.04
Putamen	−0.10	0.24†	0.23 †
Globus pallidus	0.07	0.29*	0.50***
Thalamus	−0.14	0.12	0.22†
Mesencephalon	0.19	0.28*	0.09
Pons	0.20	0.29*	0.15
Medulla oblongata	0.32*	0.23†	0.14
Hippocampus	−0.15	0.19	0.25*
Cortex gyrus hippocampus	−0.19	0.28*	0.08
Cortex gyrus cinguli	0.02	−0.14	0.13
Cortex gyrus frontalis	−0.01	−0.07	0.15
Cortex gyrus occipitalis	0.05	0.02	0.17

† $p < 0.10$; * $p < 0.05$; ** $p < 0.01$; *** $p < 0.001$; $N = 40$.

On summarizing the findings about normal ageing and monoamine metabolism, it is evident that there is reduced activity of the enzymes TH and DOD. In line with these findings it has also been shown that in high age there are reduced levels of NA and DA in post-mortem brain material. 5-HT-levels seem to be reduced in cortical areas but increased in the brain stem in relation to age. The levels of 5-HIAA, both in brain tissue and in CSF, and the levels of HVA in CSF are increased in high age. These findings are somewhat contradictory. The reduced enzyme activity and the reduced levels of active amines in brain tissue indicate a reduced metabolism with age. The increased levels of acid metabolites, especially in CSF, may indicate the opposite but may also indicate a reduced outward transport. Outward transport of the metabolites is an active process and this may be slowed down in high age.

B. Monoamines in Dementia of Alzheimer Type

In view of the widespread degeneration in the brains from patients with dementia of Alzheimer type it is considered unlikely that a single neurotransmitter would selectively be affected (Dayan, 1974). At present, there are results which indicate that not only the monoaminergic systems but also the acetyl-cholinergic system in the brain are disturbed. I will here discuss the investigations in which monoamine metabolism and dementia have been studied.

The original finding was of reduced levels of HVA in basal ganglia in patients with dementia (Gottfries and coworkers, 1965). Later, the concentration of HVA was estimated in the caudate nucleus, the putamen, and the globus pallidus in a group of patients with dementia of Alzheimer type, carefully diagnosed, and in a control group (Gottfries and coworkers, 1968, 1969). The delimination of the dementia group was made at autopsy and the degree of dementia was measured post-mortem on a rating scale. The results showed that in the pre-assumed dementia group there was a significantly lower concentration of HVA in the investigated areas. The levels of HVA were related to the degree of dementia according to the rating scale. The results indicated that the higher the degree of intellectual impairment the lower were the levels of HVA. No reduced levels of HVA were found in a multi-infarct dementia group which was also investigated. When the dementia disorders were split into a group of patients with senile dementia with onset above 65 years of age, and a group of patients with Alzheimer's disease with onset before the age of 65, the Alzheimer group had the significantly lower levels of HVA (Fig. 2 and Table 3) (Gottfries and coworkers,

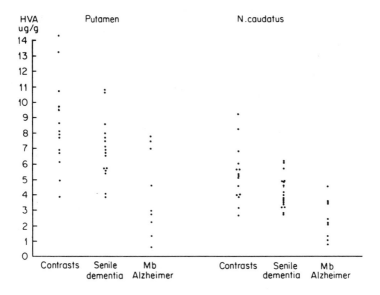

Figure 2. HVA values in μg g^{-1} tissue in nucleus caudatus and putamen in three groups: contrasts (cases with no signs of dementia before death), senile dementias, and cases with Mb Alzheimer. From Gottfries and coworkers, (1968); reproduced by permission of Excerpta Medica

Table 3. Mean value (M) and standard deviation (S.D.) for HVA in putamen and in nucleus caudatus in three groups, contrasts (cases with no signs of dementia before death), senile dementias, and cases with Mb Alzheimer. From Gottfries and coworkers (1968); reproduced by permission of Excerpta Medica

	Contrasts A			Senile dementia B			Mb Alzheimer C			p		
	n	M	S.D.	n	M	S.D.	n	M	S.D.	A/B	A/C	B/C
HVA in putamen	15	8.74	3.04	16	6.86	2.00	9	3.96	2.74	0.05	0.001	0.025
HVA in caudatus	15	5.14	1.81	17	3.94	1.09	9	2.16	1.28	0.025	0.001	0.01

1968). In post-mortem investigations performed later, significantly lower levels of DA and NA were found in groups of patients with dementia of Alzheimer type as compared to age-matched controls (Gottfries and coworkers, 1976; Adolfsson and coworkers, 1979). In this investigation, also, the reduced levels of HVA in the caudate nucleus and the putamen could be verified (Fig. 3). In the investigation by Adolfsson and coworkers (1979) the level of NA in brain tissue was correlated to the degree of dementia and significant negative correlation was found, which means that the lower the NA levels in the brain the more pronounced is the intellectual impairment.

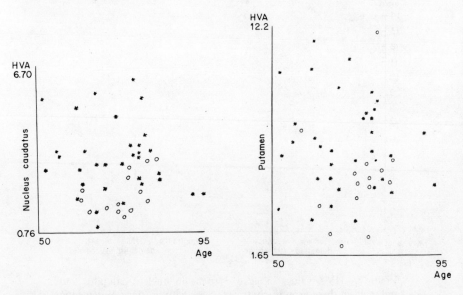

Figure 3. Homovanillic acid (HVA) (μg g^{-1} wet tissue net weight) in the caudate nucleus and in the putamen. The values are related to age. *, cases with no known psychiatric or neurologic disease; o , cases with dementia of Alzheimer type

In an on-going Swedish investigation, from which preliminary data were reported by Carlsson (1978), reduced levels of DA, 3-methoxy-tyramine, HVA, NA, and 5-HT were found (Table 4). In this investigation MHPG was also estimated and, surprisingly enough, increased levels were found in the group of dementias as compared to age-matched controls. In the caudate nucleus there was an almost 50 % reduction of both DA and 5-HT.

Table 4. Levels of monoamines and metabolites (means ± S.E.M. nmol g^{-1}) in the caudate nucleus of cases with senile dementia and of control cases with no known neuropsychiatric disorder (data from an on-going Swedish study) (Carlsson, 1978)

	Controls (n = 17)	Senile dementia (n = 15)
Dopamine	15.8[a] ± 0.90	8.5 *** ± 1.62
3-Methoxytyramine	6.6[a] ± 0.34	4.7 ** ± 0.99
Homovanillic acid	22.7 ± 1.37	15.1 ** ± 1.59
Noradrenaline	0.16 ± 0.012	0.12 * ± 0.014
MHPG	0.10 ± 0.018	0.18 * ± 0.028
5-HT	0.51 ± 0.043	0.25 *** ± 0.040
5-HIAA	1.88 ± 0.15	1.90 ± 0.028
Age (years)	72.8 ± 1.90	75.7 ± 1.93

[a] n = 54; * p < 0.05; ** p < 0.01; *** p < 0.001.

Investigation of CSF have also been performed in patients with dementia disorders of Alzheimer type (Gottfries and coworkers, 1969, 1970; Gottfries and Roos, 1973, 1976). In these investigations it has been shown that both HVA and 5-HIAA are reduced as compared to age-matched control groups (Fig. 4). In the investigation by Gottfries and coworkers (1974), a probenecid loading test was performed in patients with Alzheimer's disease and the results from this investigation also indicate a reduced metabolism of DA and 5-HT (Table 5).

Bowen and coworkers (1974) have studied the activity of DOD in post-mortem investigations from different brain regions. The patients included in the investigation suffered from senile dementia and were matched with controls. The

Table 5. 5-Hydroxyindoleacetic acid (5-HIAA) and homovanillic acid (HVA) in cerebrospinal fluid before, and increase after, probenecid loading test

Group	N	5-HIAA (ng ml^{-1})		HVA (ng ml^{-1})	
		Initial value (mean ± S.D. and variance)	Increase after probenecid (mean ± S.D. and variance)	Initial value (mean ± S.D. and variance)	Increase after probenecid (mean ± S.D. and variance)
Alzheimer's disease (age 57–73 yrs)	15	35.13 ± 13.48 (23–66)	22.53 ± 27.42 (12–93)	21.53 ± 16.58 (0–68)	49.93 ± 44.80 (13–135)
Controls (age 71–81 yrs) (Gottfries and coworkers, 1971)	25	40 ± 12 (N.S.)	–	60 ± 32 ($p < 0.01$)	–
Controls (age 59–94 yrs)	7	–	50 ± 11 ($p < 0.05$)	–	140 ± 25 ($p < 0.001$)

The values are compared to controls by Student's t-test.

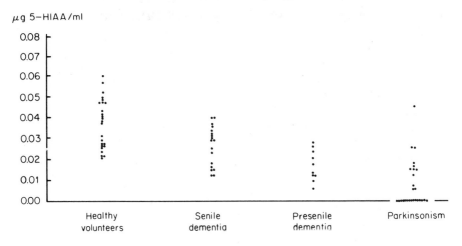

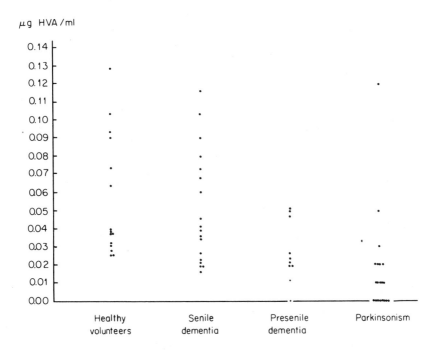

Figure 4. Homovanillic acid (HVA) and 5-hydroxyindoleacetic acid (5-HIAA) in cerebrospinal fluid from healthy volunteers, senile dementias, pre-senile dementias (Alzheimer's disease), and patients with **Parkinsonism**. From Gottfries and coworkers (1969); reproduced by permission of the International Society of Neurochemistry Ltd

results indicated that there was a reduction of the DOD activity by 70–90 % in the demented patients. These findings were later questioned as it was found that agonal status, especially when prolonged and associated with broncopneumonia, had a marked influence on this enzyme activity (Bowen and coworkers, 1976).

In order to gain information about monoamine metabolites in the CNS it is also permissible to study the activity in degrading enzyme systems. MAO is the main deaminating enzyme for the monoamines. As noted above, the activity of this enzyme has been shown to increase with age. A group of 11 patients with Alzheimer's disease were investigated for their activity of MAO in platelets. MAO was determined with β-phenylethylamine and tryptamine as substrate, and it was shown that the Alzheimer group had significantly higher MAO activity with both these substrates as compared to age-matched controls (Gottfries and coworkers, 1979).

MAO in brain tissue was also estimated in a group of patients with dementia of Alzheimer type ($n = 19$) and in a control group ($n = 17$) of the same age range. From this investigation it was evident that MAO (β-phenylethylamine) was significantly increased in the hippocampus, cortex, and caudate nucleus. MAO (tryptamine) and MAO (serotonin), however, were not significantly increased in the brain tissue from demented patients (Adolfsson and coworkers, 1979). Different interpretations can be put forward to explain the increased MAO activity in the aged brain and in demented brains. One is that there are changes in membrane structures. Since MAO is partly dependent on the composition of its membranous environment for its activity (Oreland and Ekstedt, 1972; Houslay and Tipton, 1976), such an increased rate of alteration in membrane structure may explain the increased MAO activity in Alzheimer patients. Thus, the more pronounced the changes in membrane composition the greater the increase in MAO activity. Another explanation for the increased MAO activity may be that, as a consequence of an accelerated decrease of protein-degrading enzyme activity, there is a reduced breakdown of the enzyme MAO itself. This explanation has been suggested for the increase in MAO in the ageing rat heart (Della Corte and Callingham, 1977). A further explanation is that MAO-B (determined with β-phenylethylamine as substrate) is localized to the glial cells, while MAO-A (determined with serotonin and partly with tryptamine as substrate) is localized to the neurons. In the aged brain and in the dementias there is glial cell proliferation. The increased MAO-B activity, therefore, reflects an increased glial content in the brain tissue. This interpretation would then also explain why only MAO-B is increased and not MAO-A. One objection to this explanation, however, is that MAO-B in platelets is also increased which cannot, of course, be explained by the glial cell proliferation.

In view of the increased MAO activity in platelets it may be concluded that dementia of Alzheimer type is a systemic disease, localized not only to the central nervous system but also to peripheral organs.

It may be questioned whether studies of neurotransmitters or their metabolites outside the CNS can give valid information about the turnover in brain tissue. In an investigation by Fisher (1972) the urinary excretion of HVA was studied and found to be decreased in a group of demented patients as compared with controls.

It has been suggested that ageing and dementia disorders may be related to deficiency in folic acid and vitamin B_{12} (Read and coworkers, 1965; Hurdle and Picton Williams, 1966; Carney, 1967; Shulman, 1967). The rate-limiting step in the synthesis of catecholamines and serotonin is hydroxylation of the amino acids and, as folate is the coenzyme of this process (Kaufman and Friedman, 1965; Gal and coworkers, 1966; Grahame-Smith, 1967), a deficiency of folate could be the cause of the disturbed monoamine turnover. Shaw and coworkers (1971) made an investigation of patients with dementia disorders but the results were disappointing. The authors found it unlikely that lack of folate in the demented patients is a significant factor in the amine metabolism. Bowers and Reynolds (1972) also investigated CSF for its content of folate and acid monoamine metabolites and could not find any relationship between these biochemical variables.

II. DEMENTIA DISORDERS AND PARKINSONISM

Patients with Parkinson's disease are at greater risk of dementia than the general population. Greenfield and Bosanquet (1953) and Hakim and Mathieson (1978) reported morphological changes of the type seen in Alzheimer's disease. Increased amounts of senile plaques and fibrillary tangles, as well as granule vacuolar degeneration, have been seen in brains from Parkinsonian cases. Radiological evidence of cerebral atrophy (Selby, 1968) has also been reported. Clinical investigations have shown that in Parkinsonism there are not only motor symptoms but also symptoms of dementia. In various clinical reports 12–53 % of patients with Parkinsonism have shown intellectual impairment (Pollock and Hornabrook, 1966; Mindham, 1970; Celesia and Wanamaker, 1972). This finding has, however, not been generally confirmed (Coppen and coworkers, 1972). It is of interest to notice that on the island of Guam there is a disease in which Parkinsonism and intellectual impairment are always combined. Careful clinical studies have also demonstrated motor disturbances of the Parkinson type in no less than 61 % of patients with Alzheimer's disease (Pearce, 1974).

As early as 1959 Carlsson suggested that DA was a transmitter in the CNS and that it could be involved in Parkinson's syndrome. In 1960, Ehringer and Hornykiewicz showed that the DA content of the caudate nucleus and putamen was reduced in Parkinson's disease, and already in 1961 Birkmayer and Hornykiewicz had reported a beneficial effect on Parkinsonian akinesia when the patients were treated with L-dopa.

As reported above, there is a disturbed metabolism of dopamine in patients with dementia of Alzheimer type. In fact, the levels of HVA in the CSF (Gottfries and coworkers, 1969) in subjects with Alzheimer's disease are almost as low as those found in patients with Parkinsonism. A natural question is why patients with Alzheimer's disease do not show such serious motor disturbances as the Parkinsonian patients do. It must be borne in mind, however, that in Parkinsonism—either true Parkinson's disease or the Parkinsonian type—many of the main symptoms such as tremor and akinesia are signs of an overfunction of the cholinergic system rather than an underfunction of the dopaminergic system (Hornykiewicz, 1968). In senile dementia and Alzheimer's disease there are findings indicating a reduced activity in cholinergic functions, also. Perhaps the reduced dopaminergic and cholinergic activities in the brains of the patients with senile dementia and Alzheimer's disease can still balance each other, but on a lower level than normal.

To summarize the findings about monoamine metabolism and dementia disorders of Alzheimer type, there are findings of reduced activity of DOD in these patients, although these findings have been questioned. There are reduced levels of DA, NA, 5-HT, and HVA in brain tissue. In CSF, base levels as well as probenecid loading tests have shown signs of reduced activity in dopaminergic and serotoninergic systems. Of interest, also, is that in old age and in dementia of Alzheimer type there is an increase of MAO activity. Dementia patients have higher MAO activity both in platelets and in brain tissue as compared to aged-matched controls.

In an on-going Swedish investigation (Carlsson, 1978) not only were there found reduced levels of monoamines, but also a reduced activity of choline acetyltransferase (CAT) in the same tissue samples. This indicates that all these biogenic amines, and of course also other transmitters, may be involved in the syndrome of senile dementia.

It can, of course, be discussed whether the findings made in ageing and dementia disorders have any pathogenetic importance or are only epiphenomena secondary to other degenerative changes in the brain. In the investigations by Gottfries and coworkers (1968) and Adolfsson and coworkers (1979) there were significant correlations between the degree of intellectual impairment and the reduction of the levels of HVA and NA. It can be added that when a senile dementia group was compared with a multi-infarction group for their HVA levels in brain tissue, the senile dementias had significantly lower HVA levels although those groups were demented to the same degree.

As mentioned in the introduction, not all psychic functions are vulnerable to age. It is also clinically well known that the symptoms in dementia of Alzheimer type may vary. The loss of memory of course dominates the picture but very often these patients also show signs of disturbed mood, loss of drive, and motor symptoms. One important question arises: do the degenerative processes in senile dementia affect all neurons or preferentially certain types? Can different components in the syndrome of senile dementia be specificially linked to loss of individual transmitters? In a pharmacological study (Drachman and Leavitt, 1974) it was shown that the cholinergic system is involved in age-related memory disturbances in human subjects. It is also clinically known that intoxication by anticholinergic drugs may cause confusion and treatment with physostigmine may quickly, although only temporarily, clear the confused mind. In psychiatric research there are many data which support the hypothesis that disturbed NA and 5-HT metabolism may cause affective disorders. The relation between disturbances of DA metabolism and motor disturbances is also well known from the findings in Parkinson's disease.

III. INVESTIGATIONS WITH SUBSTITUTION THERAPY IN DEMENTIA OF ALZHEIMER TYPE

In investigations by Gottfries and coworkers (1968) and Adolfsson and coworkers (1979) there were significant correlations between the degree of intellectual impairment and the reduction of the levels of catecholamines. Rather surprisingly, there was no correlation between motor impairment and reduced levels of catecholamines or their metabolites. This is in contrast to the findings in Parkinson's disease, where the degree of DA deficiency can to some extent be correlated to rigidity and akinesia (Bernheimer and coworkers, 1973). Motor impairment in the dementia patients was rated in the same way as intellectual impairment by a rating scale which was constructed for the ward staff. The rating scales did not, however, exclusively measure rigidity and akinesia but also included the dyspractic component. This may explain the lack of correlation.

The above-mentioned findings indicate that the metabolism of dopamine may be of importance not only for motor functions but also for intellectual functions. In an individual case reported by Ghosh (1976) α-methyldopa caused forgetfulness. The treatment model of L-dopa in Parkinson's disease is well known and it seems natural to employ the same kind of substitution treatment in patients with dementia of Alzheimer type. Some investigations have already been performed. In 1970, Van Woert and coworkers noticed that six patients with dementia symptoms included in a study of Parkinsonian patients also improved mentally when treated with L-dopa. However, when four patients with dementia of Alzheimer type were more systematically treated with L-dopa, no positive effect could be recorded. Parkes and coworkers (1974) treated eight patients with senile dementia with L-dopa without noting any benefit from the treatment. A more systematic investigation was published in 1977 (Kristensen and coworkers) in which 18 out-patients with pre-senile dementia were treated with L-dopa, according to the double-blind technique. After six months' treatment no significant effect was shown either on a broad spectrum of psychiatric items or on cognitive functioning. Lewis and coworkers (1978), however, treated senile dementia patients with L-dopa, also according to the double-blind technique, and this group could report significant improvement in the L-dopa-treated patients. The patients were rated on a behaviour rating scale and both 'communication' and 'continence' improved significantly. An intellectual rating scale was also used and according to this the L-dopa-treated group improved significantly. In an investigation by Adolfsson and coworkers (1978), patients with dementia disorders of Alzheimer type were treated with L-dopa and the dopamine-agonist bromocriptine. This investigation was an open trial. The patients were carefully diagnosed and the pharmacodynamic response to the treatment was followed by repeated lumbar punctures. Ten patients were treated for four weeks with L-dopa. A significant improvement in several psychological functions was seen, especially visiospatial functions. No positive effects on memory functions were observed. Ratings by the ward staff showed better psychomotor and motor functions. Biochemical investigation of the CSF showed a significant increase in base-line HVA concentration during treatment and a trend towards lower 5-HIAA concentrations. MHPG concentrations were slightly, though not significantly, higher after four weeks' treatment. Eight patients completed eight weeks' treatment with bromocriptine; three patients became confused; this was reversible after dose adjustment. No positive results could be registered in tests and rating scales or by clinical evaluation during the bromocriptine treatment.

One of the great problems when making treatment trials of this kind on patients with dementia disorders is the selection of patients. It is difficult to delimit a group of patients with dementia of Alzheimer type on clinical grounds.

As discussed above, it is not only the catecholamine systems which are affected in dementia of Alzheimer type but also the 5-HT system. Tryptophane deficiency and psychiatric symptoms are described in two diseases: pellagra and carcinoidosis (Lehmann, 1972). Tryptophane-malabsorption in L-dopa-treated Parkinsonian patients is also described by the same author (Lehmann, 1973). The author describes individual cases in which mental symptoms in patients with Parkinsonism have improved when the patients were treated with tryptophane. It would be of interest to study the effect of substitution therapy with tryptophane in patients with dementia of Alzheimer type.

IV. PICK'S DISEASE

The clinical differentiation of Alzheimer's and Pick's diseases is difficult. Pick's disease is also a progressing dementia, in which localized cerebral atrophy is found. The atrophy, however, has quite a different pattern from that seen in Alzheimer's disease, and the histological changes are also different in these two diseases. The cell loss in Pick's disease is not only found in cortical grey matter but also in white matter and basal ganglia (Jervis, 1971). Affected neurons show swelling and pallor with loss of the intracytoplasmic Nissl bodies (Braunmühl, 1958).

There are few investigations concerning the monoamine metabolism in Pick's disease. Guard and coworkers (1976) investigated a series of 17 patients with pre-senile dementias and the investigation included the probenecid test. In 13 patients with Alzheimer's disease the turnover rate of HVA and 5-HIAA was diminished as compared to normals but the difference was not significant. In four patients with Pick's disease, the turnover rate of HVA was comparable to that of normals, whereas the turnover rate of 5-HIAA was not significantly decreased.

V. JAKOB–CREUTZFELDT'S DISEASE

In a case with Jakob–Creutzfeldt's disease, investigations on cerebrospinal fluid and brain tissue showed disturbances of the monoamine metabolism (Brun and coworkers, 1971). The levels of the catecholamines were seriously decreased. Probenecid tests suggested a low dopamine turnover. As Jakob–Creutzfeldt's disease is believed to have a viral aetiology, it can be questioned whether virus infection could be responsible for the impairment of the monoamine metabolism.

VI. HUNTINGTON'S CHOREA

The most striking findings in the brains of patients with Huntington's chorea are marked atrophy in the basal ganglia, especially in the neostriatum. There is also evident atrophy in the cerebral cortex.

On the search for biochemical disturbances in Huntington's chorea, most of the interest has been focussed on the biogenic amines in the basal ganglia and many proofs have been given of the important role of DA (Chase, 1973). Also, γ-aminobutyric acid has been reported to be decreased in correspondence with the reduced glutamic acid decarboxylase in the basal ganglia of patients with Huntington's chorea (Bird and coworkers, 1973; Perry and coworkers, 1973). This is interesting because GABA seems normally to decrease the effect of DA in the basal ganglia and drugs with a strong dopaminergic receptor-blocking effect have been reported to ameliorate the symptoms of Huntington's chorea. In CSF studies, slightly reduced levels of HVA and 5-HIAA have been reported (Aquilonius and Sjöström, 1971; Curzon and coworkers, 1972; Chase, 1973).

Bernheimer and Hornykiewicz (1973) reported normal levels of NA and 5-HT in the basal ganglia, thalamus, hypothalamus, substantia nigra, mid-brain, and floor of the fourth ventricle in patients with Huntington's chorea. With the exception of a low concentration of DA and HVA in the caudate nucleus, the levels of DA and HVA were within normal limits. Against this background the authors suggest that a relation between dopaminergic activity in the caudate nucleus and the putamen-pallidus in hypokinetic-hypotonic syndrome (Huntington's chorea) is different from that in hypokinetic-rigid syndrome

(Parkinson's disease). In the Huntington's chorea patient, the concentration of DA-HVA is reduced in the caudate nucleus, while in Parkinson's disease the concentration of DA-HVA is most reduced in the putamen-pallidus. Different regions of the brains from patients with Huntington's chorea were investigated by Mattsson and coworkers (1974). In their five cases, striatum degeneration with nerve cell loss, and gliosis and varying cortical atrophy dominated the pathological findings. A low concentration of HVA was found in the caudate nucleus. Low concentrations of 5-HT in the hippocampus and frontal cortex were also recorded in this investigation.

Conclusions from the amine studies in Huntington's chorea must be drawn with care. The number of patients in the series is small and individual variations rather large. However, there seems to be good evidence for a reduced dopamine metabolism within the basal ganglia complex. 5-HT neurons seem to play a certain role in the genesis of the disease (Mattsson and Persson, 1974), and a direct finding of reduced 5-HT levels in the hippocampus and frontal cortex is therefore of interest. The reduced 5-HT levels should, perhaps, be interpreted principally as being more associated with the psychiatric symptom, dementia, which is a part of the Huntington's chorea syndrome.

REFERENCES

Adolfsson, R., C. G. Gottfries, L. Oreland, B. E. Roos, and B. Winblad (1978). Reduced levels of catecholamines in the brain and increased activity of monoamine oxidase in platelets in Alzheimer's disease: therapeutic implications, in R. Katzman, R. D. Terry and K. L. Bick (Eds), *Alzheimer's disease: senile dementia and related disorders* (Aging, Vol. 7) pp. 441–451, Raven Press, New York.

Adolfsson, R., C. G. Gottfries, L. Oreland, Å. Wiberg, and B. Winblad (1979). Increased platelet and brain MAO activity in dementia disorders of the Alzheimer type. To be published.

Algeri, S., M. Bonati, N. Brunello, F. Ponzio, G. Stramentinoli, and M. Gualano (1978). Biochemical changes in central catecholaminergic neurons of the senescent rats, in P. Deniker, C. Radouco-Thomas and A. Villeneuve (Eds), *Neuro-Psychopharmacology, Proceedings of the Tenth Congress of the Collegium International Neuro-Psychopharmacologicum*, Quebec, July 1976, Vol. 2, pp. 1647–54, Pergamon Press, Oxford and New York.

Aquilonius, S. M. and R. S. Sjöström (1971). Cholinergic and dopaminergic mechanisms in Huntington's Chorea, *Life Sci.*, **10**, 405–14.

Bernheimer, H., W. Birkmayer, O. Hornykiewicz, O. Jellinger, and F. Seitelberger (1973). Brain dopamine and the syndromes of Parkinson and Huntington, *J. Neurol. Sci.*, **20**, 415–55.

Bernheimer, H. and O. Hornykiewicz (1973). Brain amines in Huntington's Chorea, in *Advances in Neurology*, **1**, 525–31. Raven Press, New York.

Bird, E. D., J. Barnes, L. L. Iversen, E. G. Spokes, A. V. P. Mackay, and M. Shepherd (1977). Increased brain dopamine and reduced glutamic acid decarboxylase and choline acetyl transferase activity in schizophrenia and related psychoses, *Lancet*, *ii*, 1157–1159.

Bird, E. D., A. V. P. MacKay, C. N. Rayner, and L. L. Iversen (1973). Reduced glutamic-acid-decarboxylase activity of post mortem brain in Huntington's Chorea, *Lancet, i,* 1090–1092.

Birkmayer, W. and O. Hornykiewicz (1961). Der L-3-4-Dioxyphenyl alanin(=DOPA)-Effekt bei der Parkinson-Akinese. *Wien. Klin. Wochenschr.,* **45**, 787–788.

Bowen, D. M., R. H. A. Flack, P. White, C. B. Smith, and A. N. Davison (1974). Brain-decarboxylase activities as indices of pathological change in senile dementia, *Lancet, i,* 1247–1249.

Bowen, D. M., C. B. Smith, P. White, and A. N. Davison (1976). Neurotransmitter-related enzymes and indices of hypoxia in senile dementia and other abiotrophies, *Brain,* **99**, 459–496.

Bowers, M. B. and F. A. Gerbode (1968). Relationship of monoamine metabolites in human cerebrospinal fluid to age, *Nature, London,* **219**, 1256–1257.

Bowers, M. B. and E. H. Reynolds (1972). Cerebrospinal-fluid folate and acid monoamine metabolites, *Lancet, ii,* 1376.

Braunmühl, A., von (1958). Alterserkrankungen des Zentralnervensystems, O. Lubarsch, F. Henke und R. Rössle *Handbuch, spez. path. Anat.* XIII/1A, pp. 337–539, Springer Verlag, Berlin.

Brun, A., C. G. Gottfries and B. E. Roos (1971). Studies of the monoamine metabolism in the central nervous system in Jakob Creutzfeldt disease, *Acta Neurol. Scand.,* **47**, 642–645.

Carlsson, A. (1959). The occurrence, distribution and physiological role of catechol-amines in the nervous system, *Pharmacol. Rev.,* **11**, 490–493.

Carlsson, A. (1978). The impact of catecholamine research on medical science and practice. Lecture given at the *Fourth International Catecholamine Symposium,* Asilomar, California, September 17–22, 1978.

Carlsson, A., B. Falck, and N. Å. Hillarp (1962). Cellular localization of brain monoamines, *Acta Physiol. Scand.,* **56**. Suppl. 196:1.

Carlsson, A. and B. Winblad (1976). Influence of age and time interval between death and autopsy on dopamine and 3-methoxytyramine levels in human basal ganglia, *J. Neural. Transm.,* **38**, 271–276.

Carney, M. W. P. (1967). Serum folate values in 423 psychiatric patients, *Br. Med. J.,* **4**, 512–516.

Celesia, G. G. and W. M. Wanamaker (1972). Psychiatric disturbances in Parkinson's disease, *Dis. Nerv. Syst.,* **33**, 577–583.

Chase, T. N. (1973). Biochemical and pharmacologic studies of monoamines in Huntington's Chorea, in *Advances in Neurology* 1, 533–549, Raven Press, New York.

Coppen, A. (1967). The biochemistry of affective disorders, *Brit. J. Psychiat.,* **113**, 1237–1264.

Coppen, A., M. Metcalfe, J. D. Carroll, and J. G. L. Morris (1972). Levadopa and L-tryptophan therapy in Parkinsonism, *Lancet, i,* 654.

Cote, L. J. and L. T. Kremzner (1974). Changes in neurotransmitter systems with increasing age in human brain, *Abstracts of the American Society of Neurochemistry,* p. 83.

Curzon, G., J. Gumpert and D. Sharpe (1972), Amine metabolites in the cerebrospinal fluid in Huntington's Chorea, *J. Neurol. Neurosurg. Psychiatry,* **35**, 514–519.

Dayan, A. D. (1974). The brain, ageing, and dementia, *Psychol. Med.,* **4**, 349–352.

Della Corte, L. and B. A. Callingham (1977). The influence of age and adrenalectomy on rat heart monoamine oxidase, *Biochem. Pharmacol.,* **26**, 407–415.

Drachman, D. A. and J. Leavitt (1974). Human memory and the cholinergic system, *Arch. Neurol.,* **30**, 113–121.

Ehringer, H. and O. Hornykiewicz (1960). Verteilung von Noradrenalin im Dopamin (3-hydroxy-tyramin) im Gehirn des Menschen und ihre Verhalten bei Erkrankungen des extrapyramidalen Systems, *Klin. Wochenschr.*, **38**, 1236–1240.

Finch, C. E. (1973). Catecholamine metabolism in the brains of ageing male mice, *Brain Res.*, **52**, 261–276.

Fisher, R. H. (1972). The urinary excretion of homovanillic acid and 4-hydroxy-3-methoxy mandelic acid in the elderly demented, *Geront. Clin.*, **14**, 172–175.

Gal, E. M., J. C. Armstrong and B. Ginsberg (1966). The nature of *in vitro* hydroxylation of L-tryptophan by brain tissue, *J. Neurochem.*, **13**, 643–654.

Gottfries, C. G., R. Adolfsson, L. Oreland, B. E. Roos and B. Winblad (1979). Monoamines and their metabolites and monoamine oxidase activity related to age and to some dementia disorders. In Crooks, J. and Stevenson, I. H. (Eds) *Drugs and the elderly. Perspectives in geriatric clinical pharmacology*. Proceedings of a symposium held in Ninewells Hospital, University of Dundee, on 13–14 September 1977, pp. 189–197, MacMillan, London.

Gottfries, C. G., I. Gottfries, B. Johansson, R. Olsson, T. Persson, B. E. Roos, and R. Sjöström (1971). Acid monoamine metabolites in human cerebrospinal fluid and their relations to age and sex, *Neuropharmacology*, **10**, 665–672.

Gottfries, C. G., I. Gottfries, and B. E. Roos (1968). Disturbances of monoamine metabolism in the brains from patients with dementia senilis and Mo Alzheimer, *Excerpta Medica International Congress Series*, No. 180, 310–312.

Gottfries, C. G., I. Gottfries, and B. E. Roos (1969). The investigation of homovanillic acid in the human brain and its correlation to senile dementia, *Brit. J. Psychiatry*, **115**, 563–574.

Gottfries, C. G., I. Gottfries, and B. E. Roos (1970). Homovanillic acid and 5-hydroxyindoleacetic acid in cerebrospinal fluid related to rated mental and motor impairment in senile and presenile dementia, *Acta Psychiatr. Scand.*, **46**, 99–105.

Gottfries, C. G., L. Oreland, Å. Wiberg, and B. Winblad (1975). Lowered monoamine oxidase activity in brains from alcoholic suicides, *J. Neurochem.*, **25**, 667–673.

Gottfries, C. G. and B. E. Roos (1973). Acid monoamine metabolites in cerebrospinal fluid from patients with presenile dementia (Alzheimer's disease), *Acta Psychiatr. Scand.*, **49**, 257–263.

Gottfries, C. G. and B. E. Roos (1976). Monoamine metabolites in cerebrospinal fluid (CSF) in patients with organic presenile and senile dementias, *Aktuel. Gerontol.*, **6**, 37–42.

Gottfries, C. G., B. E. Roos, and B. Winblad (1974), Determination of 5-hydroxytryptamine, 5-hydroxyindoleacetic acid and homovanillic acid in brain tissue from an autopsy material, *Acta Psychiatr. Scand.*, **50**, 496–507.

Gottfries, C. G., B. E. Roos and B. Winblad (1976). Monoamine and monoamine metabolites in the human brain post mortem in senile dementia, *Aktuel. Gerontol.*, **6**, 429–435.

Gottfries, C. G., A. M. Rosengren, and E. Rosengren (1965). The occurrence of homovanillic acid in human brain, *Acta Pharmacol. Toxicol.*, **23**, 36–40.

Grahame-Smith, D. G. (1967). The biosynthesis of 5-hydroxytryptamine in brain, *Biochem. J.*, **105**, 351–360.

Greenfield, J. G. and F. D. Bosanquet (1953). The brainstem lesions in Parkinsonism, *J. Neurol. Neurosurg. Psychiatry*, **16**, 213–226.

Guard, O., B. Renaud, and G. Chazot (1976). Métabolisme cérébral de la dopamine et de la sérotonine au cours des maladies d'Alzheimer et de Pick. Etude dynamique par le test au probénécide, *Encephale*, **II**, 293–303.

Hachinski, V. D., N. A. Lassen, and J. Marshall (1974). Multi-infarct dementia. A cause of mental deterioration in the elderly, *Lancent, ii,* 207.

Hakim, A. M. and G. Mathieson (1978). Basis of dementia in Parkinson's disease, *Lancet, ii,* 729.

Hornykiewicz, O. (1968). Gegenwärtiger Stand der biochemisch-pharmakologischen Erforschung des extrapyramidal-motorischen Systems, *Pharmakopsychiatr. Neuropsychopharmakol.,* **1**, 6–17.

Houslay, M. D. and K. F. Tipton (1976). Multiple forms of monoamine oxidase: fact and artifact, *Life Sci.,* **19**, 467–478.

Hurdle, A. D. F. and T. C. Picton Williams (1966). Folic acid deficiency in elderly patients admitted to hospital, *Brit. Med. J.,* **2**, 202–205.

Jervis, G. A. (1971). Pick's disease, in J. Minckler (Ed.) *Pathology of the nervous system,* pp. 1395–1404, McGraw-Hill, New York.

Kaufman, S. and S. Friedman (1965). Dopamine-β-hydroxylase, *Pharmacol. Rev.,* **17**, 71–100.

Kristensen, V., M. Olsen, and A. Theilgaard (1977). Levodopa treatment of presenile dementia, *Acta Psychiatr. Scand.,* **55**, 41–51.

Larsson, T., T. Sjögren, and G. Jacobson (1963). Senile dementia. A clinical, sociomedical and genetic study. *Acta Psychiatr. Scand.,* Suppl. 167.

Lehmann, J. (1972). Mental and neuromuscular symptoms in tryptophan deficiency, *Acta Psychiatr. Scand.,* Suppl. 237.

Lehmann, J. (1973). Tryptophan malabsorption in levodopa-treated Parkinsonian patients. Effect of tryptophan on mental disturbances, *Acta Med. Scand.,* **194**, 181–189.

Lewis, C., B. R. Ballinger, and A. S. Presly (1978). Trial of levodopa in senile dementia, *Brit Med. J.,* **1**, 550.

Livrea, P., N. di Reda, A. de Blasi, and A. Bertolino (1978). Homovanillic acid (HVA) and 5-hydroxyindoleacetic acid (5-HIAA) in human brain areas at autopsy. Effect of predeath conditions with special attention to the state of consciousness and metabolic diseases. Submitted for publication to *Acta Neurol.* (Napoli).

Lloyd, K. and O. Hornykiewicz (1970). Occurrence and distribution of L-dopa decarboxylase in the human brain, *Brain Res.,* **22**, 426–428.

MacLean, R., W. J. Nicholson, C. M. B. Pare, and R. S. Stacey (1965). Effect of monoamineoxidase inhibitors on the concentrations of 5-hydroxytryptamine in the human brain, *Lancet, ii,* 205–208.

Mattsson, B., C. G. Gottfries, B. E. Roos, and B. Winblad (1974). Huntington's chorea: pathology and brain amines, *Acta Psychiatr. Scand.,* Suppl. 255, 269–277.

Mattsson, B. and S. Å. Persson (1974). Cerebrospinal fluid homovanillic acid and 5-hydroxyindoleacetic acid in Huntington's chorea, *Acta Psychiatr. Scand.,* Suppl 255, 245–260.

McGeer, E. G. and P. L. McGeer (1973). Some characteristics of brain tyrosine hydroxylase, in A. J. Mandell (Ed.) *New concepts in neurotransmitter regulation,* pp. 53–69, Plenum Press, New York.

McGeer, E. G., P. L. McGeer, and S. A. Wada (1971). Distribution of tyrosine hydroxylase in human and animal brain. *J. Neurochem.,* **18**, 1647–1658.

Mindham, R. H. S. (1970). Psychiatric symptoms in Parkinsonism, *J. Neurol. Neurosurg. Psychiatry,* **33**, 187.

Oreland, L. and B. Ekstedt (1972). Soluble and membrane-bound pig liver mitochondrial monoamine oxidase: thermostability, tryptic digestability and kinetic properties, *Biochem. Pharmacol.,* **21**, 2479–2488.

Pare, C. M. B., D. P. H. Young, K. Price, and R. S. Stacey (1969). 5-hydroxytryptamine, noradrenaline, and dopamine in brainstem, hypothalamus and caudate nucleus of

234 *Biochemistry of Dementia*

controls and patients committing suicide by coalgas poisoning, *Lancet, ii*, 133–135.

Parkes, J. D., C. D. Marsden, J. E. Rees, G. Curzon, B. D. Kantamaneni, R. Knill-Jones, A. Akbar, S. Das, and M. Kataria (1974). Parkinson's disease, cerebral arteriosclerosis, and senile dementia, *Q. J. Med.*, New Series, XLIII, No. 169, 49–61.

Pearce, J. (1974). Letter: Mental changes in Parkinsonism, *Brit. Med. J.*, **2**, 445.

Perry, T. L., S. Hansen, and M. Kloster (1973). Huntington's chorea: Deficiency of gamma-aminobutyric acid in brain, *New Engl. J. Med.*, **288**, 337–342.

Pollock, M. and R. W. Hornabrook (1966). The prevalence, natural history and dementia of Parkinson's disease, *Brain*, **89**, 429.

Read, A. E., K. R. Gough, J. L. Pardoe, and A. Nicholas (1965). Nutritional studies on the entrants to an old people's home, with particular reference to folic-acid deficiency, *Br. Med. J.*, **2**, 843–848.

Robinson, D. S., J. M. Davis, A. Nies, R. W. Colburn, J. N. Davis, H. R. Bourne, W. E. Bunney, D. M. Shaw, and A. J. Coppen (1972). Ageing, monoamines, and monoamine oxidase levels, *Lancet, i*, 290–291.

Robinson, D. S., T. L. Sourkes, A. Nies, L. S. Harris, S. Spector, D. L. Bartlett, and I. S. Kaye (1977). Monoamine metabolism in human brain, *Arch. Gen. Psychiatry*, **34**, 89–92.

Schildkraut, J. J. (1965). The catecholamine hypothesis of affective disorders: A review of supporting evidence, *Am. J. Psychiatry*, **122**, 509–522.

Selby, G. (1968). Cerebral atrophy in Parkinsonism, *J. Neurol. Sci.*, **6**, 517–559.

Shaw, D. M., D. A. Macsweeney, A. L. Johnson, R. O'Keeffe, D. Naidoo, D. M. Macleod, S. Jog, J. M. Preece, and J. M. Crowley (1971). Folate and amine metabolites in senile dementia: a combined trial and biochemical study, *Psychol. Med.*, **1**, 166–171.

Shulman, R. (1967). A survey of vitamin B_{12} deficiency in an elderly psychiatric population, *Br. J. Psychiatry*, **113**, 241–251.

Van Woert, M. H., G. Heninger, U. Rathey, and M. B. Jr Bowers (1970). L-Dopa in senile dementia, *Lancet, i*, 573–574.

Weil-Malherbe, H. (1972). The biochemistry of affective disorders, in A. Lajtha (Ed.) *Handbook of neurochemistry (Vol. 7): Pathological chemistry of the nervous system*, pp. 371–416, Plenum Press, New York.

Short Reports

Human Brain Angiotensin Converting Enzyme: Age-related Changes in Substantia Nigra and Alterations in Neuropsychiatric Disorders

ALBERTO ARREGUI, ANGUS V. P. MACKAY, LESLIE L. IVERSEN, and ERNEST G. SPOKES

MRC Neurochemical Pharmacology Unit,
Medical School, Hills Road, Cambridge, U.K.

The angiotensin converting enzyme (ACE) is a dipeptidyl peptidase (EC 3.4.15.1) which, in the peripheral tissues, converts the inactive decapeptide angiotensin-I to the active octapeptide angiotensin-II by removal of the carboxyl end-group His-Leu. The same enzyme is also known to inactivate bradykinin (Soffer, 1976). ACE activity is present in mammalian brain and is unevenly distributed (Yang and Neff, 1972; Arregui and coworkers, 1977), with the highest activities in human brain occurring in the corpus striatum (Arregui and coworkers, 1977) and in the substantia nigra (Arregui, Emson, and Spokes, 1978). We have recently suggested, on the basis of results obtained in animal and human studies, that a substantial part of the ACE activity in substantia nigra may be localized to nerve terminals of striatonigral neurons (Arregui, Emson, and Spokes, 1978).

We have measured ACE activity in several brain areas obtained post-mortem from control subjects, from Huntington's disease cases and from psychotic patients dying with hospital diagnosis of schizophrenia. We have found a reduction of the activity of ACE in striatal and nigral areas of Huntington's disease, and in the pars reticulata of substantia nigra of schizophrenic patients in whom the onset of disease occurred between the ages of 15 and 24 years, but no reduction of ACE activity in schizophrenia-like patients or in late-onset schizophrenics. In addition, a significant age-related decrease of ACE activity has been found in substantia nigra reticulata of the control population but not in other areas.

Cases of Huntington's disease were confirmed by neuropathology. Clinical assessement of the case histories of the psychotic patients was carried out as

Correspondence to Dr. A. Arregui, Department of Neurology, The Johns Hopkins Hospital, Baltimore, MD 21205, U.S.A.

described previously (Bird and coworkers, 1977). Briefly, two independent psychiatrists categorized the patients into 'schizophrenia' and 'schizophrenia-like' illness, according to research diagnostic criteria which include those of Wing, Cooper and Sartorius (1974). Angiotensin converting enzyme was measured in total homogenates of brain samples as described by Yang and Neff (1972), using the artificial substrate Hip-His-Leu at 1 mM concentration in the presence of 1 mM p-chloromercuribenzoate.

Samples of Huntington's disease cases showed a reduction of ACE activity in the striatal and nigral areas (Table 1). When the values from the psychotic population as a whole were examined, no significant differences were seen except in the pars reticulata of substantia nigra, where ACE activity was significantly reduced when compared to the control group (controls: 103 ± 5, $n = 40$; psychotics: 86 ± 5, $n = 51$; means $\pm$ S.E.M.; $p < 0.02$ by two-tailed t-test). When the psychotic population was subdivided into patients with 'schizophrenia' and 'schizophrenia-like' illnesses, the reduction in ACE activity in pars reticulata was seen to exist only in the 'schizophrenia' group and, furthermore, within this group reduced activity was seen only in those patients in whom onset of disease had occurred between the ages of 15 and 24 years (Table 1). The values from patients with 'schizophrenia-like' illness, in whom the onset of illness had been between the ages of 15 and 24 years, did not differ from those of the control group (Table 1). No changes in ACE activity were observed in the same 'schizophrenia' patients in nucleus accumbens, caudate nucleus, pars compacta (Table 1), or in cerebellar cortex, basal pons, cerebral cortex, thalamus (data not shown).

As illustrated in Fig. 1, ACE activity in the control pars reticulata had a significant decrease with age. This decrease with age at death was not found in any of the other brain regions so far examined. In view of this, the data from the pars reticulata was further analysed according to age at death (Table 2). No significant differences from age-matched controls were observed in the 'schizophrenia-like' group in any of the 'age of death' subdivisions. However, the values in the Huntington's disease and 'schizophrenia' groups showed reduced ACE activity both in the 20–50 years and the 50–70 years age groups. The mean $\pm$ S.D. ages at death for the control, Huntington's disease, and schizophrenia groups was 61.5 ± 19.3 yr, 54.0 ± 11.1 yr, and 49.0 ± 18.0 yr, respectively; we may, therefore, be underestimating the reduction in ACE activity in these two disease entities, since ACE activity normally decreases with age (Fig. 1).

The present results show a clear reduction of ACE activity in the striatal and nigral areas in Huntington's disease. In addition, they also show a clear reduction of ACE activity in one particular brain region, pars reticulata of substantia nigra, in post-mortem brain samples from patients with early-onset schizophrenia. Unfortunately, little is known about the functional significance of ACE activity in mammalian brain, in particular in the striatonigral system. Since the converting enzyme is also capable of degrading bradykinin (Soffer, 1976), its

Table 1. Angiotensin converting enzyme activity in brain areas of control and Huntington's disease patients, and of psychotic patients according to age of onset of disease

	Caudate Nucleus		Nucleus Accumbens		Nigra Reticulata		Nigra Compacta	
Controls	257 ± 18	(24)	150 ± 12	(25)	103 ± 5	(40)	56 ± 6	(32)
Huntington's disease	108 ± 25****	(8)	109 ± 12*	(16)	24 ± 5***	(10)	29 ± 5**	(10)
Schizophrenia: onset 15–24 years	237 ± 25	(12)	182 ± 25	(7)	64 ± 10**	(13)	67 ± 16	(12)
Schizophrenia: onset > 24 years	235 ± 24	(17)	128 ± 16	(9)	97 ± 6	(19)	84 ± 14	(16)
Schizophrenia-like: onset 15–24 years	245 ± 37	(6)	128 ± 23	(5)	98 ± 16	(7)	67 ± 15	(7)
Schizophrenia-like: onset > 24 years	228 ± 23	(10)	123 ± 12	(10)	91 ± 11	(12)	$64 - 7$	(10)

Significance by two-tailed t-test: * $p < 0.02$; ** $p < 0.005$; *** $p < 0.001$, when compared to controls.
Enzyme activity: pmol His-Leu per min per mg tissue ± S.E.M. (n).

Table 2. Activity of angiotensin enzyme in pars reticulata of control subjects and of Huntington's disease and psychotic patients according to age of death

	20–50 years		Age at death groups 50–70 years		More than 70 years	
Controls	125.3 ± 12.9	(9)	109.9 ± 7.4	(15)	84.9 ± 6.3	(16)
Huntington's disease	18.8 ± 3.2***(5)		28.3 ± 9.4****(5)		None	
Schizophrenia	65.0 ± 15.7**	(7)	85.5 ± 8.4*	(16)	92.8 ± 9.5	(9)
Schizophrenia-like	90.9 ± 15.4	(8)	94.3 ± 11.9	(9)	102.5 ± 27.5	(2)

Significance by two-tailed t-test: * $p < 0.05$; ** $p < 0.02$; *** $p < 0.001$, when compared to controls. Enzyme activity: pmol His-Leu per min per mg tissue ± S.E.M. (n).

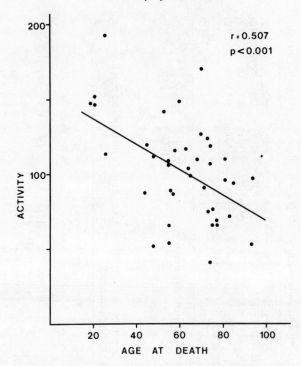

Figure 1. Age-related decrease of angiotensin converting
enzyme activity in the pars reticulata of substantia nigra
of the control population. Activity: pmol His-Leu per min
per mg tissue

function in CNS may not be restricted to the angiotensin system, and it is possible
that it may be involved in the regulation of other CNS peptides. Our previous
findings (Arregui, Emson, and Spokes, 1978) suggest that the bulk of ACE
activity in the substantia nigra is neuronally located, possibly in nerve terminals
of striatonigral neurons. The reduction of about 50 % in ACE activity in pars
reticulata in patients with early-onset schizophrenia (when compared to age-
matched controls) can be compared with the 80 % reduction in ACE activity
observed in patients with Huntington's disease who, in addition, also have
reduced ACE activity in caudate nucleus, putamen, globus pallidus, and pars
compacta (Arregui and coworkers, 1977; Arregui, Emson, and Spokes, 1978).

It is of interest to note that patients with Huntington's disease not infrequently
present with, or develop during the course of their illness, a psychotic syndrome
resembling schizophrenia (Bruyn, 1971). The selective reduction in ACE activity
in a postulated striatonigral neuronal pathway in both Huntington's disease and
schizophrenia suggests some possible biochemical similarities in these
conditions.

The reason for the observed age-related decrease in ACE activity in the substantia nigra reticulata of the control population is unclear. However, recent work in this laboratory shows that under conditions of chronic hypoxia in the rat (breathing 10 % oxygen for three weeks) there is a 70 % decrease of ACE activity in the substantia nigra and a 35 % decrease in the striatum (Arregui, Barer, and Iversen, unpublished observations). It is thus possible, for example, that local tissue hypoxia produced in arterial boundary zones may be responsible for the age-related decrease of ACE activity.

Despite the lack of information on the functional role of ACE in the CNS the present finding of reduced enzyme activity in a selected group of patients with schizophrenia helps support the notion that schizophrenia, as presently defined, is not a single homogeneous condition but, rather, a group of conditions in which different causal factors may lead to a final common syndrome (Richter, 1976).

REFERENCES

Arregui, A., J. P. Bennett, E. D. Bird, H. I. Yamamura, L. L. Iversen, and S. H. Snyder (1977). *Ann. Neurol.*, **2**, 294–8.

Arregui, A., P. C. Emson, and E. G. Spokes (1978). *Eur. J. Pharmacol.*, **52**, 121–4.

Bird, E. D., E. G. Spokes, J. Barnes, A. V. P. MacKay, L. L. Iversen, and M. Shepherd (1977). *Lancet*, **2**, 1157–9.

Bruyn, G. (1971). In P. J. Vinken and G. Bruyn (Eds) *Diseases of the Basal Ganglia*, North-Holland, Amsterdam. pp. 298–378.

Richter, D. (1976). In D. Kemali, G. Bartholini, and D. Richter (Eds) *Schizophrenia Today*, Pergamon Press, Oxford. pp. 71–83.

Soffer, R. L. (1976). *Ann. Rev. Biochem.*, **45**, 73–94.

Wing, J. K., J. E. Cooper, and N. Sartorius (1974). *The Measurement and Classification of Psychiatric Symptoms*, Cambridge University Press, London.

Yang, H. -Y. T. and N. H. Neff (1972). *J. Neurochem.*, **19**, 2443–50.

Factors Affecting Synaptosomal Oxygen Uptake at Critical Oxygen Tensions

H. Wise*, M. J. Parry**, G. G. Lunt†, and H. S. Bachelard*

* Department of Biochemistry, St Thomas's Hospital Medical School, London, SE1 7EH, U.K.
** Pfizer Central Research, Pfizer Ltd, Sandwich, Kent, U.K.
†Department of Biochemistry, University of Bath, Bath, BA2 7AY, U.K.

Appreciable changes occur in local cerebral Po_2 without concomitant changes in ATP production, even at mild degrees of hypoxia at which signs of changed cerebral functioning are first evident. Siesjö and coworkers (1974) have suggested that the functional effects of moderate hypoxia may represent a failure in transmission rather than in energy supply. Since oxygen is required by a variety of enzymes necessary for both energy production—the cytochrome oxidase system—and for transmitter synthesis—tyrosine and tryptophan hydroxylases—synaptosomal oxygen uptake has been studied at low oxygen tensions.

Rat cerebral cortex synaptosomes were prepared by the method of Bradford and coworkers (1975) and oxygen uptake measured at $30\,°C$ in Krebs-phosphate medium using a Rank oxygen electrode. Previous work (Wise, Bachelard, and Lunt, 1978) has indicated that synaptosomes placed in media with a low oxygen concentration (14 μmol), show a rate of oxygen uptake that is steady until 6 μmol O_2 when it falls off sharply.

When synaptosomes were pre-incubated at $30°C$ for 35 min in an open vessel and subsequently placed in media of reduced oxygen tension (14 μmol), variations in the rate of oxygen uptake were observed according to the nature of the pre-incubation conditions and the medium constituents (see Table 1). Under conditions of no pre-incubation, synaptosomal oxygen uptake was increased in response to glucose (10 mmol) or bovine serum albumin (BSA 3.3 mg ml^{-1}). Pre-incubation using a shaking water-bath also gave these responses, although at much reduced general rates of oxygen uptake. If pre-incubation was performed in a non-shaking water-bath, the control rates remained similar but the response to glucose was absent and BSA significantly reduced the rate of oxygen uptake.

Although pre-incubation in the absence of added glucose or BSA, under shaking and non-shaking conditions, significantly increased the proportion of

242

Table 1. The effect of varying conditions on synaptosomal oxygen uptake at low oxygen tensions

Condition	Oxygen uptake (μmol O_2 per h per 100 mg)	Significance level compared to:	
		Control Krebs	Own control
Control:			
Krebs	15.49(3.70)		
Glucose (10 mmol)	26.64(6.03)	$p < 0.01$	
BSA (3.3 mg ml^{-1})	35.53(3.92)	$p < 0.001$	
Glucose + BSA	47.09(8.94)	$p < 0.001$	
Pre-incubation, non-shaking:			
Krebs	13.88(4.18)	N.S.	
Glucose (10 mmol)	15.70(2.22)	N.S.	N.S.
BSA (3.3 mg ml^{-1})	5.80(1.76)	$p < 0.01$	$p < 0.01$
Glucose + BSA	11.16(3.08)	N.S.	N.S.
Pre-incubation, shaking:			
Krebs	7.28(2.01)	$p < 0.05$	
Glucose (10 mmol)	11.60(2.05)	$p < 0.05$	$p < 0.05$
BSA (3.3 mg ml^{-1})	13.50(4.01)	N.S.	$p < 0.05$
Glucose + BSA	20.84(6.93)	N.S.	$p < 0.01$

Results expressed as mean (S.D.) of 4–6 experiments. Values taken when the Po_2 had reached 7 μmol after starting at an initial Po_2 of 14 μmol. All additions of glucose and BSA are made to the oxygen electrode chamber and are not present during the pre-incubations. Control tissue kept on ice.

free to occluded lactate dehydrogenase when compared to tissue kept on ice, there was no difference between the two forms of pre-incubation. The presence of glucose during the pre-incubation resulted in a further increase in the proportion of free lactate dehydrogenase activity.

Although the presence of both glucose and BSA resulted in increased rates of oxygen uptake when there was no pre-incubation, these rates were maintained more with glucose than with BSA as the oxygen tension fell.

The effects of BSA on synaptosomal oxygen uptake may reflect the marked affinity of albumin for free fatty acids which are known to be released during ischaemic anoxia (Galli and coworkers, 1978). The composition of the released fatty acid pool in ischaemic anoxia is characterized by high levels of arachidonic acid and stearic acid and thus closely resembles that of brain diglycerides and phosphatidylinositol (Galli and coworkers, 1978). Bazan (1970) has shown that the ratio of total saturated to total unsaturated fatty acids liberated after decapitation, suggests a predominance in the hydrolysis of the β-fatty acid bond of phosphoglycerides, indicating phospholipase A_2 activity. Even when a lipolytic activation also takes place, the major portion of the liberated free fatty acids arises from molecules other than triglycerides.

The ischaemic condition produces mainly unsaturated long chain fatty acids

(Bazan, 1970), such as oleic acid, which have been shown to be more potent uncouplers of oxidative phosphorylation than saturated ones. Chan and Higgins (1978) have shown that the washing of isolated mitochondria with BSA can increase their respiratory control index (RCI), with proportionally more unsaturated fatty acids being removed by the BSA and a consequent higher percentage of saturated fatty acids retained by the mitochondria.

It would be expected that fatty acids, acting as uncouplers, would stimulate respiration; however, in our experiments BSA increased oxygen uptake. This could be due to binding of the free fatty acids which have been shown to lower oxygen uptake in mitochondria (Lochner, Kotzé, and Gevers, 1976), possibly by causing the leakage of essential cofactors such as NAD, cytochrome c, and acetyl-coenzyme A.

Our experiments indicated that the stimulation of synaptosomal oxygen uptake by BSA could be repeated using a preparation of fatty acid-free BSA. However, a Ca^{2+}-free medium also mimicked these results (see Table 2). These results suggest that the BSA may be exerting its effects by sequestering Ca^{2+} ions and this is being looked into further.

Table 2. The effect of various media on synaptosomal oxygen uptake at low oxygen tensions

Condition	Oxygen uptake (μmol O_2 per h per 100 mg)	Significance level compared to control
Krebs control	22.69 (2.65)	
BSA (3.3 mg ml^{-1})	32.96 (4.92)	$p < 0.01$
Fatty acid-free BSA (3.3 mg ml^{-1})	34.49 (6.79)	$p < 0.01$
Ca^{2+}-free (containing 1 mmol-EGTA)	36.81 (7.64)	$p < 0.01$

Results expressed as mean (S.D.) of 5–6 experiments. Values taken when the Po_2 had reached 7 μmol after starting at an initial Po_2 of 14 μmol. Addition of BSA made to the oxygen electrode chamber.

Further experiments have been initiated to study the release of free fatty acids under hypoxic conditions. By blowing a variable mixture of N_2 and air over the surface of a stirred suspension of synaptosomes while in the oxygen electrode chamber, the Po_2 can be kept fairly constant at 14μmol and below. After 10 minutes' incubation at 30°C, the tissue is rapidly separated from the medium by a filtration system using a combination of Whatman GF/B and GF/F glass-fibre filters in a Swinny adaptor connected to a syringe. The free fatty acids are then extracted and their methyl esters monitored by GLC. Preliminary results indicate the presence of palmitic, stearic, oleic, and arachidonic acid plus two unidentified slow-running compounds. Arachidonic acid is the predominant form. After 10 minutes of hypoxia, there is an indication of an overall increase in the relative proportions of palmitic, stearic, and oleic acids with a decrease in the relative proportion of arachidonic acid. Arachidonic acid is the precursor of prostaglandins of the PG_2 series; it has been suggested that prostaglandin liberation during ischaemic anoxia of various tissues may contribute, by vasodilatation, to increase blood flow (Galli and coworkers, 1978). This may reflect a biochemical response of the tissue to hypoxia to improve blood flow and, therefore, the availability of nutrients.

ACKNOWLEDGEMENT

H. Wise is supported by an SRC-CASE studentship.

REFERENCES

Bazan, N. G. (1970). *Biochim. Biophys. Acta*, **218**, 1–10.
Bradford, H. F., D. G. Jones, H. K. Ward, and J. Booher (1975). *Brain Res.*, **90**, 245–259.
Chan, S. H. P. and E. Higgins (1978). *Can. J. Biochem.*, **56**, 111–116.
Galli, C., C. Spagnuolo, L. Sautebin, and G. Galli (1978). *Proc. 2nd Meeting Eur. Soc. Neurochem.*, pp. 271–284.
Lochner, A., J. C. N. Kotzé, and W. Gevers (1976). *J. Mol. Cell. Cardiol.*, **8**, 465–480.
Siesjö, B. K., H. Johannsson, B. Ljunggren, and K. Norberg (1974). In F. Plum (Ed.) *Brain Dysfunction in Metabolic Disorders*, Res. Publ. Ass. Nerv. Mental Dis., Vol. 53, Raven Press, New York.
Wise, H., H. S. Bachelard and G. G. Lunt (1978). *Proc. 2nd Meeting Eur. Soc. Neurochem.*, p. 303.

On the Polypeptide Composition of Mammalian Neurofilaments

ROBIN THORPE, BRIAN H. ANDERTON

Department of Biochemistry, St. George's Hospital Medical School,
Cranmer Terrace, London, SW17 0RE

JIM COHEN, S. SELVENDRAN, and

M.R.C. Neuroimmunology Project, Department of Zoology,
University College London, Gower Street, London, WC1E 6BT, U.K.

PETER WOODHAMS

M.R.C. Development Neurobiology Unit, Institute of Neurology,
33 John's Mews, London, WC1N 2NS, U.K.

Neurofilaments from different sources have been reported to be composed of a variety of apparently unrelated polypeptides. Those from two invertebrate giant nerve fibres have prominent polypeptides with molecular weights of 200 000 and 65 000 for squid axons (Lasek and Hoffman, 1976) and 152 000 and 160 000 for *Myxicola* (Gilbert, Newby, and Anderton 1975). Mammalian neurofilaments are not obviously similar to either of the above: those from peripheral nerve have polypeptides with chain weights of approximately 200 000, 150 000 and 70 000 (Micko and Schlaepfer, 1978a, b), whereas those from brain have been claimed to be composed principally of a 50 000 mol. wt species (Davison and Winslow, 1974; Yen and coworkers, 1976) although other minor components are present. A major difficulty encountered when assigning polypeptides to the neurofilaments is the obvious contamination of isolated mammalian neurofilaments with other particulate material (Anderton, Ayers, and Thorpe, 1978). Preparations both from peripheral nerve and brain contain aggregated filaments with entrapped membranous material, but those from brain contain two clearly distinguishable types of aggregate: tightly and loosely packed bundles of 10 nm filaments (Fig. 1), neither of which has been positively identified as neurofilamentous. It has been suggested, however, that the tight bundles are glial filaments and the loosely packed filaments are neurofilaments (DeVries, Norton, and Raine, 1972; Shelanski and coworkers, 1971); our observation that peripheral nerve contains only the loosely packed form is consistent with this proposition and,

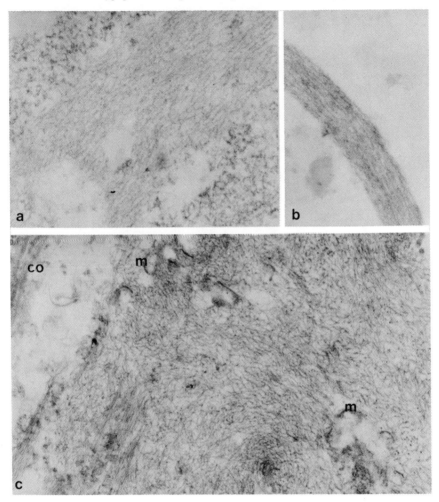

Figure 1. Electron micrographs of: (a) loosely packed brain 10 nm filaments; (b) part of a tight bundle of brain 10 nm filaments; (c) rat sciatic nerve neurofilaments. All × 38 350; m, membranes; co, collagen

consequently, we prefer to refer to the brain preparations as brain 10 nm filaments rather than brain neurofilaments (Anderton, Ayers, and Thorpe, 1978).

We have compared by sodium dodecyl sulphate (SDS)-gel electrophoresis the polypeptides of sciatic nerve axoplasm with isolated brain 10 nm filaments from rat and from rabbit (Fig. 2). The polypeptides which have been identified as originating from sciatic nerve neurofilaments are identified by the letter 'n' (Micko and Schlaepfer, 1978a) and other polypeptides known to be either

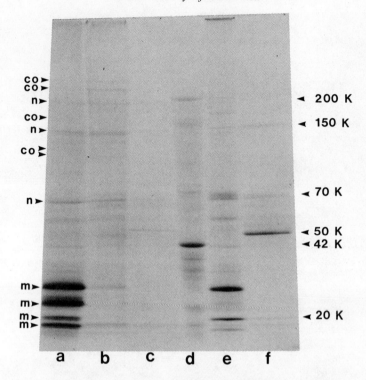

Figure 2. SDS-gel electrophoresis of: (a) myelinated rat sciatic nerve; (b) rat sciatic nerve demyelinated axonal material; (c) rat brain 10 nm filament preparation; (d) rabbit skeletal muscle myofibrils (main bands, myosin heavy chain; mol. wt 200 000 and actin mol. wt 42 000); (e) myelinated rabbit sciatic nerve; (f) rabbit brain 10 nm filament preparation. Mol. wt values are shown on the right-hand side; co, collagen; m, myelin-associated polypeptides; n, neurofilament polypeptides

Figure 3. Immunofluorescence on 8 μm frozen sections of rat brain and peripheral nerve. (a) Cerebellum stained with antiserum to whole brain 10 nm filaments. In addition to axonal staining of the perisomatic Purkinje cell baskets (B), the radial Bergmann glial fibres are strongly positive (serum diluted down to 1:40); this antiserum showed a slight non-specific activity against blood vessels (BV) even after absorption with brain 10 nm filaments. (b) Cerebellum stained with antiserum to the 210 000 mol. wt polypeptide. Purkinje cell baskets are brightly positive (serum diluted down to 1:40) but glial staining is absent. Axons are also seen in the granular layer and above the Purkinje cells in the lower part of the molecular layer where, in this sagittal section, they are seen running transversely across the axis of the folium. (c) Transverse section of sciatic nerve, showing intra-axonal staining with antiserum to the 210 000 mol. wt polypeptide (diluted 1:40). (d) Control cerebellar section stained with antiserum to the 210 000 mol. wt polypeptide pre-absorbed with brain 10 nm filaments. Scale bar = 100 μm

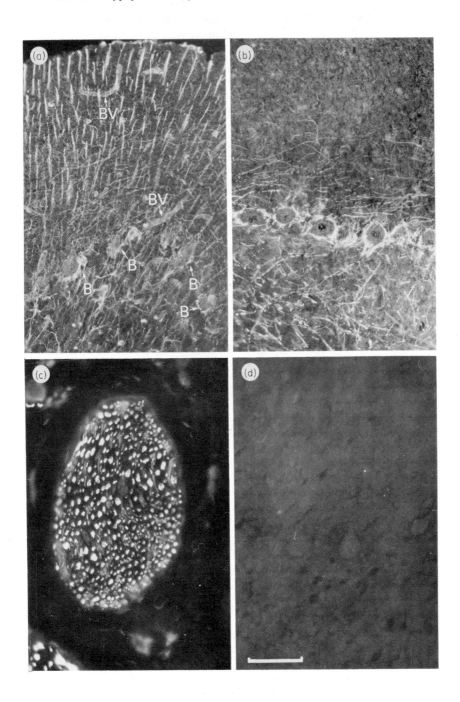

collagen or myelin components are identified with letters 'co' or 'm' (Micko and Schlaepfer, 1978a, 1978b). It is apparent that the triplet of neurofilament polypeptides of 200 000, 150 000, and 70 000 mol. wt in sciatic nerve migrate with three corresponding components present in brain 10 nm filaments, but that the major 50 000 mol. wt polypeptide in the brain preparation does not possess a counterpart in sciatic nerve axoplasm.

Antisera to bovine brain 10 nm filaments and to bovine brain 210 000 and 155 000 mol wt polypeptides (corresponding to 200 000 and 150 000 mol. wt of rat since there are species differences in mol. wt) have been produced in rabbits. The antisera have been tested by indirect immunofluorescence on cryostat sections of rat cerebellum and on primary cultures of dissociated rat cerebellum. The brain 10 nm filament antiserum labels both neurons and astrocytes in the cultures, as well as sections of the cerebellum. Fig. 3a illustrates the staining pattern on sections of cerebellum where the Bergmann glial fibres are strongly fluorescent and, in addition, there was staining of basket cell processes which surround the Purkinje cell bodies. The antisera to the 210 000 and 155 000 mol. wt polypeptides gave identical staining patterns which were neuron-specific. These results are illustrated in Fig. 3b, in which it can be seen that the basket cell processes were labelled by the anti-210 000 mol. wt but the parallel Bergmann glia in the molecular layer were not revealed. The anti-210 000 and anti-155 000 mol. wt reagents also labelled the axons in transverse sections of rat sciatic nerve (Fig. 3c). The brain 10 nm filament antiserum gave similar results with sciatic nerve but the non-axonal areas also showed some weak staining.

The 200 000 and 150 000 mol. wt polypeptides thus appear to be specifically located in neurons of both the central and peripheral nervous systems. Possibly, the 70 000 mol. wt component will also be found to have only a neuronal distribution, but so far we have not obtained an antiserum to this polypeptide. The antiserum to the whole brain 10 nm filament preparation contains antibody to the 50 000 mol. wt polypeptide as well as against some of the higher molecular-weight triplet components (Anderton and coworkers, in preparation) and this could explain the mixed neuronal and astrocyte staining pattern obtained with this antiserum if the 50 000 mol. wt polypeptide partially arises from glial 10 nm filaments. We have also shown that the 50 000 mol. wt material is heterogeneous, apparently composed of at least three separable polypeptide species (Thorpe and coworkers, 1979). We conclude, therefore, that the higher molecular-weight triplet of polypeptides are probable neurofilament components, and that the 50 000 mol. wt material is, at least partially, of glial origin. Liem and coworkers (1978) have recently made a similar suggestion and found that the polypeptide triplet is shared between 10 nm filaments from brain and spinal cord. These workers suggested that the 50 000 mol. wt component consisted largely of proteolytic degradation products of the triplet polypeptides and our findings are not inconsistent with this proposition (Thorpe and coworkers, 1979).

Our results are pertinent to investigations on neurofibrillary tangles found in the brain of patients with dementia of the Alzheimer type. Until now, workers in this field have assumed that mammalian neurofilaments are composed of the 50 000 mol. wt polypeptide (Iqbal and coworkers, 1977) discussed above and this now appears to be an erroneous assumption. Preliminary studies with our antisera have demonstrated that human neurofilaments cross-react with bovine and rat neurofilament proteins, and it will be interesting to see if the antisera label neurofibrillary tangles in pathological tissue.

ACKNOWLEDGEMENT

This work was supported in part by a grant from the Medical Research Council to B. H. Anderton.

REFERENCES

Anderton, B. H., M. Ayers, and R. Thorpe (1978). *FEBS Lett.*, **96**, 159–63.
Davison, P. F. and B. Winslow (1974). *J. Neurobiol.*, **5**, 119–33.
DeVries, G. H., W. T. Norton and C. S. Raine (1972). *Science*, **175**, 1370–2.
Gilbert, D. S., B. J. Newby, and B. H. Anderton (1975). *Nature*, **256**, 586–9.
Iqbal, K., I. Grundke-Iqbal, H. M. Wisniewski, and R. D. Terry (1977). *J. Neurochem.*, **29**, 417–24.
Lasek, R. J. and P. M. Hoffman (1976). In R. Goldman, T. Pollard, and J. Rosenbaum (Eds) *Cell Motility*, Vol. 3, Cold Spring Harbor Laboratories, Cold Spring Harbor, New York, pp. 1021–49.
Liem, R. K. H., S.-H. Yen, G. D. Salomon, and M. L. Shelanski (1978). *J. Cell Biol.*, **79**, 637–45.
Micko, S. and W. W. Schlaepfer (1978a). *J. Neurochem.*, **30**, 1041–9.
Micko, S. and W. W. Schlaepfer (1978b). *Anal. Biochem.*, **88**, 566–72.
Shelanski, M. L., S. Albert, G. H. DeVries, and W. T. Norton (1971). *Science*, **174**, 1242–5.
Thorpe, R., A. Delacourte, M. Ayers, C. Bullock, and B. H. Anderton (1979). *Biochem. J.* **181**, 275–284.
Yen, S.-H., D. Dahl, M. Schachner, and M. L. Shelanski (1976). *Proc. Nat. Acad. Sci. U.S.A.*, **73**, 529–33.

Factors Influencing Cerebral Blood Flow, CMR-oxygen and CMR-glucose in Dementia Patients

SIEGFRIED HOYER

Department of Pathochemistry and General Neurochemistry,
University of Heidelberg, D-6900 Heidelberg, West Germany

It has previously been assumed that the most important pathophysiological disturbance in dementia was a decreased cerebral blood flow due to an arteriosclerosis of the brain vessels. However, neuropathological findings in dementia patients have revealed that about 60 % of pre-senile and senile dementia cases showed degenerative changes, but that only 20–25 % had cerebrovascular and 15–20 % had both degenerative and cerebrovascular changes in brain tissue (Tomlinson, Blessed, and Roth, 1970; Jellinger, 1976). Furthermore, studies of cerebral blood flow (and metabolism) in unselected demented patients showed no uniform variations (Shieve and Wilson, 1953; Hoyer, 1969, 1970; O'Brien, 1972). It could thus be assumed that pathophysiological variations other than cerebral blood flow alone were associated with dementia symptoms and were possibly responsible for them. In a research programme of dementia, carried out over a period of several years, we therefore investigated cerebral blood flow (CBF), CMR-oxygen (CMR_{O_2}) and CMR-glucose (CMRGL) in various types and various degrees of dementia and with different durations.

MATERIAL AND METHODS

A total of 294 dementia patients of both sexes, aged from 40 to 83 years, were included in the study. Demented patients due to head injuries, brain tumours, brain infarctions, brain infections, endogenous and exogenous intoxications were excluded from the investigations. The patients were separated into degenerative and cerebrovascular (multi-infarct) dementias by means of standard neuropsychiatric methods with partial support by means of the ischaemic score (Hachinski and coworkers, 1975). Psychometric tests such as the AMP-rating scale system (Scharfetter, 1972; Helmchen, 1975), served to determine the degree of dementia and to group dementia symptoms as clusters which could be

252

assigned into mild to moderate (clusters I–III) and severe (clusters IV–VII) syndromes.

Cerebral blood flow was measured by means of the Kety–Schmidt technique (Kety and Schmidt, 1948) as modified by Bernsmeier and Siemons (1953). Blood samples were taken from the femoral artery and from the internal jugular bulb by means of motor syringes over 10 minutes under steady-state conditions of arterial blood pressure, in normocapnia and in normoxemia. An extracerebral contamination of the mixed cerebral venous blood was avoided by the low extraction rate of the blood of 1 ml min^{-1} and the exact position of the needle in the internal jugular bulb. In arterial and mixed cerebral venous blood we measured the oxygen volumes by means of gas chromatography (Weinhardt, Quadbeck, and Hoyer, 1972) and the glucose concentrations by the hexokinase reaction. For statistical calculations the analysis of variance of a two-way design, the t-test and the Bartlett-test were used.

RESULTS

Investigations in 115 out of the 294 demented patients showed that the distribution curves of cerebral blood flow, CMR_{O_2} and CMR_{GL} were abnormal. There were at least two major groups of patients. In one group CBF and CMR_{O_2} were generally decreased. Clinically, these patients showed more cerebrovascular (multi-infarct) disturbances. In the other group, CBF and CMR_{O_2} were almost in a normal or only slightly decreased range. Clinically, these patients suffered more from a degenerative dementia. A similar correlation could not be found in CMR_{GL} (Hoyer and coworkers, 1975) (Fig. 1a–c). Based

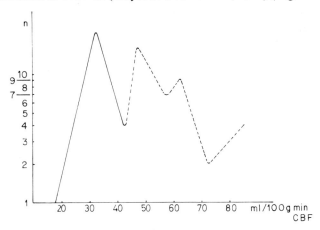

Figure 1(a) Distribution curve of cerebral blood flow (CBF) in 115 dementia patients. Multi-infarct dementias (continuous line) showed a mean CBF of $\leq$ 40 ml per 100 g per min; Alzheimer patients (broken line) a mean CBF of 40 ml per 100 g per min

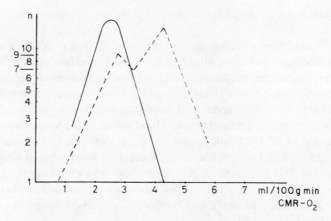

(b) Distribution curves of CMR_{O_2} in the same patients as in
(a). CMR_{O_2} was decreased in multi-infarct dementias (continuous line) and was near normal in Alzheimers (broken
line); CBF as in (a)

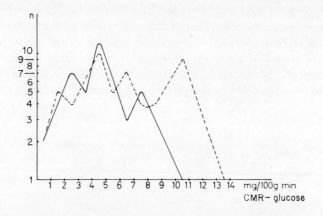

(c) Distribution curves of CMR_{GL} in the same groups of
patients as in (a) and (b). CMR_{GL} was either decreased, or
normal, or increased in both types of dementia (continuous
line, multi-infarcts; broken line, Alzheimer patients). CBF as
in (a)

on a psychometric design, Hachinski and coworkers (1975) arrived at the same
results as far as cerebral blood flow was concerned. Thus, distinct morphological
changes in the brain tissue seem to influence brain blood flow and metabolism.

In 94 out of the 294 dementia patients we studied the influence of the duration
of the disease on brain blood flow and metabolism. A dementia with an

anamnesis of less than 2 years was designated as 'initial', one with an anamnesis of 2–10 years as 'intermediate', and one with an anamnesis longer than 10 years as 'chronic'. In the initial phase, both CBF and $CMRo_2$ were not markedly disturbed in both the degenerative and the multi-infarct dementia. But $CMRGL$ was decreased in the degenerative and increased in the cerebrovascular group, demonstrating an imbalance between oxygen and glucose: in degenerative dementia a glucose deficit and in multi-infarct dementia a 'surplus' of glucose. In the intermediate phase of the dementia process, CBF and metabolism decreased markedly in both dementia groups. In chronic dementia brain blood flow and metabolism diminished to a common pathologically low level in both groups. At this level brain blood flow and metabolism were sufficiently high to meet the needs of the brain (Hoyer, 1978a, 1978b) (Fig. 2).

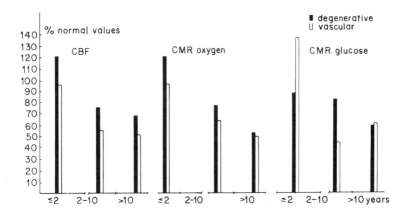

Figure 2. CBF, CMR-oxygen and CMR-glucose expressed as percentages of normal values in dementia due to degenerative and vascular (multi-infarct) brain diseases at different times of the disease

In 85 out of the 294 dementia patients we correlated CBF, $CMRo_2$ and $CMRGL$ with the degree of dementia symptoms as measured by the AMP-rating scale system. In mild to moderate dementia symptoms (clusters I–III) brain blood flow and metabolism were only slightly or moderately decreased. In severely demented patients with amnestic (cluster V) and hypoactive (cluster VII) dementia, CBF and metabolism were more markedly decreased than in the mild and moderate forms. However, severely demented patients with confusion (cluster IV) and hyperactive dementia (cluster VI) showed seemingly normal or only subnormal values of CBF and metabolism. But the deviation of blood flow and the metabolic data were large in these patients, thus indicating that an increased (pathological) activity of the brain could either be associated with pathologically increased or decreased brain blood flow and metabolism which might be supposed to be elevated above normal in non-atrophic brains, while in atrophic brains these parameters were decreased. Thus, no correlations exist between the degree of psychiatric impairment in dementia and the degree of decreases in CBF and metabolism. On the other hand, one might conclude that in pre-senile and senile dementia a clear correlation exists between the deranged functional state of the brain and its disturbed blood flow and metabolism (Hoyer, 1978c) (Fig. 3).

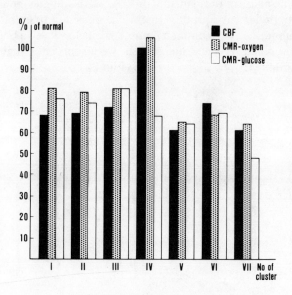

Figure 3. Relationship between psychiatric impairment expressed as clusters based on the *AMP*-rating scale system, and blood flow and metabolism of the brain

CONCLUSION

At least three factors seem fundamentally to influence the quality and quantity of the variations in brain blood flow and metabolism in pre-senile and senile dementia:

    (i) The morphological variation in brain tissue.
   (ii) The duration of dementia symptoms.
  (iii) The type of psychiatric impairment.

REFERENCES

Bernsmeier, A. and K. Sierhons (1953). *Pflügers Arch. Ges. Physiol.*, **258**, 149–62.
Hachinski, V. C., L. D. Iliff, E. Zilkha, G. H. Du Boulay, V. L. McAllister, J. Marshall,

R. W. Ross Russell, and L. Symon (1975). *Arch. Neurol.*, **32**, 632–7.

Helmchen, H. (1957). In H. Hippius (Ed.) *Assessment of Pharmacodynamic Effects in Human Pharmacology.* Stutgart; Schattauer, Stuttgart. pp. 87–134.

Hoyer, S. (1969). In M. Brock, C. Fieschi, D. H. Ingvar, N. A. Lassen, and K. Schürmann (Eds) *Cerebral Blood Flow.* Springer-Verlag, Berlin. pp. 235–6.

Hoyer, S. (1970). *Dtsch. Z. Nervenheilk.*, **197**, 285–92.

Hoyer, S. (1978a). In R. Katzman, R. D. Terry, and K. L. Bick (Eds) *Alzheimer's Disease: Senile Dementia and Related Disorders.* Raven Press, New York. pp. 219–226.

Hoyer, S. (1978a). In R. Katzman, R. D. Terry, and K. L. Bick (Eds) *Alzheimer's Disease: Senile Dementia and Related Disorders.* Raven Press, New York. pp. 219–226.

Hoyer, S. (1978b). *Nervenarzt*, **49**, 201–7.

Hoyer, S., G. Krüger, and F. Weinhardt (1978). In *Proc. 9th Int. Salzburg Conf. on Cerebral Vascular Disease.*

Hoyer, S., K. Oesterreich, F. Weinhardt, and G. Krüger (1975). *J. Neurol.*, **210**, 227–37.

Jellinger, K. (1976). *Acta Neurol. (Belg.)*, **76**, 83–102.

Kety, S. S. and C. F. Schmidt (1948). *J. Clin Invest.*, **27**, 476–83.

O'Brien, M. D. (1972). In J. S. Meyer, M. Reivich, H. Lechner, and O. Eichhorn (Eds) *Research on the Cerebral Circulation.* C. C. Thomas, Springfield, Illinois. pp. 287–90.

Scharfetter, C. (1972). *Das AMP-System.*, 2nd edn, Springer-Verlag, Berlin.

Schieve, J. F., and W. P. Wilson (1953). *Amer. J. Med.*, **15**, 171–4.

Tomlinson, B. E., G. Blessed, and M. Roth (1970). *J. Neurol. Sci.*, **11**, 205–42.

Weinhardt, F., G. Quadbeck, and S. Hoyer (1972). *Z. prakt. Anästh.*, **6**, 337–47.

Glycolytic Enzymes from Human Autoptic Brain Cortex: Normally Aged and Demented Cases

P. Iwangoff, R. Armbruster, A. Enz, W. Meier-Ruge, and P. Sandoz,

*Department of Preclinical Research,
Sandoz Ltd, Basel, Switzerland*

In earlier investigations (Iwangoff and coworkers, 1977) significant age-dependences were detected for the following enzyme activities in autoptic human brain cortex and putamen: an increase of soluble hexokinase (sHK), a decrease of phosphofructokinase (PFK) and phosphoglycerate mutase (PGM). However, the great majority of glycolytic enzyme activities did not show age-related differences in either part of the brain.

A rough classification of the cases according to their clinical records was carried out. This study, which differentiated between sudden death and prolonged agonal state, showed a more significant negative correlation of PFK activity with age in the group of sudden death cases than in the total of all cases (Iwangoff and coworkers, 1979). In agreement with the findings of Bird, Gale, and Spokes (1977), PFK activities measured from cases with long agony, e.g. pneumonia, were considerably lower than those from cases with sudden death. Subdivision according to agonal state did not reveal additional information on the observed increase in sHK and decrease in PGM.

Autoptic human brain material of temporal lobe from cases of dementia and normal controls was obtained from Professor J. A. N. Corsellis and Dr D. Bowen (London). The senile dementia cases were divided into two groups: (a) senile dementia of the 'Alzheimer's' type (non-vascular, NVA), and (b) senile dementia of the 'Alzheimer's' type combined with (at least moderate) atherosclerotic lesions (VAS).

The number of cases and the average age (*aa*) for the different groups was: NVA: $n = 15$, $aa = 80.7$ years; VAS: $n = 10$, $aa = 85.4$ years; controls: $n = 18$, $aa = 74.7$ years. The average post-mortem delay until isolation and refrigeration of the tissue was between 14 and 16 hours. The activity of glycolytic enzymes was determined in accordance with the literature (Bücher, Luh, and Pette, 1964) in

258

the supernatant fraction obtained after centrifugation from the homogenates of the temporal lobe.

In autoptic brain tissue from demented cases, in comparison with normally-aged controls, the decrease in enzymatic activity in sHK, PFK, and PGM is reinforced. The differences between all Alzheimer cases (NVA and VAS) and the controls are significant ($p < 0.05$) for all three enzymes (values calculated in relation to wet weight). For the single groups NVA and VAS, only the decrease in PGM is significant (Fig. 1a–c). In addition, some other glycolytic enzymes which are not age-dependent in normal brain cortex show significantly reduced activity in NVA but not in VAS samples: phosphoglucose isomerase (PGI), aldolase (ALD), triosephosphate isomerase (TIM) (Fig. 2), lactate dehydrogenase (LDH). Thus, the destructive effects on glycolytic enzymes are more pronounced in brain tissue from cases with NVA than from those with VAS. The LDH of VAS cases even shows an increase, although this is not significant. On the other hand, glucose-6-phosphate dehydrogenase, an enzyme which is indirectly related to the glycolytic chain, is increased under conditions of both types of Alzheimer senile dementia.

In comparison with normal ageing in human autoptic brain tissue, senile dementia of Alzheimer's type induces more pronounced dysfunctions of the glycolytic pathway. The deactivation of sHK, PFK, and PGM is reinforced under both vascular and non-vascular Alzheimer conditions. Many of our cases—particularly those of senile dementia of the Alzheimer type—were reported to have died from bronchopneumonia, which is known to decrease considerably PFK in autoptic human brain (Bird, Gale, and Spokes, 1977, Iwangoff and coworkers, in press). Therefore, the considerable loss of PFK activity can, but need not be, the crucial step in the difference between controls and the cases of senile dementia of the Alzheimer's type. However, the decrease in some enzymes—PGI, ALD, PGM, TIM, and LDH—particularly under NVA conditions, seems to be much more specific for Alzheimer's dementia. With normal ageing, these enzymes do not show differences due to age when measured in human autoptic brain tissue, and most of them do not decrease under post-mortem delay conditions (Iwangoff and coworkers, in press). Broncho-pneumonia induces only a very slight insignificant decrease in activity of these enzymes.

Earlier results (Iwangoff and coworkers, 1979) indicated a significant re-duction in glycolytic capacity in human autoptic brain with age. The reduction is reinforced by senile dementia of the Alzheimer's type, especially NVA con-ditions. According to Siesjö and Rehncrona (Chapter 6) and Blass and coworkers (Chapter 7) hypoxia may lead to the decrease in glycolytic function. This impairment of glycolysis in NVA may be the reason for some conditions of cerebral insufficiency. It may induce disturbances of transmitter meta-bolism, particularly of the cholinergic system (Gibson, Shimada, and Blass, 1978).

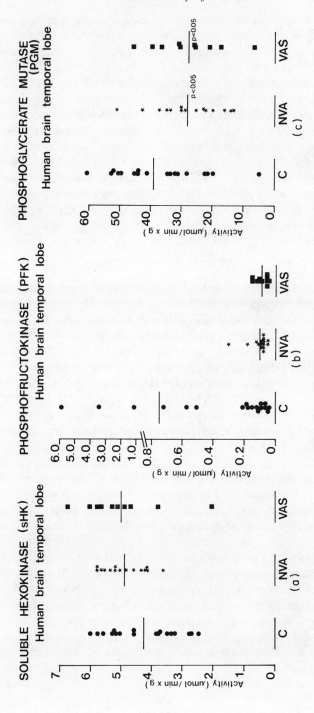

Figure 1. Activity of (a) sHK, (b) PFK, and (c) PGM in autoptic human temporal lobe: controls and cases senile dementia of the 'Alzheimer's type. NVA, Cases with senile dementia of the Alzheimer's type (non-vascular); VAS, Cases with senile dementia of the Alzheimer's type with (at least moderate) atherosclerotic lesions For sHK, PFK and PGM: VAS + NVA significantly different from controls by student's *t*-test

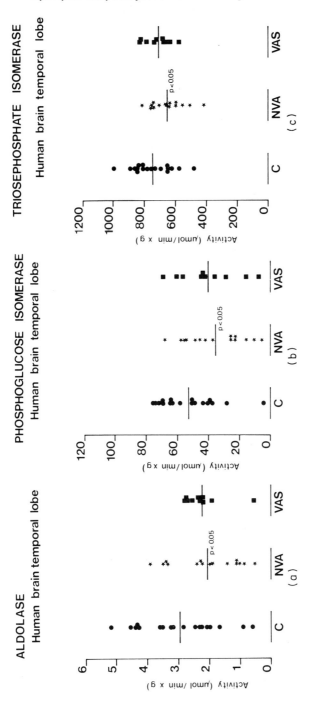

Figure 2. Activity of (a) ALD, (b) PGI, and (c) TIM in autoptic human temporal lobe: controls and cases of senile dementia of the 'Alzheimer's' type. Abbreviations as for Fig. 1

On the other hand, the reduction of glycolytic activity may be the result, rather than the cause, of the loss of neuronal function.

REFERENCES

Bird, E. D., J. S. Gale, and E. G. Spokes (1977). *J. Neurochem.*, **29,** 539–45.

Bücher, T., W. Luh, and D. Pette (1964). *Handbuch der Physiol.- und Patholog.-Chemischen Analyse von Hoppe–Seyler und Thierfelder*, 10th edn, vol. VIA, Springer-Verlag, Berlin.

Gibson, G. E., M. Shimada, and J. P. Blass (1978). *J. Neurochem.*, **31,** 757–60.

Iwangoff, P., R. Armbruster, and A. Enz (1977). *Z. Physiol. Chem.*, **358,** 254.

Iwangoff, P., A. Enz, R. Armbruster, H. Emmenegger, A. Pataki, and P. Sandoz (In press). *Akt. Gerontol.*

Iwangoff, P., K. Reichlmeier, A. Enz, and W. Meier-Ruge (1979). *Interdisciplinary Topics in Gerontology*, Vol. 15, Karger, Basel. pp. 13–33.

Biochemistry of Dementia
Edited by P. J. Roberts
© 1980 John Wiley & Sons Ltd.

Chapter 11

Summary: Dementia—Its Biochemistry and Prospects for a Rational Pharmacological Approach

PETER J. ROBERTS

Department of Physiology and Pharmacology, School of Biochemical and Physiological Sciences, University of Southampton, Southampton, U.K.

'Dementia', if taken in its widest sense, encompasses a range of conditions including the more unusual diseases such as Huntington's chorea which, although rare, has been extensively studied biochemically, and a number of possible animal models for the disease have been developed. This volume, however, is concerned primarily with the clinical, histopathological, and neurochemical changes which are associated with dementia of old age, and those occurring more rarely (approximately 1 person in 10 000) in the younger patient.

As might be anticipated, any severe destructive process involving the central nervous system is likely to result in marked functional impairment, such as is characteristic of dementia. Thus, a number of disease processes have been shown to be associated with dementia, in particular, Alzheimer's disease, Jakob–Creutzfeldt disease, white matter infarcts, ischaemic disease, arteriosclerosis, etc. In cases of pre-senile dementia, the majority of patients have cerebral atrophy which cannot be attributed to a known predisposing cause, e.g. arteriosclerosis and is, therefore, considered to be probably of Alzheimer's origin.

Alzheimer's disease is associated with severe atrophy, particularly of the cerebral cortex and hippocampus. The cerebral cortex becomes occupied by vast numbers of senile plaques (up to 50 % of cortical volume). These plaques consist of swollen synaptic terminals, axonal in origin and containing dense round or oval bodies, frequently filled with neurofibrillary tangles (helically wound pairs of neurotubules made up of abnormal protein). Between these may be found microglia, astrocytes, and a mass of amyloid. In the hippocampus are seen particularly dramatic changes, with severe granulovacuolar degeneration.

Generally speaking, the severity of these degenerative changes is very much greater in the pre-senile as opposed to the senile demented patient.

I. ARE THESE PATHOLOGICAL CHANGES UNIQUE TO DEMENTIA?

Certainly this does not seem to be so, and elderly patients may be found to have plaques without presenting any clinical evidence of dementia. However, the reverse situation does not hold and there is a good correlation between histopathological and clinical appearance. It does seem likely, from the available evidence, that these changes associated with dementia are occurring at least to some degree in normal brain during the process of normal ageing. A fundamental question to be answered, therefore, is: to what extent, if any, is dementia an acceleration of normal senescence, or are the two processes mutually exclusive and merely sharing some of the ultrastructural changes? Obviously, accurate diagnosis of dementia is critical and this can now be performed with considerable reliability (although not to say that this is generally the case) by means of fairly simple psychological tests of orientation and memory. The demented patient is frequently forgetful, unable to concentrate, shows decreased mental agility, and may be disorientated.

II. CEREBRAL BLOOD FLOW IN DEMENTIA

Do vascular lesions cause, or even predispose towards dementia? Blood flow frequently does decrease to a variable extent in dementia. However, since blood flow and metabolic status are intimately linked to each other, this finding may be merely a reflection of a lesser metabolic requirement. Of course, it is possible that in a small number of dements, such as in the hypertensive patient where vascular occlusion has occurred, this link might become dissociated. Thus, vasodilator drugs might be of some therapeutic value where the brain's needs are not being met, although these and reconstructive arterial surgery appear unlikely to be of much general value in the treatment of dementia.

III. A BIOCHEMICAL LESION?

Since the advent of highly sensitive assays for neurotransmitters, their associated synthetic and degradative enzymes and, of course, their receptors, neurochemists and pharmacologists have been infatuated with the concept of specific biochemical lesions and hence the development of unitary hypotheses to account for the clinical manifestations of a number of neurological diseases. Certainly in the case of Parkinson's disease, we know that certain discrete populations of dopaminergic neurons degenerate, and classical replacement therapy in the form of the immediate transmitter precursor, L-dopa, can successfully be undertaken. Although it is clearly vital to investigate as many biochemical parameters as possible in dementia, to propose a single neurotransmitter hypothesis, which might be controlled in an analogous manner to Parkinsonism, appears unrealistic.

What biochemical changes occur in dementia? A major problem here relates to the source and type of biological material under investigation. It is possible to assay the concentrations of neurotransmitter metabolites in cerebrospinal fluid and thus obtain indirect estimates of brain function. More usually, however, one relies upon brains obtained from dead patients; biopsy material is not likely to be abundant since its removal from the patient is ethically justifiable only when there is some possibility that the dementia might be reversible. Post-mortem material itself provides enormous variability and the aim is to obtain age-matched control material which has been handled in essentially the same manner, i.e. this must take proper account of terminal hypoxia of the patient, time of death, sampling procedures, storage conditions, time of delay until assay, etc. Invariably, these patients, particularly if institutionalized, are likely to have received extensive medication, which in itself may effect a whole variety of neurochemical changes.

Secondly, the use of dead material precludes the investigation of metabolic function, neurotransmitter release, and inactivation mechanisms, and the determination of labile constituents such as peptides, a number of enzymes, and possibly also some receptors. What kinds of approach are possible? One obviously considers animal models, but the difficulty here lies in the fact that we do not know whether dementia has any direct parallel in other species. Secondly, how might we expect a demented rat or mouse to manifest its condition behaviourally? The models that are currently available have been selected on their ability to mimic particular facets of the pathological changes seen in dementia. Alzheimer's disease produces very wide changes in the brain, and no single agent will produce all of these. Scrapie (slow viral) infection in mice results in the accumulation of plaques. A second model involves the addition to normal cells of micropore-filtered extracts from the tip of temporal lobes of patients who had suffered from Alzheimer's disease. This has been found to induce the characteristic perihelical filaments, and would appear to suggest that an infective agent may be involved in the aetiology of the disease. The final model which results in the induction of neurofibrillary tangles is the use of high concentrations of aluminium, a substance which has a variety of neurotoxic effects such as the induction of seizures, and has, in fact, been extensively used for producing models of focal epilepsy. How closely these animal models are related to the clinical situation remains to be seen. However, these are the best that the basic scientist has to date for bringing dementia to the laboratory bench. The way is now clear for detailed comparative biochemical evaluation of these models.

IV. DO ANY NEURONAL SYSTEMS DEMONSTRATE A SPECIAL VULNERABILITY IN DEMENTIA?

One of the most striking findings described in this volume is the marked loss of choline acetyltransferase (CAT) in autopsy samples from Alzheimer brains. This appears to be particularly marked in the acetylcholine-rich areas, the hippocampus, the amygdala, and temporal and parietal lobes of the cortex, but without any obvious involvement of other cholinergic systems such as in the caudate/putamen. This loss of CAT is consistent with a loss of pre-synaptic terminals and cholinergic cell bodies; the use of muscarinic receptor probes (e.g. ^{3}H-quinuclidinyl benzilate) suggest that the post-synaptic sites are not affected. The Alzheimer patient frequently exhibits deficits of short-term memory, a function that has long been tentatively linked to cholinergic activity in the hippocampus. Replacement therapy for a specific hippocampal cholinergic lesion should, theoretically, be feasible. Unfortunately, treatment with the precursor choline fails to effect any marked improvement in clinical symptoms. This is perhaps not entirely unexpected, for severe degenerative changes may deplete most of the terminals which accumulate and utilize the choline. On the other hand, application of cholinergic agonists such as arecoline, or the anticholinesterase drug, physostigmine, might be anticipated as being more likely to produce beneficial responses. The clinical trials have, however, yielded highly equivocal results. With physostigmine, some patients improve, while others exhibit a marked worsening of their condition. An added complication associated with cholinesterase inhibition relates to the cellular localization of the enzyme, since it is also widely found pre-synaptically, and in dementia its loss tends to parallel the loss of cholinergic neurons. Somewhat surprisingly, denervation supersensitivity of post-synaptic receptors, which would be expected to enhance the response to exogenously applied cholinergic agonists, does not seem to develop. Lecithin has also been investigated clinically, as described in this volume but, once again, except in the earliest stages of the disease, the substance appeared to be largely ineffective.

Notwithstanding the meagre success attained with cholinergic drugs so far, there is little doubt of a major cholinergic involvement, since the loss of CAT activity correlates extremely well with both plaque formation and psychiatric assessment of severity of the condition.

A number of other neurotransmitter systems have been investigated and a variety of changes have been reported to occur in dementia; for example, Reisine and coworkers (*Brain Res.*, **159**, 477–481 (1978)) found that, while the cholinergic system was extensively affected, other cell types also degenerated, in particular, those which were modulated by the GABA system in the caudate nucleus and the frontal cortex and the dopamine system in the caudate nucleus. GABA binding to its receptor has also been reported to decrease by 50 % in Alzheimer's disease and serotonin receptors may also be depleted. One major point to be considered in relation to GAD, however, is the sensitivity of this enzyme to post-mortem changes, and special care is needed when interpreting such data. The likely involvement of other transmitters in dementia, particularly the biogenic amines, has been described in this volume, and it would therefore seem undeniable that while particularly dramatic effects may be detected on the cholinergic systems, many other transmitters, including those not yet extensively investigated in this respect, such as the peptides which are intimately involved in behavioural responses, are likely to be involved.

Consideration must also be given to possible impairment of neuronal energy metabolism in the demented brain. In some patients there is undoubtedly a decreased cerebral venous blood flow associated with moderately decreased oxygen uptake (CMR_{O_2}) and glucose utilization. Whether oxygen deficit may lead to neuronal damage in dementia is unknown. Neurons, however, are particularly vulnerable due to their high metabolic requirement compared with, say, astrocytes. What are likely to be the consequences of a modest impairment of carbohydrate metabolism? As little as a 10% impairment is likely to produce major changes in the synthesis of those transmitters such as ACh, GABA, glutamate, and aspartate, which are most intimately linked to the TCA cycle. Because of their compartmentalized metabolism with preferential synthesis from glucose, mild hypoxia or reduced glucose availability is rapidly reflected in decreased transmitter levels; axonal conduction is unimpeded and synaptic failure occurs. These possibilities raise the whole question of cause and effect in relation to the biochemical changes occurring. If brain function is impaired as a consequence of cell death, dependent upon, let us say for argument, an infective agent or a kainic acid – like neurotoxicity due to hyperactivity of glutamatergic function, transmitter synthesis will be impaired. Thus, the changes measured in post-mortem brain material would be rather as predicted, representing secondary effects rather than the primary change in dementia. At this stage, however, it would seem inadvisable to become obsessed with notoriously elusive cause–effect relationships, but rather to characterize as fully as possible the specific biochemical changes that occur in dementia. One of the major questions facing both the basic scientist and the clinician is the relationship of the normal ageing process to dementia. Even today, very little is known with certainty of the biochemical changes occurring in normal senescence. There is a wealth of evidence that there is a fundamental relationship between ageing processes and changes in neurotransmitter substances in the brain. It is far from clear, however, what proportion of these changes may be ascribed to genetic or environmental influences. Endocrine factors are likely to be of major importance. In relation to disease, many elderly patients with seemingly similar disease symptoms may exhibit very different, yet specific, abnormalities in neurotransmitter function. Thus, for any neurological disorder—and probably especially for the dementias—the problem of ultimately establishing a causal relationship between disease, behavioural patterns, and neurotransmitters will be extremely difficult.

With regard to possible prevention and therapy of dementia, this must rely heavily on experimental models and further detailed biochemical studies. The relative lack of success with cholinergic therapy bears out the complexity of the situation and if indeed one were able to treat the metabolic impairment of sick cells, their ability to synthesize and release the requisite transmitter in response to activation of a particular neuronal pathway might be significantly improved. A number of drugs have been investigated therapeutically, such as the purported stimulators of cerebral circulation and metabolism, e.g. piracetam (1-acetamido-2-pyrrolidine), hydergine, cyclandelate, and hyperbaric oxygen. However, none of these treatments has so far proved conspicuously successful.

If development of a more general model of dementia proves possible, perhaps by use of selective lesioning techniques with neurotoxic agents, such as kainic acid, the pharmacologist will then be in a strong position to examine rigorously the actions of drugs currently available, and hopefully to develop truly effective ones.

Index